Nora Henry
James Napier
Roy White

CCEA A2
LIFE & HEALTH SCIENCES

COLOURPOINT
EDUCATIONAL

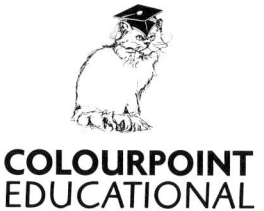

Print ISBN: 978-1-78073-245-9
eBook ISBN: 978-1-78073-335-7

First Edition
Second Impression, 2023

Layout and design: April Sky Design
Printed by: GPS Colour Graphics Ltd, Belfast

Copyright

Colourpoint Educational
An imprint of Colourpoint Creative Ltd
Colourpoint House
Jubilee Business Park
Jubilee Road
Newtownards
County Down
Northern Ireland
BT23 4YH

Tel: 028 9182 6339
E-mail: sales@colourpoint.co.uk
Website: www.colourpointeducational.com

The Authors

NORA HENRY is a teacher at a Belfast grammar school and a part-time tutor for a university education department. She works for an examining body as Chair of Examiners for A Level Chemistry and Reviser for A Level Chemistry Life and Health Sciences and GCSE Double Award Science. In addition to this text, she has written around 30 textbooks, workbooks and study guides for GCSE and A Level.

JAMES NAPIER is a former teacher at a Northern Ireland grammar school. He has written and co-written a number of Biology and Science textbooks supporting the work of students and teachers. He works for an examining body as Chief Examiner for A Level Biology. He has also published a range of Popular Science books in the areas of Genetics and Evolution. His 'non-science' charity books have raised significant amounts of money for cancer and mental health charities.

ROY WHITE taught Physics to A level for over 30 years in Belfast. He works for an examining body as Chair of Examiners for Double Award Science, Chair of Examiners for A level Life and Health Sciences, Principal Examiner for GCSE Physics and Principal Moderator for Entry Level Science. In addition to this text, he has been the author or co-author of over a dozen successful books supporting the work of science teachers in Northern Ireland.

Publisher's Note: This book has been through a rigorous quality assurance process by an independent person experienced in the CCEA specification prior to publication. It has been written to help students preparing for the A2 Life and Health Sciences specification from CCEA. While Colourpoint Educational, the authors and the quality assurance readers have taken every care in its production, we are not able to guarantee that the book is completely error-free. Additionally, while the book has been written to address the CCEA specification, it is the responsibility of each candidate to satisfy themselves that they have fully met the requirements of the CCEA specification prior to sitting an exam set by that body. For this reason, and because specifications and CCEA advice change with time, we strongly advise every candidate to avail of a qualified teacher and to check the contents of the most recent specification for themselves prior to the exam. Colourpoint Creative Ltd therefore cannot be held responsible for any errors or omissions in this book or any consequences thereof.

CONTENTS

Note: In line with feedback from teachers, this book has been written for a proposed revised version of the specification that has not yet been approved at the time of publication in 2021. Teachers and students are strongly encouraged to refer to the version of the CCEA specification that is in use at the time of teaching, and to always give precedence to the wording on the CCEA specification where there are any discrepancies.

Unit A2 2:
Organic Chemistry

1: NOMENCLATURE AND STRUCTURE IN ORGANIC COMPOUNDS

Students should be able to:

- 1.1 demonstrate an understanding that a hydrocarbon is composed of carbon and hydrogen only;
- 8.1.2 demonstrate an understanding of the terms empirical and molecular formula and the relationship between them;
- 8.1.3 represent organic molecules according to structural, skeletal, molecular and general formulae;
- 8.1.4 calculate empirical and molecular formulae using data, giving composition by mass;
- 8.1.5 demonstrate an understanding of the terms structural formulae, homologous series and functional groups;
- 8.1.6 apply International Union of Pure and Applied Chemistry (IUPAC) rules to naming organic compounds with up to six carbon atoms;
- 8.1.9 determine the possible structure and skeletal formulae of an organic molecule given its molecular formula.

Bonding in organic compounds

Organic chemistry is the study of the millions of organic compounds which contain carbon bonded by covalent bonds. Organic chemicals have a huge range of uses – in pharmaceutical drugs, cosmetics, paints, clothes and plastics. All organic compounds contain carbon. The chemistry of carbon is vast; there are in excess of ten million known carbon compounds.

Carbon can form so many compounds because:

- a carbon atom can form bonds with other carbon atoms to make chains and rings;
- a carbon atom can form single or double bonds to another carbon atom;
- a carbon atom can bond with other atoms – for example hydrogen, oxygen and chlorine.

Carbon has four electrons in its outer shell, as shown in the following diagram, and can form four covalent bonds in all its compounds by sharing the four outer shell electrons.

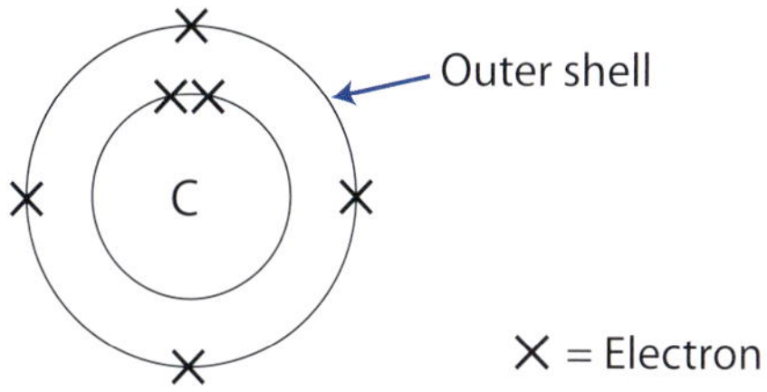

A carbon atom

A covalent bond can be represented by a line. The four bonds formed by carbon can be single bonds or, sometimes, a mixture of single bonds and double bonds as shown below.

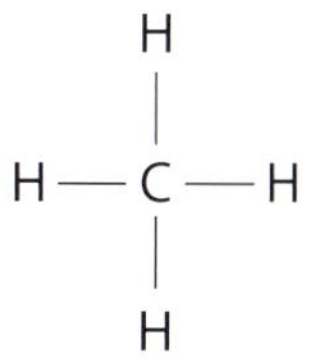

There are four single bonds from the carbon atom to the hydrogen atoms.

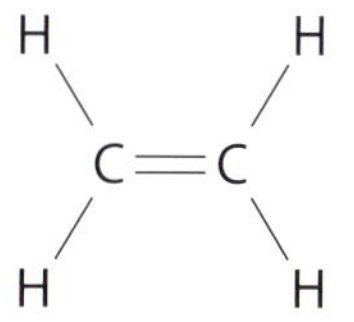

There is a double bond (two bonds) between the two carbon atoms.

Tip: When drawing organic structures count the number of bonds around carbon – there should always be four.

Homologous series

To make the study of the large number of carbon compounds more manageable, carbon compounds are divided into families called **homologous series**.

A homologous series is a family of organic compounds that have:

- **the same general formula;**
- **show similar chemical properties;**
- **show a gradation in their physical properties; and**
- **successive members differ by a 'CH_2' unit.**

Tip: A gradation in physical properties means that the physical properties change as the number of carbon atoms in the series increases. This may be an increase in boiling point for example.

You will study three homologous series in detail in this module – the alkanes, alkenes and alcohols. You also will come across carboxylic acids, halogenoalkanes and aldehydes and ketones.

In organic chemistry, compounds are named according to the **number of carbon atoms present**. A **prefix** shows the length of the carbon chain:

- **meth** means the organic compound contains **1** carbon atom in the longest carbon chain;
- **eth** means the organic compound contains **2** carbon atoms in the longest carbon chain;
- **prop** means the organic compound contains **3** carbon atoms in the longest carbon chain;
- **but** means the organic compound contains **4** carbon atoms in the longest carbon chain;
- **pent** means the organic compound contains **5** carbon atoms in the longest carbon chain;
- **hex** means the organic compound contains **6** carbon atoms in the longest carbon chain.

The name of a compound also has a **suffix** which shows the **homologous series** it belongs to:

- the suffix for alkanes is **-ane**;
- the suffix for alkenes is **-ene**;
- the suffix for alcohols is **-ol**.

You will also learn a little about the following series, so it is useful to remember their suffixes too:

- the suffix for aldehydes is **-al**;
- the suffix for ketones is **-one**;
- the suffix for carboxylic acids is **-oic acid**.

Tip: Don't mix up **-OL** which is an alcohol and **-AL** which is an aldehyde.

In the name **ethane**, the prefix **eth** tells us that the compound contains two carbon atoms in the longest carbon chain, while the suffix **-ane** tells us that it is an alkane. Similarly, in the name **pentanol**, the prefix **pent** tells us that the compound contains five carbon atoms in the longest carbon chain, while the suffix **-ol** tells us that it is an alcohol.

Worked example

What is the name of a carboxylic acid which has four carbon atoms?

Answer

4 carbon atoms — prefix **but**

carboxylic acid — suffix **-oic acid**

For acids, you need to add **-an** to the name.

The name is **butanoic acid.**

Worked example

What is the name of an alkene with three carbon atoms?

Answer

3 carbon atoms — prefix **prop**

alkene — suffix **-ene**

The name is **propene.**

General formulae

All homologous series are represented by a general formula. A general formula is one involving a variable number ***n***, which gives the number of carbon atoms present in the chain. It can be used to work out the molecular formula of any compound in the homologous series. The general formulae of some homologous series are shown in the following table.

Homologous series	General formula (*n* = number of carbon atoms)
Alkanes	C_nH_{2n+2}
Alkenes	C_nH_{2n}
Alcohols	$C_nH_{2n+1}OH$

The alkane propane has three carbon atoms, $n = 3$. The general formula is C_nH_{2n+2} so there are 8 hydrogen atoms $((2 \times 3) + 2)$ and the molecular formula is C_3H_8.

The alkene ethene has two carbon atoms, $n = 2$. The general formula is C_nH_{2n} so there are 4 hydrogen atoms (2×2) and the molecular formula is C_2H_4.

The alkane butanol has four carbon atoms, $n = 4$. The general formula is $C_nH_{2n+1}OH$ so the molecular formula is C_4H_9OH.

The alkanes and alkenes are hydrocarbons. **A hydrocarbon is a compound which contains carbon**

and hydrogen only. The alcohols are not hydrocarbons because they also contain the element oxygen.

Functional groups

The functional group is the reactive group within a compound. Each homologous series, apart from the alkanes, have a functional group, as shown in the following table.

Homologous series	Functional group
Alkanes	No functional group
Alkenes	C=C (carbon carbon double bond)
Alcohols	OH (hydroxyl group)

Molecular formulae and empirical formulae

A molecular formula is a formula which shows the actual number of atoms of each element in a molecule. The table below shows the molecular formulae of three compounds.

Compound	Molecular formula	Number of atoms present
Ethane	C_2H_6	2 atoms of C, 6 atoms of H
Chloropropane	C_3H_7Cl	3 atoms of C, 7 atoms of H, 1 atom of Cl
Ethanoic acid	$C_2H_4O_2$	2 atoms of C, 4 atoms of H, 2 atoms of O

Tip: The functional group is not shown in a molecular formula. The molecular formula shows only the simplest ratio of the atoms of each element. Thus the molecular formula of ethanol is C_2H_6O not C_2H_5OH, and the molecular formula of ethanoic acid is $C_2H_4O_2$ not CH_3COOH.

An empirical formula is a formula which shows the simplest whole number ratio of each element in a compound. The table below shows the molecular formulae of the same three compounds.

Compound	Molecular formula	Empirical formula
Ethane	C_2H_6	CH_3
Chloropropane	C_3H_7Cl	C_3H_7Cl
Ethanoic acid	$C_2H_4O_2$	CH_2O

Tip: Notice that the empirical and molecular formulae of chloropropane are the same.

Worked example

What are the molecular and empirical formulae of an alcohol with 6 carbons?

Answer

The general formula of an alcohol is $C_nH_{2n+1}OH$

In this case, $n = 6$, so

$2n + 1 = (2 \times 6) + 1 = 12 + 1 = 13$

So the general formula is $C_6H_{13}OH$

Therefore the molecular formula is $C_6H_{14}O$

Finding the molecular formula from the empirical formula

To find the molecular formula from the empirical formula the **relative formula mass** is needed. First find the mass of the empirical formula, using mass numbers from the Periodic Table. The molecular formula will then be a multiple of this, with same total mass as the relative formula mass.

Tip: Relative formula mass can be represented by the letters M_r or sometimes by the letters RFM.

Worked example

A compound has relative formula mass of 28 and empirical formula CH_2. What is the molecular formula of the compound?

Answer

A molecular formula is a multiple (n) of the empirical formula.

We know that $(CH_2)_n = 28$

Substituting the mass numbers of 12 for carbon and 1 for hydrogen gives:

$$(12 + (2 \times 1)) \times n = 28$$
$$14n = 28$$
$$n = 2$$

$(CH_2)_n = (CH_2)_2 = C_2H_4$

The molecular formula is C_2H_4

Worked example

The empirical formula of a compound is CH_2O and its relative formula mass is 60. What is the molecular formula of the compound?

Answer

We know that $(CH_2O)n = 60$

$(12 + (2 \times 1) + 16)n = 60$

$30n = 60$

$n = 2$

$(CH_2O)_n = (CH_2O)_2 = C_2H_4O_2$

The molecular formula is $C_2H_4O_2$

Calculating empirical formulae

It is possible to calculate the empirical formula of a compound using mass data or using percentage composition data. The general method is as follows:

1. Find the number of moles of **each element** in the compound using

$$\text{moles} = \frac{\text{mass}}{\text{relative atomic mass}} = \frac{\text{mass}}{A_r}$$

Tip: Relative atomic mass can be represented as A_r or RAM.

2. Find the **simplest ratio of moles**. A simple way to do this is to compare the values of moles and find the smallest value, then divide all the mole values by this smaller number.
3. If the mole values are not whole numbers, **multiply** by a number to bring to a **whole number** ensuring it is still the smallest whole number ratio.

Tip: You may find it helpful to remember the phrase "To convert mass to mole, divide by smallest, multiply 'til whole".

The next two examples demonstrate how to calculate empirical formulae using **mass data**.

Worked example

A hydrocarbon contains 1.710 g carbon and 0.287 g hydrogen. The relative formula mass of the hydrocarbon is 56. Calculate the empirical and molecular formulae of the hydrocarbon.

Answer

First calculate the number of moles of each element and then the simplest ratio of moles.

Element	C	H
Mass (g)	1.710	0.287
Moles	$\frac{1.710}{12} = 0.1425$	$\frac{0.287}{1} = 0.287$
Ratio (divide by the smallest number of moles)	$\frac{0.1425}{0.1425} = 1$	$\frac{0.287}{0.1425} = 2$

So the empirical formula is CH_2

$(CH_2)n = 56$

$(12 + (2 \times 1))n = 56$

$14n = 56$

$n = 4$

So the molecular formula is C_4H_8

Worked example

A sample of 1.16 g of a hydrocarbon contains 0.20 g of hydrogen. It has a relative molecular mass of 58. Calculate the empirical and molecular formulae of the hydrocarbon.

Answer

The mass of only one element, hydrogen, is given. However, because the compound is a hydrocarbon and made of carbon and hydrogen only, the mass of carbon can be found by subtraction:

Element	C	H
Mass (g)	1.16 – 0.20 = 0.96	0.2
Moles	$\frac{0.96}{12} = 0.08$	$\frac{0.2}{1} = 0.2$
Ratio (divide by the smallest number of moles)	$\frac{0.08}{0.08} = 1$	$\frac{0.2}{0.08} = 2.5$
Multiply by 2 to get to whole numbers	2	5

So the empirical formula is C_2H_5

$(C_2H_5)n = 58$

$((2 \times 12) + (5 \times 1))n = 58$

$29n = 58$

$n = 2$

So the molecular formula is C_4H_{10}

The next example demonstrates how to calculate empirical formulae using **percentage data**. Percentage means 'out of 100' so you can assume that the percentages represent the mass of each element in 100 g of the sample. Thereafter, carry out the calculation in the same way.

Worked example

Find the empirical formula of a compound which contains 22.2% carbon, 3.7% hydrogen and 74.1% bromine.

Answer

The percentages tell us that in a sample of 100 g of this compound there is 22.2 g of carbon, 3.7 g of hydrogen and 74.1 g of bromine

Element	**C**	**H**	**Br**
Mass (g)	22.2	3.7	74.1
Moles	$\frac{22.2}{12} = 1.85$	$\frac{3.7}{1} = 3.7$	$\frac{74.1}{80} = 0.926$
Ratio (divide by the smallest number of moles)	$\frac{1.85}{0.926} = 2$	$\frac{3.7}{0.926} = 4$	$\frac{0.926}{0.926} = 1$

So the empirical formula is C_2H_4Br

Structural formulae

A structural formula shows the arrangement of atoms in a molecule, carbon by carbon, with the attached hydrogens and functional groups, with or without showing the bonds.

For example, all of the following are valid structural formulae for ethanol. The second does not show the bond between O and H, while the third does not show any bonds and is often called a condensed structural formula.

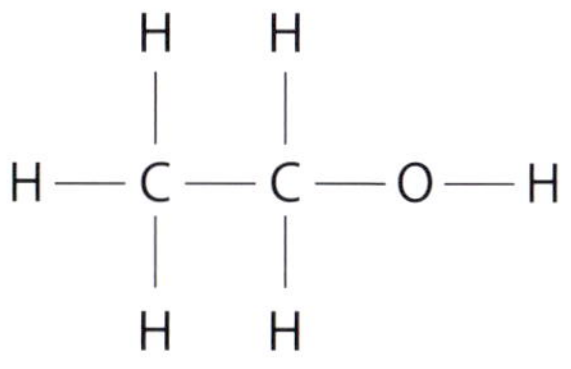

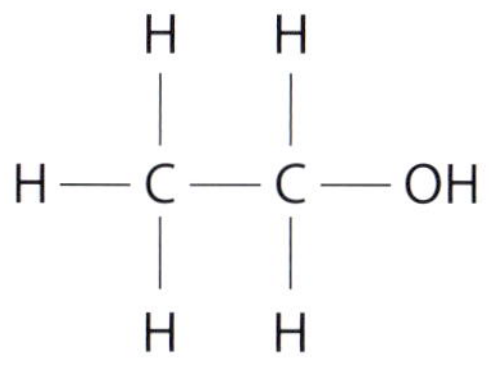

CH_3CH_2OH

Similarly, the following are two structural formulae for butane. The first shows all the bonds, while the second does not show any bonds.

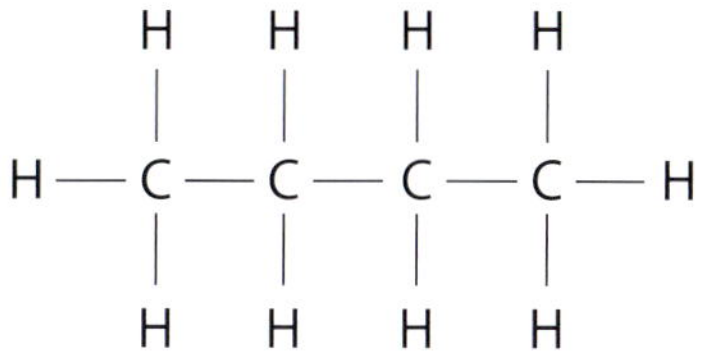

$CH_3CH_2CH_2CH_3$

Writing structural formulae and condensed structural formulae

The structural formula of butanoic acid with bonds is shown below. By looking at the vertical lines it is possible to write the structural formula without the bonds.

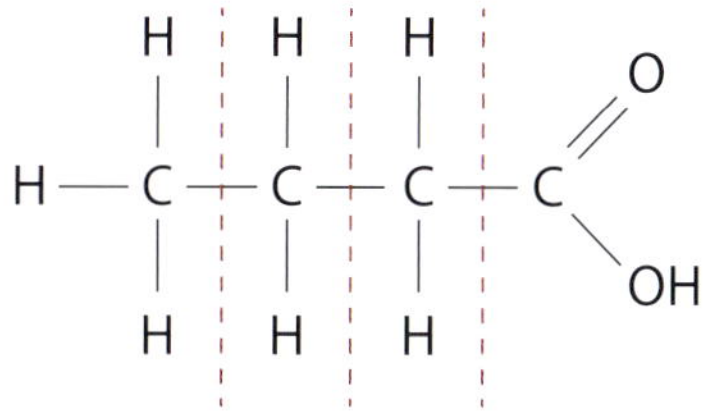

CH_3 CH_2 CH_2 COOH

$CH_3CH_2CH_2COOH$ is a structural formula without the bonds. This can be shortened further to $CH_3(CH_2)_2COOH$.

The structural formula of propan-2-ol with bonds is shown below. (The meaning of the '2' in the name will be discussed later in this chapter.) Again, by looking at the vertical lines, it is possible to write the formula showing the structure without the bonds. Note that the OH group is **shown in brackets** as it is not part of the main chain, but is bonded to a carbon atom in the middle of the chain.

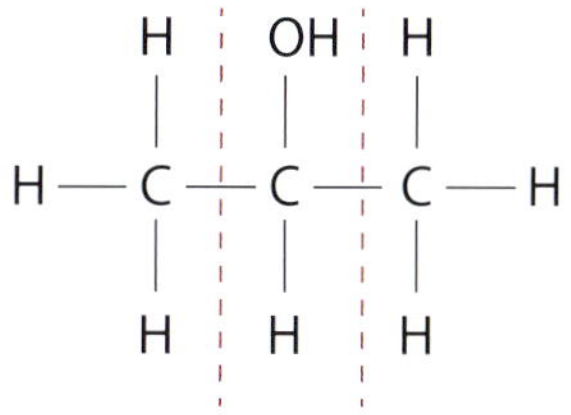

CH_3 CH(OH) CH_3

$CH_3CH(OH)CH_3$

The structural formula of 2-chloropentane with bonds is shown below, along with the condensed structural formula. No brackets are needed around chlorine because it is an atom, not a group of atoms.

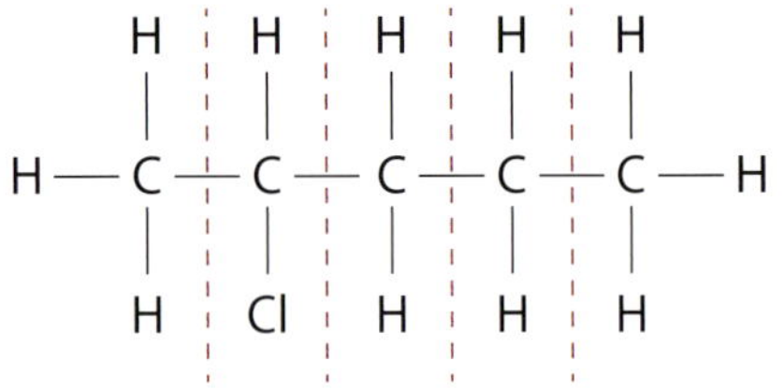

CH_3 $CHCl$ CH_2 CH_2 CH_3

$CH_3CHClCH_2CH_2CH_3$

The structural formula of 2-methylpentane is shown below, along with the condensed structural formula. Brackets are needed around CH_3 because it is a group.

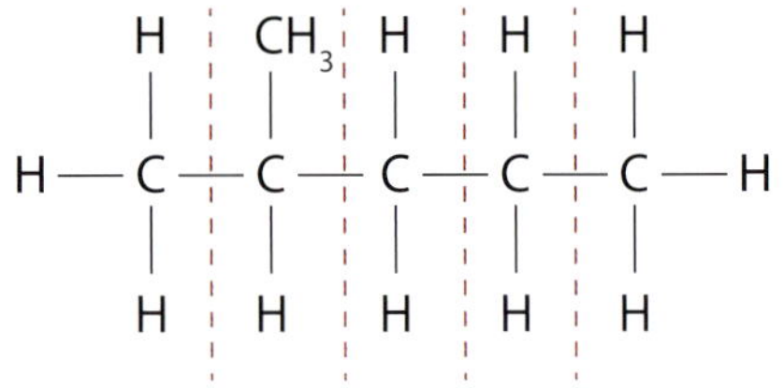

CH_3 $CH(CH_3)$ CH_2 CH_2 CH_3

The structural formula of 2-methylpropan-2-ol with bonds is shown below, along with the condensed structural formula. Note that the central carbon atom has three CH_3 groups around it, so another way of writing the formula is $(CH_3)_3COH$.

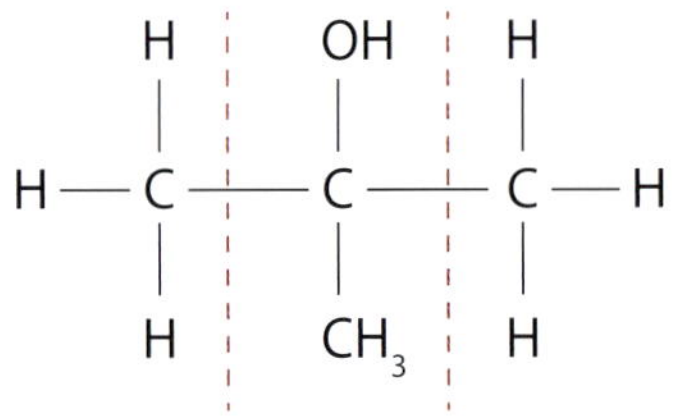

CH_3 $C(CH_3)(OH)$ CH_3

It is possible to draw a structural formula of a compound, if given its name. This is illustrated in the following two examples.

Worked example

Draw the structural formula of butane.

Answer

1. The prefix 'but' means four carbons, so first draw four carbons bonded in a row

C — C — C — C

2. Then draw in additional bonds so that each carbon has four bonds.

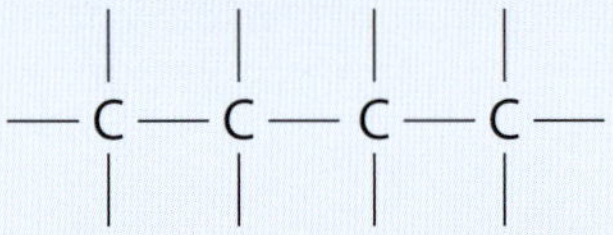

3. Now draw hydrogen atoms at the end of each bond.

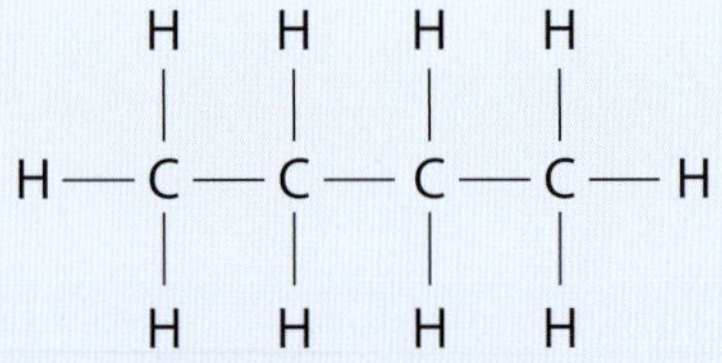

This is the structural formula. It can also be written as $CH_3CH_2CH_2CH_3$.

Worked example

Draw the structural formula of propan-2-ol.

Answer

1. The prefix 'prop' means three carbons, so draw three carbon atoms bonded in a row.

C — C — C

2. It is an alcohol and so it has the OH group. The '2' means that we draw it in position 2. (This will be discussed later in the chapter.)

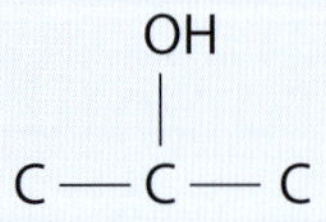

3. Now add bonds so that every carbon has four bonds.

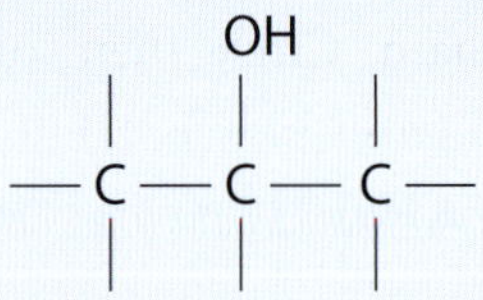

4. Add hydrogen atoms to each bond.

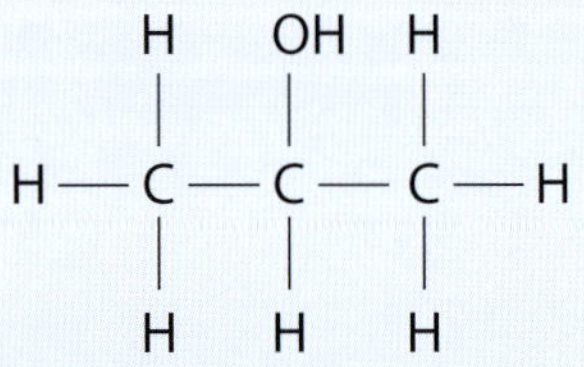

This is the structural formula. It can also be written as $CH_3CH(OH)CH_3$

Nomenclature

The rules for nomenclature (naming) of organic compounds are based on the IUPAC (International Union of Pure and Applied Chemistry) system. The correct chemical name of a compound is often called the IUPAC name. You must be able to use IUPAC rules to name organic compounds – either rings or chains – with up to six carbon atoms.

A name is made up of a prefix, a stem and a suffix. To determine the chemical name of a compound from its structural formula, use the following process.

1. Underline the **longest carbon chain** in the molecule. Count the number of carbon atoms in the longest unbranched chain and use the correct **prefix** name. For example, in the structure below the longest unbranched chain has six carbons so the prefix is 'hex'.

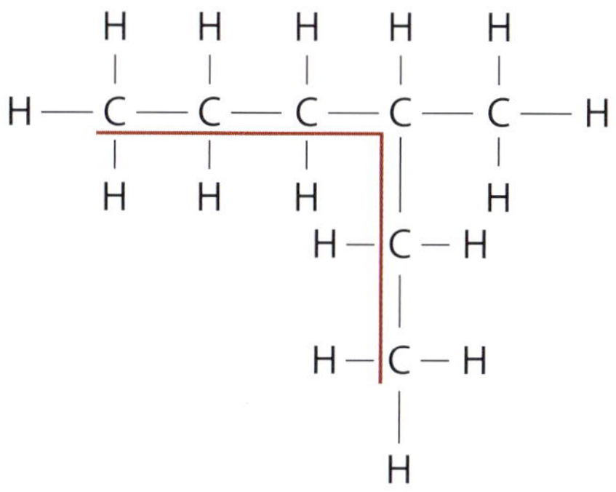

Tip: In exam questions, watch out for the longest chain not being drawn completely straight; this is there to catch you out! Always count the longest continuous chain.

2. Identify any **side groups** or **substituents**. These are groups which are attached to, but not part of, the longest chain. Circle them on the structure and give them names as shown in the table below.

Side group or substituent	Name
$-CH_3$	methyl
$-CH_2CH_3$ $(-C_2H_5)$	ethyl
$-CH_2CH_2CH_3$ $(-C_3H_7)$	propyl
–F	fluoro
–Cl	chloro
–Br	bromo
–I	iodo

The structure shown below has a 'methyl' side group on the longest chain.

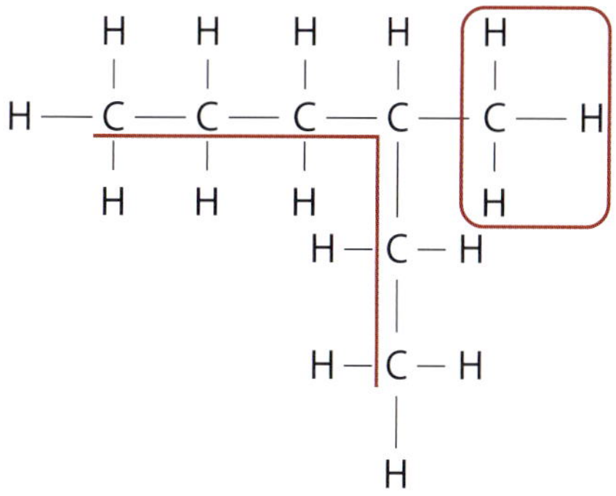

3. Identify the **suffix**. This will depend on the functional group. As you have already learned, alkanes have the suffix '-ane'; alkenes have a double bond and the suffix '-ene'; and alcohols have a hydroxyl group and the suffix '-ol'.

4. All substituents are listed **alphabetically**. For example chloro comes before methyl.

5. If there is more than one substituent group this is prefixed with di-, tri-, tetra- and so on. For example, 'dichloro' is used if there are two chlorine atoms (even if they are bonded to different carbon atoms) and trimethyl is used if there are three methyl groups (even if each is bonded to a different carbon atom). Note that the di-, tri- and tetra- prefixes **do not change the alphabetical order**. The order is based on the name of the substituent group. For example the groups in the name 'trichlorodifluoro' are correctly ordered based on the names of the substituent groups, not the prefixes 'tri-' and 'di-'.

6. Each substituent group must have a number to indicate its position on the carbon chain. This is often called a **locant number** and is placed in front of each substituent group. A separate number is needed for each substituent. Commas are used to separate the numbers. **Dichloro** requires two **locant** numbers, one for the position of each chlorine atom, for example '1,2-dichloro' or '1,1-dichloro'. You can number from **either end**, but for the correct name **the carbon atoms in the longest chain are numbered from the end that gives the lowest locant numbers**. You can't number from both ends at the same time. Note that the position of the functional group for alcohols, and alkenes and ketones must often be given.

7. Dashes are placed between numbers and letters.

8. If the compound has the carbon atoms arranged in a **ring** then the name 'cyclo' is added to the name. Cyclohexane is shown below. We will look at this in detail later.

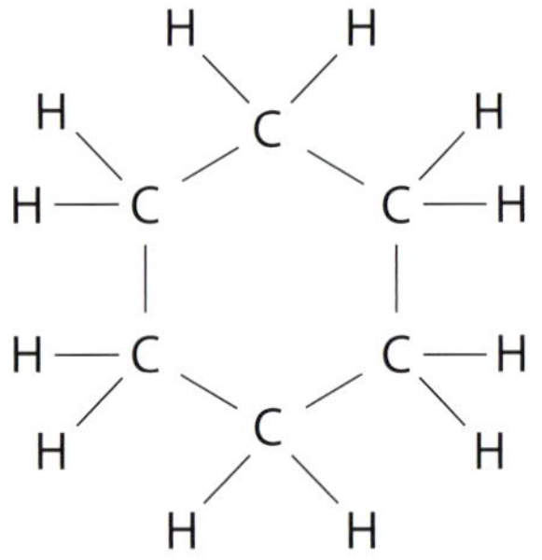

The following series of examples demonstrate how to use this process to name molecules using the IUPAC system.

Worked example

Give the IUPAC name for the molecule below.

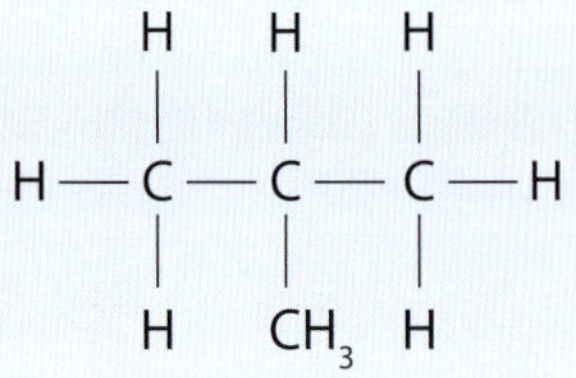

Answer

Underline and name the longest unbranched carbon chain.

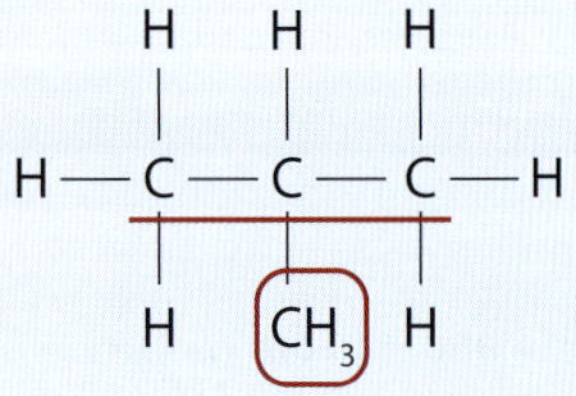

There are three carbons so the prefix is 'prop-'.

Circle the CH_3 side group. The name for this substituent is 'methyl'.

The methyl group is on carbon 2.

So the IUPAC name is 2-methylpropane.

Worked example

Give the IUPAC name for the molecule below.

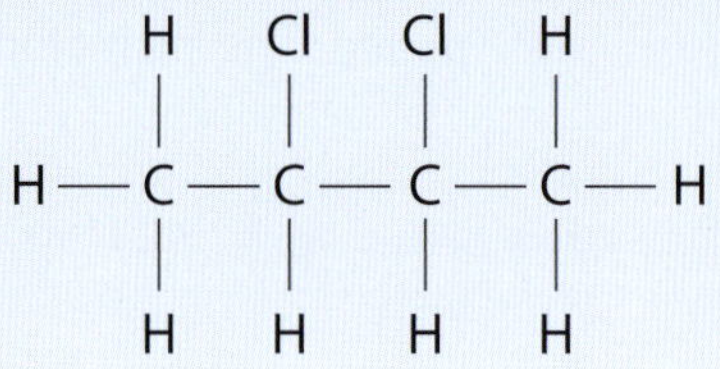

Answer

Underline and name the longest unbranched carbon chain.

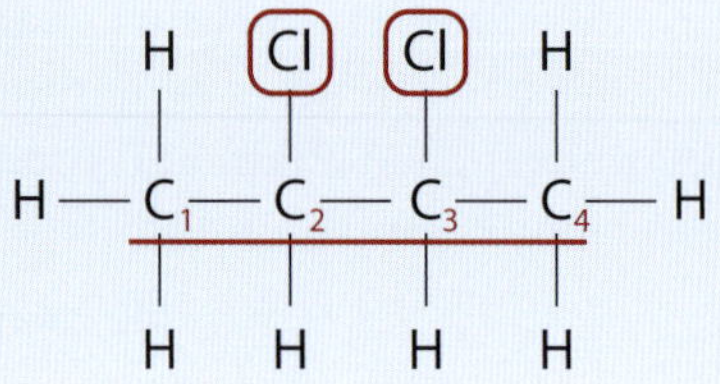

There are four carbons so the prefix is 'but-'.

There are two chloro side groups, so the name for these substituents is 'dichloro'.

The chloro groups are on carbon 2 and carbon 3.

So the IUPAC name is 2,3-dichlorobutane.

> **Tip:** Number the carbon atoms, as shown above. This makes it easier to see where the side groups are attached.

Worked example

Give the IUPAC name for the molecule below.

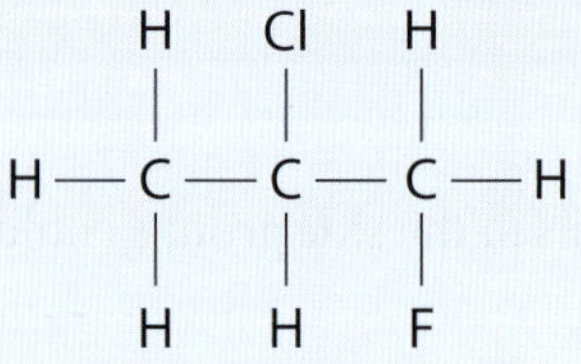

Answer

Underline and name the longest unbranched carbon chain.

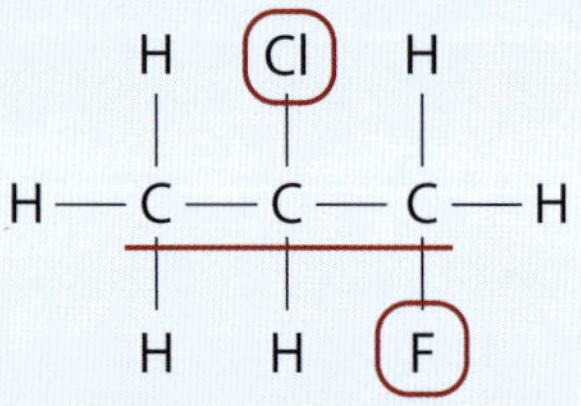

There are three carbons so the prefix is 'prop-'.

There are two side groups, and the name for these substituents are 'chloro' and 'fluoro'.

The positions of the side groups could be 2 and 3 or 1 and 2, depending on which end you count from. However, we should use the lowest combination which is 1,2.

The names of the side groups should appear in alphabetical order.

So the IUPAC name is 2-chloro-1-fluoropropane.

Worked example

Give the IUPAC name for the molecule below.

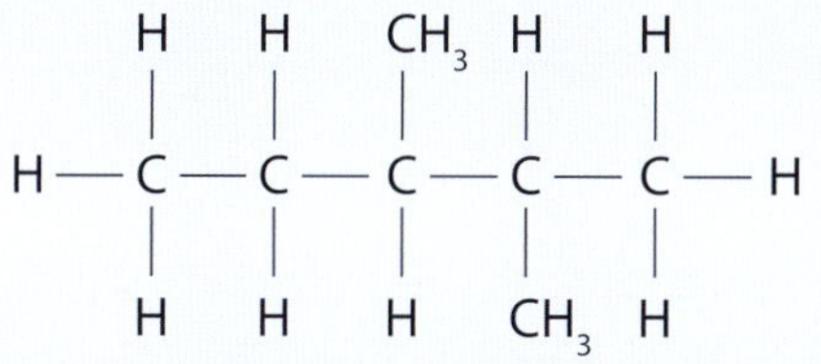

Answer

Underline and name the longest unbranched carbon chain.

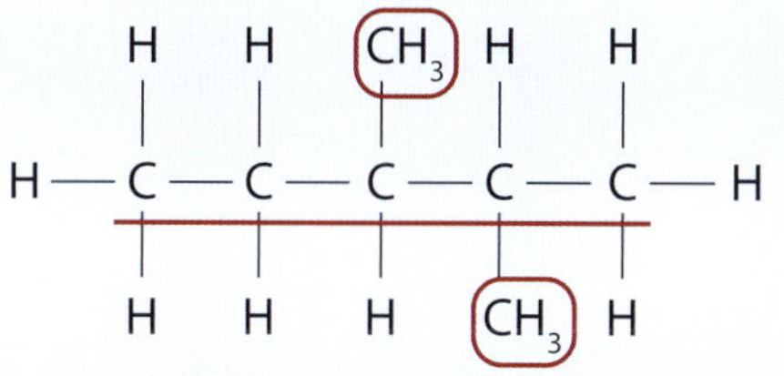

There are five carbons so the prefix is 'pent-'.

There are two methyl side groups, so the name for these substituents is 'dimethyl'.

The positions of the side groups could be 2 and 3 or 3 and 4. However, the lowest combination is 2,3.

So the IUPAC name is 2,3-dimethylpentane.

Worked example

Give the IUPAC name for the molecule below.

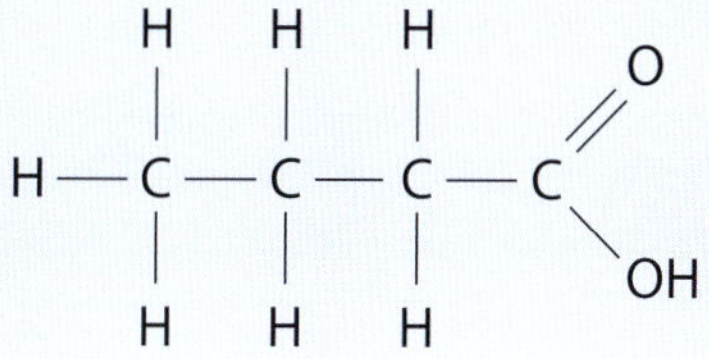

Answer

Underline and name the longest unbranched carbon chain. There are four carbons so the prefix is 'but-'.

There is a functional group, COOH, so the name ends in '-oic acid'.

So the IUPAC name is butanoic acid.

Worked example

Give the IUPAC name for the molecule below.

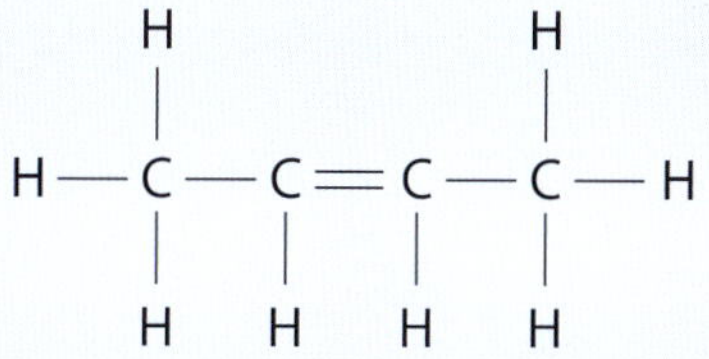

Answer

Underline and name the longest unbranched carbon chain. There are four carbons so the prefix is 'but-'.

There is a functional group C=C, so the name ends in '-ene'.

The position of the functional group is needed. It is between carbon 2 and 3, so we choose the lowest number, which is 2.

So the IUPAC name is but-2-ene.

Worked example

Give the IUPAC name for the molecule below.

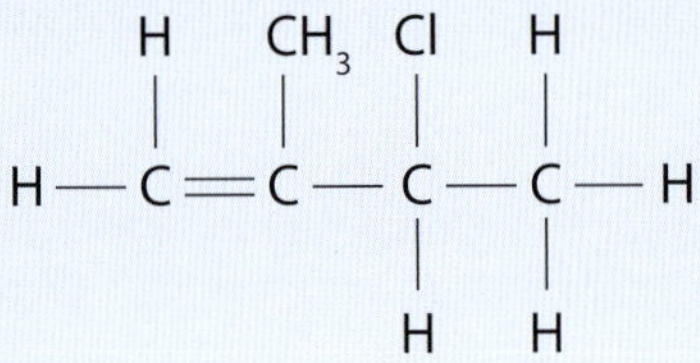

Answer

Underline and name the longest unbranched carbon chain. There are four carbons so the prefix is 'but-'.

There is a functional group C=C, so the name ends in '-ene'.

The functional group is between carbon 1 and 2 so choose the lowest number, which is 1.

The side groups are 'methyl' (position 2) and 'chloro' (position 3).

Remember that the substituent names should appear in alphabetical order.

So the IUPAC name is 3-chloro-2-methylbut-1-ene.

Worked example

Give the IUPAC name for the molecule below.

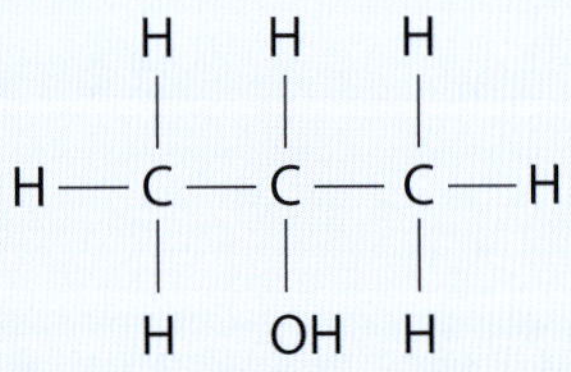

Answer

Underline and name the longest unbranched carbon chain. There are three carbons so the prefix is 'prop-'.

There is a functional group OH, so the name ends in '-ol'.

Give the position of functional group, which is 2.

So the IUPAC name is propan-2-ol.

Tip: A common error is to name this compound prop-2-anol which is incorrect.

Worked example

Give the IUPAC name for the molecule below.

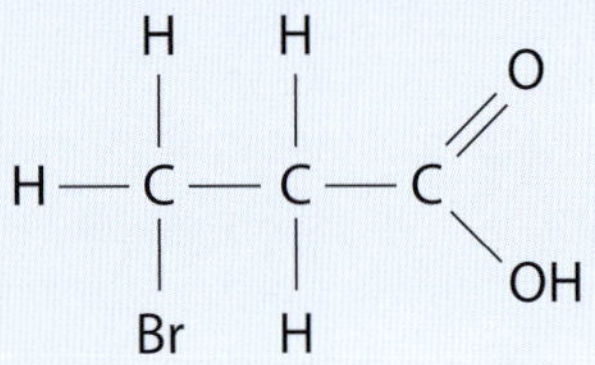

Answer

Underline and name the longest unbranched carbon chain. There are three carbons so the prefix is 'prop-'.

There is a functional group COOH, so the name ends in '-oic acid'.

For acids the COOH is always the first carbon in the chain.

There is a side group 'bromo' on carbon 3.

So the IUPAC name is 3-bromopropanoic acid.

Worked example

Give the IUPAC name for the molecule below.

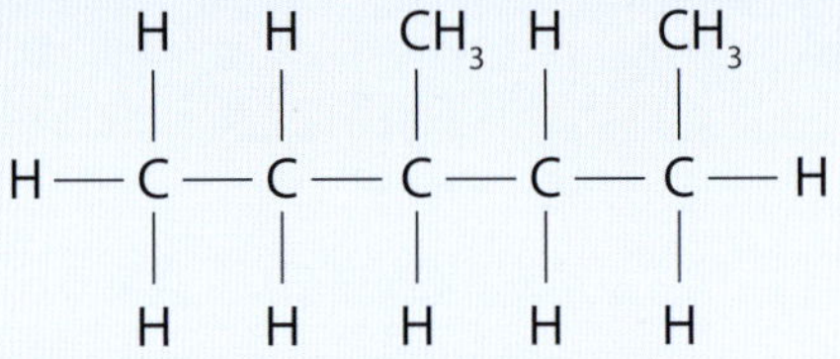

Answer

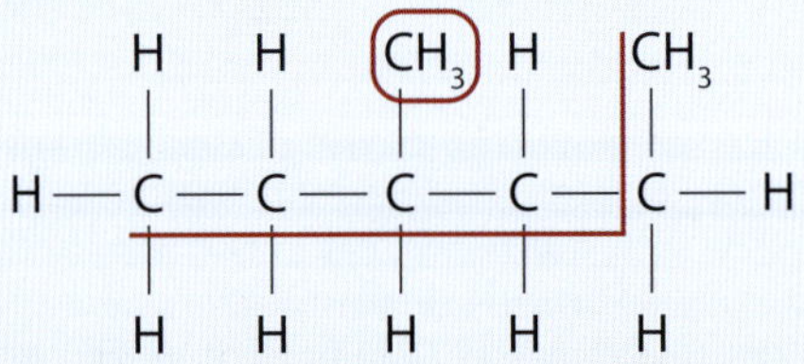

Underline and name the longest unbranched carbon chain. There are six carbons so the prefix is 'hex-'.

There is one CH_3 side group, so the substituent name is 'methyl'.

The methyl group is on carbon 3.

So the IUPAC name is 3-methylhexane.

Tip: Always watch out for a methyl group on the end of a chain – it will usually be part of the longest unbranched chain.

Worked example

Give the IUPAC name for the molecule below.

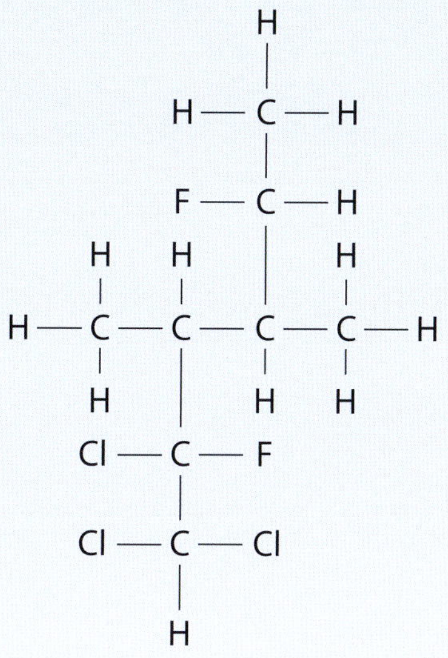

Answer

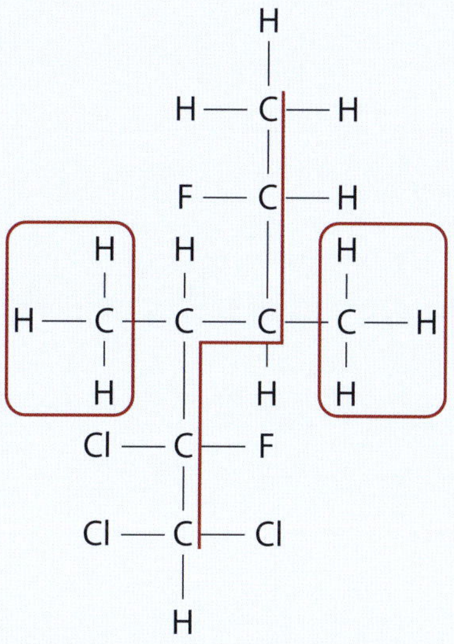

Underline and name the longest unbranched carbon chain. There are two methyl side groups (circled) so this is named 'dimethyl'. There are six carbons so the prefix is 'hex-'.

There are three chlorine side groups, 'trichloro'; and two fluorine side groups, 'difluoro'.

The positions of the side groups are 1,1,2 or 6,6,5 for trichloro; 2,5 or 2,5 for difluoro; and 3,4 or 3,4 for dimethyl. So choose the lowest numbers.

Ensure the substituents are in alphabetical order, ignoring the prefix. The correct order is: trichloro, difluoro, dimethyl.

So the IUPAC name is 1,1,2-trichloro-2,5-difluoro-3,4-dimethylhexane.

Worked example

Give the IUPAC name for the molecule below.

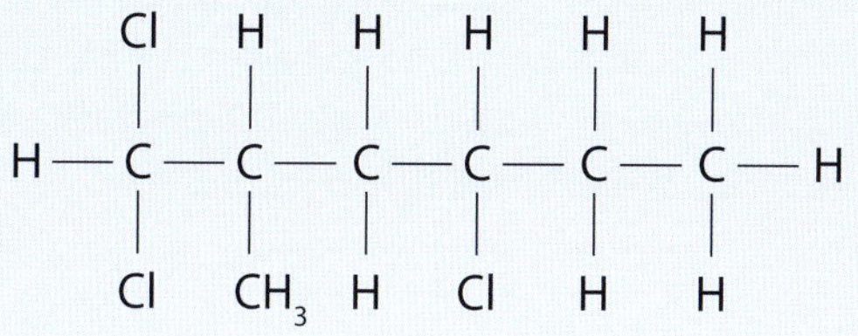

Answer

Name the longest unbranched carbon chain. There are six carbons, so the prefix is 'hex-'.

There is one CH_3 side group, 'methyl'; and three chloros are also attached, 'trichloro'.

The methyl group is on carbon 2 and the trichloro is on carbons 1, 1 and 4.

So the IUPAC name is 1,1,4-trichloro-2-methylhexane. Note the alphabetical order of substituents.

Tip: For trichloro you need to give three numbers, as the position of each chlorine must be given. Note that it is written in alphabetical order: chloro and then methyl.

Worked example

Give the IUPAC name for the molecule below.

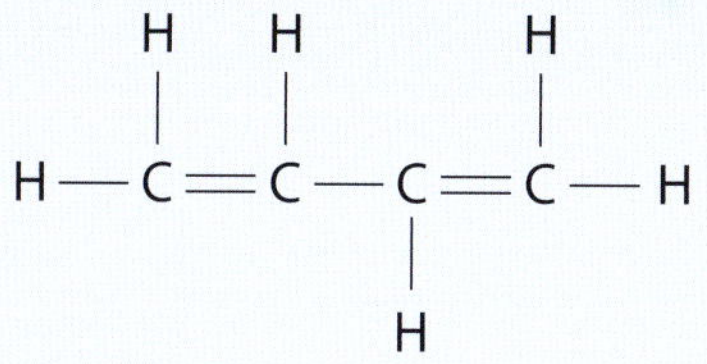

Answer

Underline and name the longest unbranched carbon chain. There are four carbons, so the prefix is 'but-'.

There are two double bonds – this is written 'diene'.

Give the position of both double bonds: they are at positions 1 and 3.

For dienes the stem name gets an extra 'a'.

So the IUPAC name is buta-1,2-diene.

Skeletal formulae

These are bare stick-like drawings which just show the carbon skeleton, with hydrogen atoms removed and functional groups present. Each carbon–carbon bond is shown as a line. The skeletal formula of 2-methylbutane is shown below.

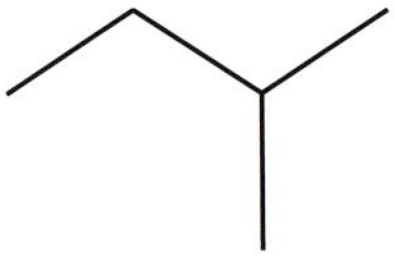

In a skeletal formula there is a carbon atom **at each junction** between bonds in a chain and at **the end** of each bond (unless there is something else there already, such as the -OH group in an alcohol.)

> **Tip:** Remember that, although they are not visible, hydrogen atoms are attached to each carbon to make the total number of bonds on that carbon up to four.

To draw a skeletal formula, follow these steps:

1. Draw the structural formula.
2. Draw the formula without any hydrogen atoms (or their bonds) apart from those in any functional groups. Include the functional groups.
3. Now draw each carbon as a junction between lines.

Worked example

Draw the skeletal formula of butane:

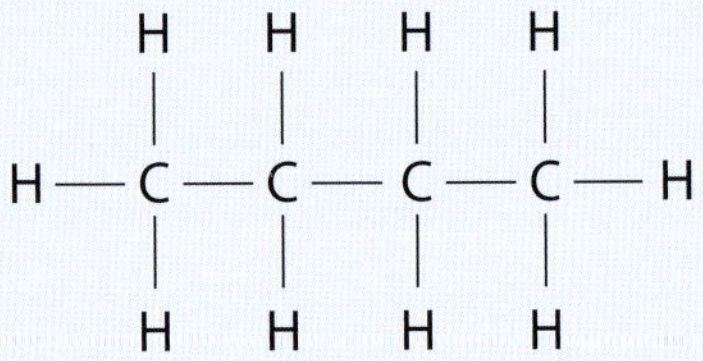

Answer

Removing all the hydrogens, this becomes:

C – C – C – C

Now draw each carbon either as a junction between bonds, or at the end of a bond.

So the skeletal formula is:

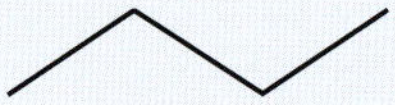

Worked example

Draw the skeletal formula of propan-1-ol:

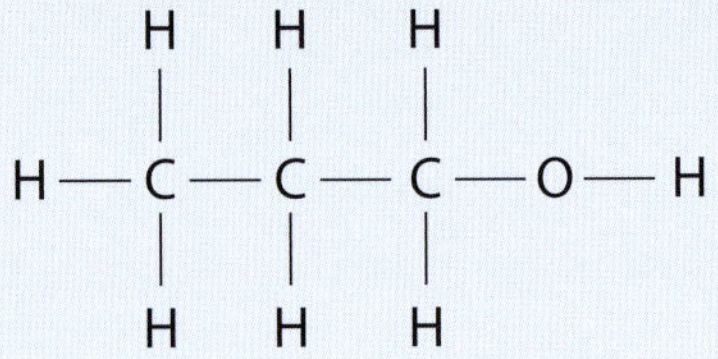

Answer

Removing all hydrogens, this becomes:

C – C – C – OH

So the skeletal formula is:

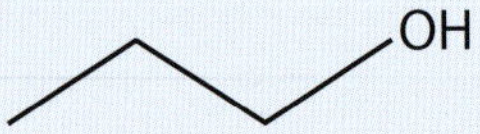

Worked example

Draw the skeletal formula of pent-2-ene:

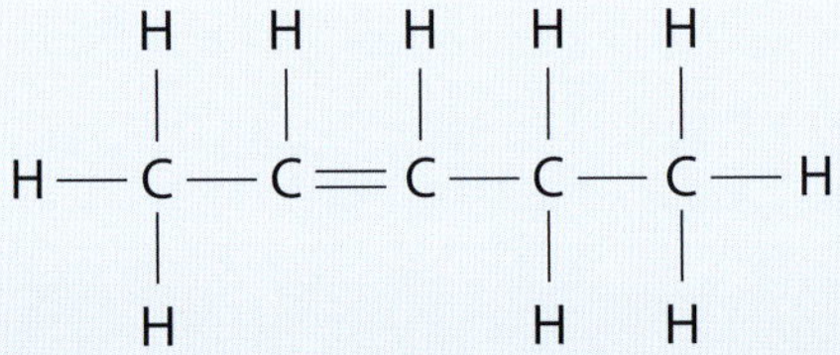

Answer

Removing all the hydrogens, this becomes:

C—C=C—C—C

So the skeletal formula is:

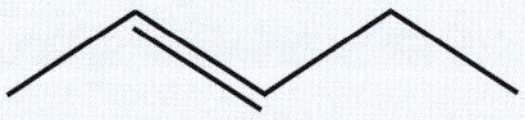

Worked example

Draw the skeletal formula of ethanoic acid:

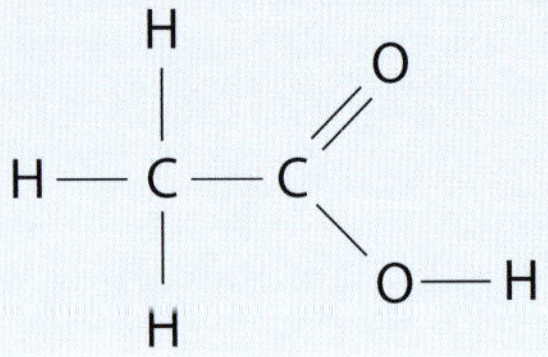

Answer

Removing the hydrogens, this becomes:

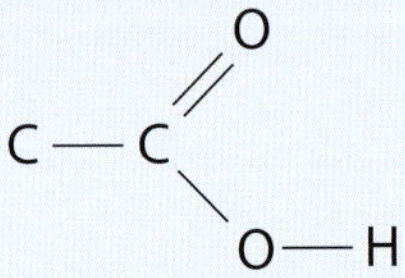

So the skeletal formula is:

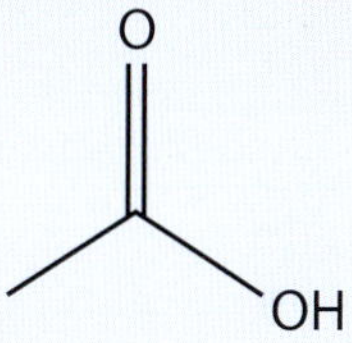

Worked example

Draw the skeletal formula of 2-methylpropane:

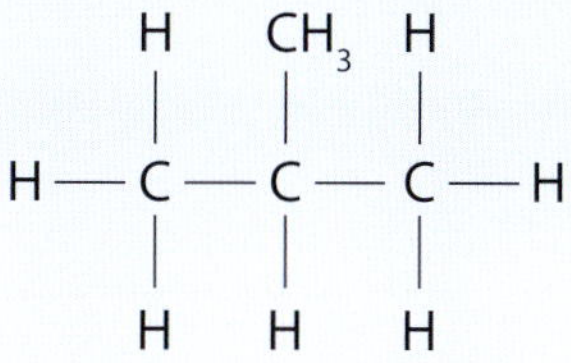

Removing the hydrogens, this becomes:

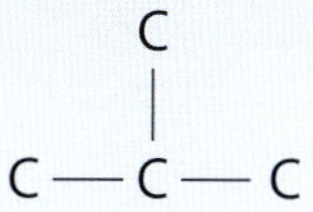

So the skeletal formula is:

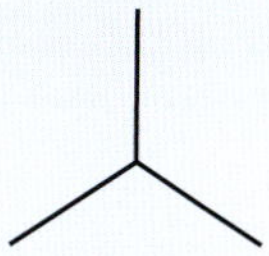

Tip: Do not make the mistake of placing a CH_3 on this skeletal formula because the line pointing up represents the CH_3 side group.

The following table shows some further examples.

Name	Skeletal formula	Structural formula
butan-2-ol	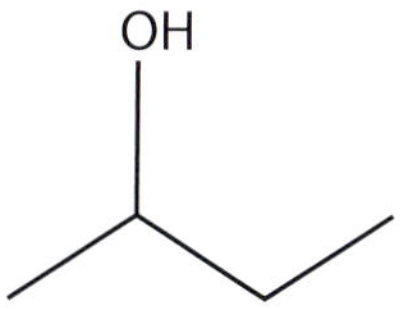	$CH_3CH(OH)CH_2CH_3$
pent-1-ene	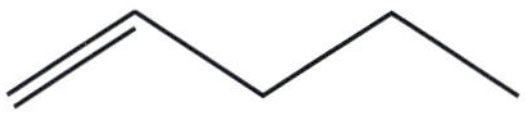	$CH_2{=}CHCH_2CH_2CH_3$
methanoic acid	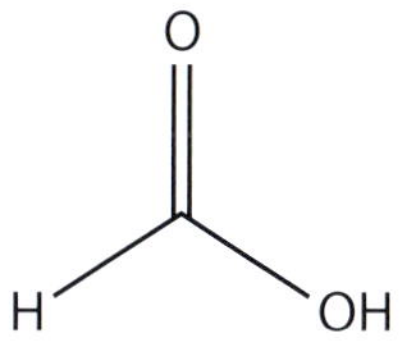 Note: a hydrogen atom must be placed at the end of the chain to show that there is only one carbon in the molecule.	HCOOH
cyclopentane	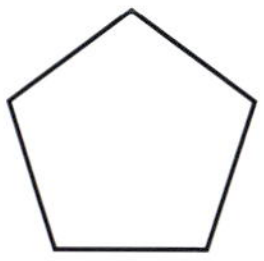	C_5H_{10}

Questions

1. Copy and complete the following table.

n	Name of alkane	Molecular formula	Name of alkene	Molecular formula
2				
3				
6				

[3]

2. Copy and complete the following table.

Homologous series	General formula	Name of functional group	Hydrocarbons (yes/no)?
alkanes		[redacted]	
alkenes			
alcohols			

[3]

3. Copy and complete the following table.

	Name	Molecular formula	Name of functional group
Alkane with 1 carbon	methane	CH_4	none
Alkene with 3 carbons			
Alcohol with 3 carbons			
Alkene with 2 carbons			
Alkane with 5 carbons			
Alcohol with 1 carbon			
Alkane with 6 carbon atoms			

[6]

4. Some data relating to the homologous series of alkanes is shown in the table below.

Name of alkane	Melting point / °C	Boiling point / °C	Structural formula
methane	–186	–164	CH_4
ethane	–183	–89	CH_3CH_3
propane	–160	–42	$CH_3CH_2CH_3$
butane	–138	–1	$CH_3CH_2CH_2CH_3$

(a) State the general formula of the alkanes. [1]
(b) State one piece of evidence from the structural formula column that shows that the alkanes are part of a homologous series. [1]
(c) Suggest other evidence from the table that shows that the alkanes are a homologous series. [2]
(d) Suggest the molecular formula for an alkane which contains 7 carbon atoms. Suggest how its boiling point compares to that of butane. [2]

5. Write the empirical formula for each of the following compounds.
   (a) C_5H_{10}
   (b) CH_3CH_2OH
   (c) C_3H_8
   (d) CH_4
   (e) C_6H_6
   (f) CH_3COOH

6. (a) A compound has the empirical formula CH_2O and M_r 120. What is the molecular formula? [1]
   (b) What is the molecular formula of a compound which has the empirical formula C_2H_6O and a relative formula mass of 46? [1]
   (c) State the definitions of empirical formula and molecular formula. [2]

7. A hydrocarbon contains 2.88 g of carbon and 0.36 g hydrogen. What is the empirical formula of the hydrocarbon? [3]

8. Calculate the empirical formula for a compound containing 81.8% carbon and 18.2% hydrogen. [3]

9. An alcohol has the composition by mass shown in the table below. The relative formula mass of the alcohol is 204. Calculate its empirical and molecular formula.

Element	% of element by mass
C	70.6
H	13.7
O	15.7

[4]

10. 1.29 g of a hydrocarbon contained 1.08 g of carbon. The relative formula mass of the hydrocarbon is 86.
   (a) Determine the empirical formula of the hydrocarbon [3]
   (b) Determine the molecular formula of the hydrocarbon. [1]

11. Find the empirical formula of a compound which contains 24.0% carbon 66.5% fluorine, 1.5% hydrogen and 8.0% oxygen. [3]

12. For each of the following:
   - draw a structural formula showing all the bonds,
   - write a condensed structural formula without any bonds,
   - draw a skeletal formula.

   (a) butane
   (b) propene
   (c) butan-2-ol
   (d) 2-methylpropane
   (e) 2-chloropropane
   (f) 3-methylhexane
   (g) 2,4-dimethylpentane
   (h) pent-2-ene
   (i) 2-methylhex-2-ene

[30]

13. Give the IUPAC name for each of the following. compounds

(a)

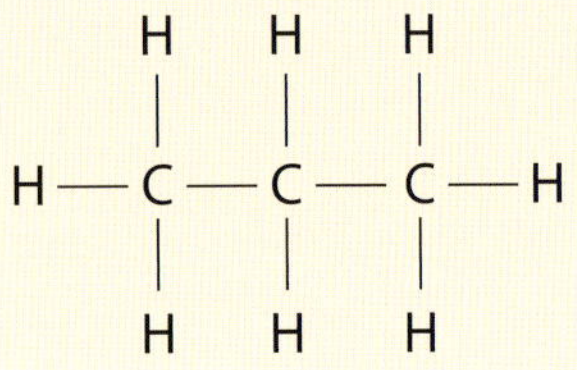

(b)

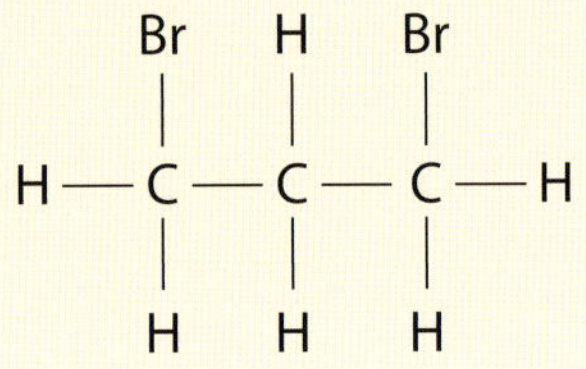

(c)

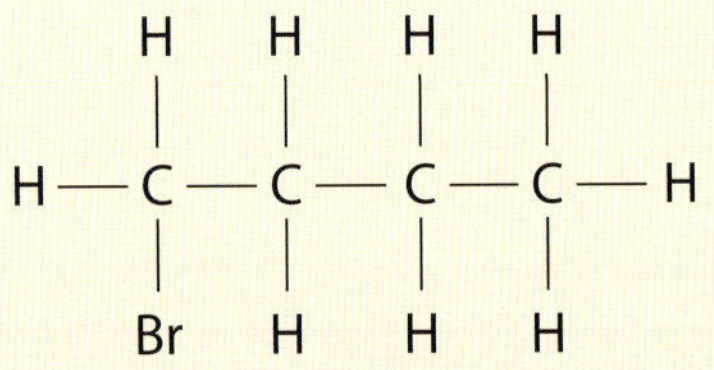

(d)

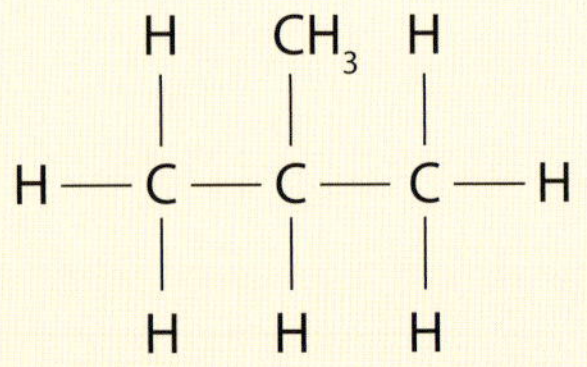

(e)

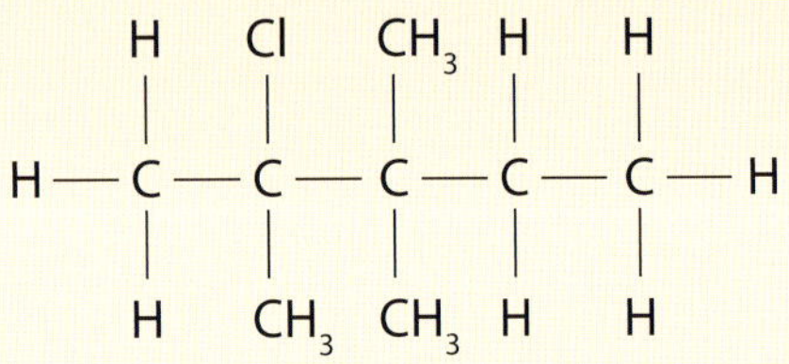

(f)

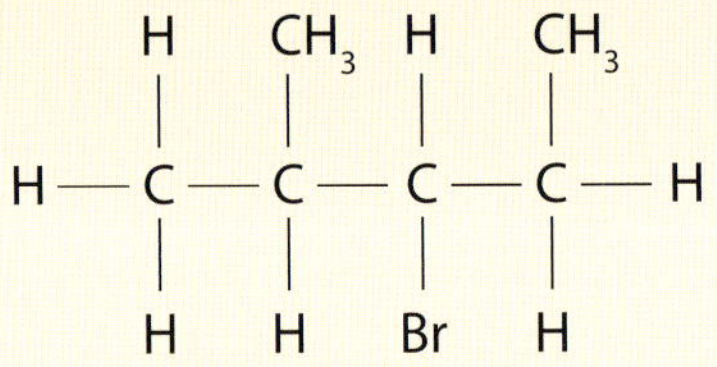

(g)

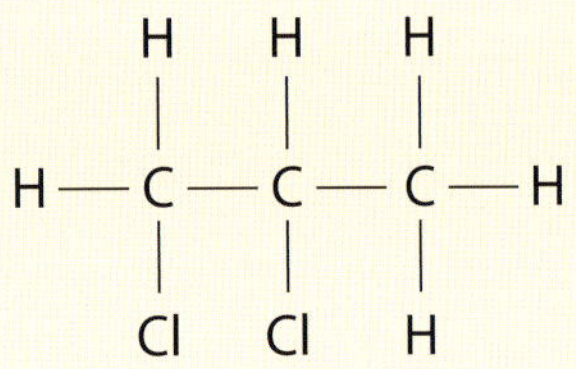

(h)

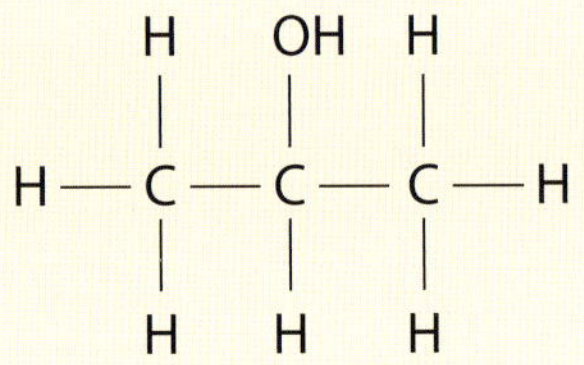

(i)

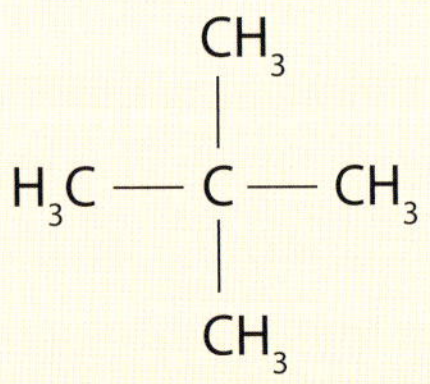

(j)

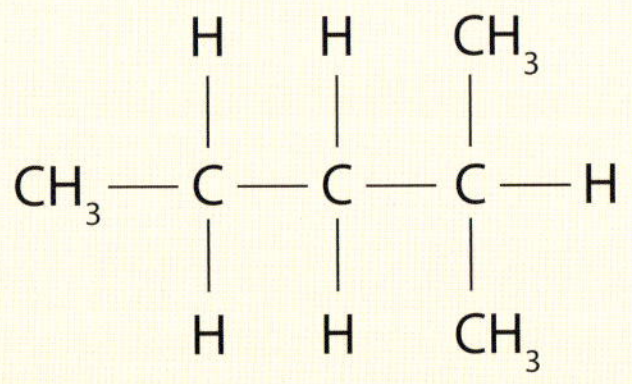

(k)

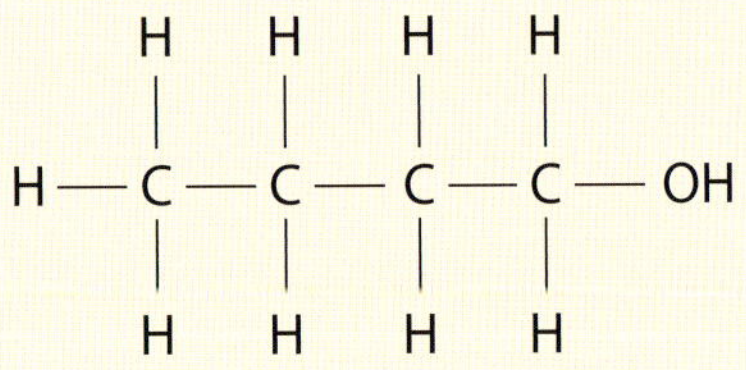

(l)

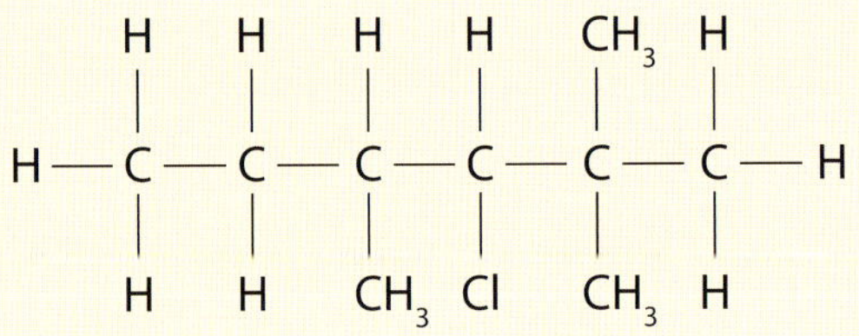

(m)

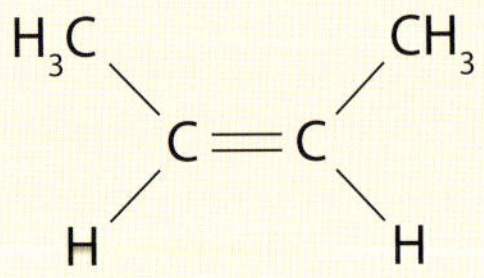

(n)

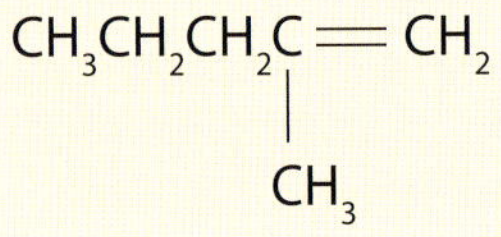

(o) 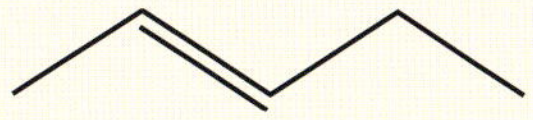	(p) 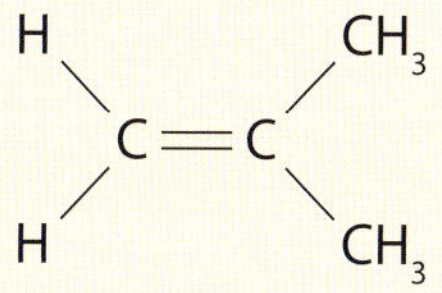
(q) 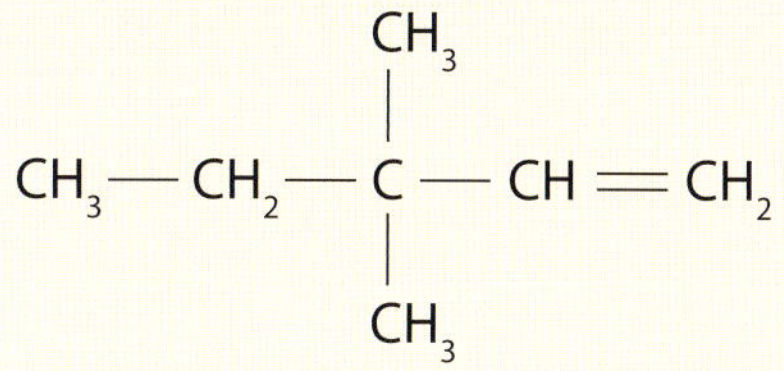	(r) 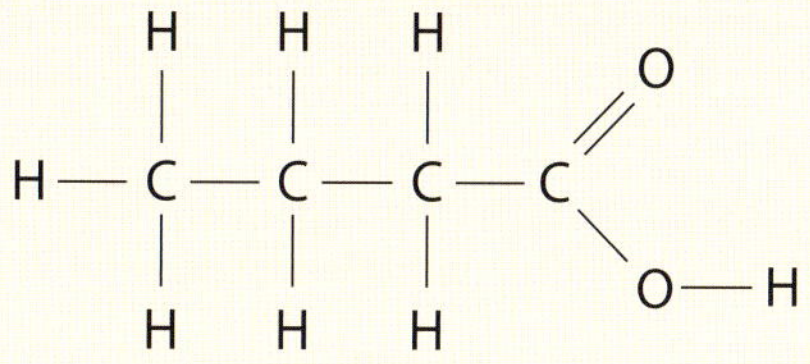
(s) $CH_2CBrCH_2CH_3$	(t) $(CH_3)_2CHOH$

[20]

2: ALKANES

Students should be able to:

- **8.2.1** write the general formula for alkanes as C_nH_{2n+2};
- **8.2.2** demonstrate an understanding and explain that alkanes and cycloalkanes are saturated compounds;
- **8.2.3** recall the structural and molecular formulae for alkanes with up to six carbon atoms;
- **8.2.5** apply IUPAC rules to naming alkanes with up to six carbon atoms;
- **8.1.8** describe and explain structural isomerism for aliphatic compounds containing up to six carbon atoms.
- **8.2.4** demonstrate an understanding that alkane fuels are obtained from the fractional distillation, cracking and reforming of crude oil;
- **8.2.6** describe the following reactions using balanced symbol equations:
  - the combustion of alkanes in both limited and plentiful supplies of air; and
  - the substitution reactions between methane and halogens (mechanism not required);
- **8.2.7** state that pollutants including carbon monoxide, oxides of nitrogen and sulfur, carbon particulates and unburned hydrocarbons are formed during the combustion of alkane fuels;
- **8.2.8** discuss the environmental problems associated with spillage and combustion of hydrocarbons.
- **8.2.9** demonstrate an understanding of how using a catalytic converter solves some problems caused by vehicle emissions by allowing the conversion of unburnt hydrocarbons to carbon dioxide and water, of carbon monoxide to carbon dioxide and of NO_x to nitrogen;
- **8.2.10** demonstrate an understanding of the use of alternative fuels, including alcohol and biodiesel derived from renewable sources such as plants, comparing these with non-renewable fossil fuelsl;
- **8.1.7** classify reactions for molecules up to six carbon atoms long as addition, elimination, substitution, oxidation, reduction, hydrolysis or polymerisation [Note: some of these reaction types are explained in later chapters.]

Introduction to alkanes

Alkanes are a homologous series with the general **formula** C_nH_{2n+2}. Alkanes are **saturated** hydrocarbons.

Saturated means that a molecule contains only single C-C bonds and no C=C or C≡C bonds.

Tip: Remember that a hydrocarbon is a molecule that contains carbon and hydrogen only.

The table below shows the first six straight chain alkanes.

Number of carbon atoms (*n*)	Name	Molecular formula	Structural formula	Skeletal formula
1	methane	CH_4	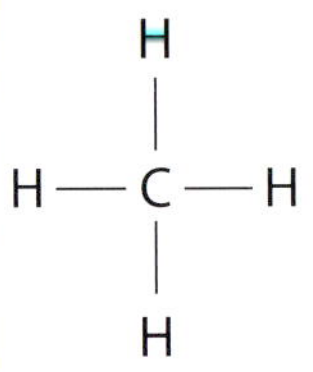	No skeletal formula
2	ethane	C_2H_6	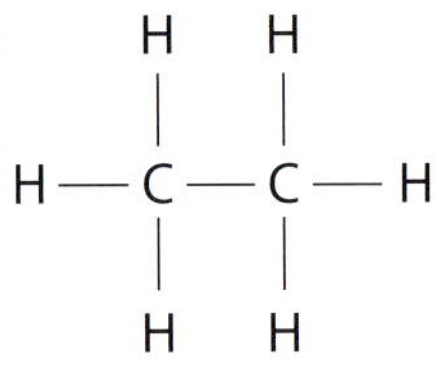	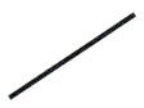

Number of carbon atoms (*n*)	Name	Molecular formula	Structural formula	Skeletal formula
3	propane	C_3H_8	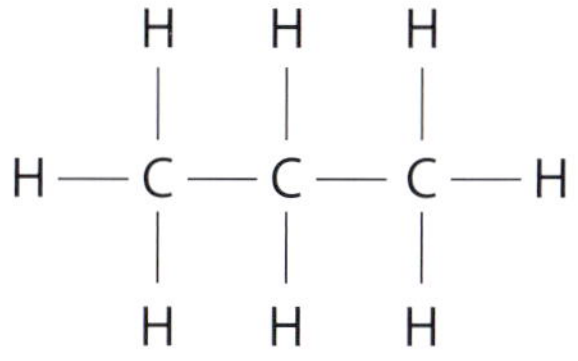	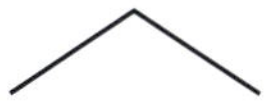
4	butane	C_4H_{10}	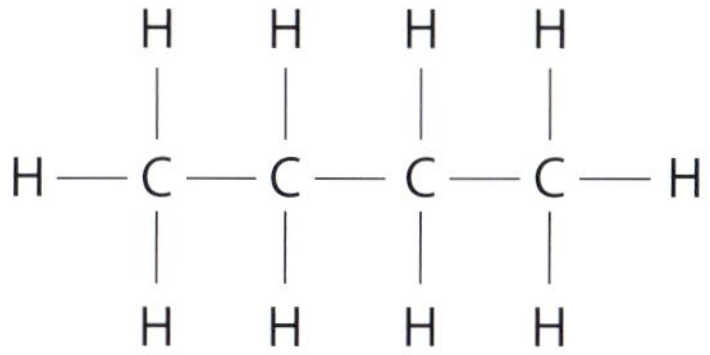	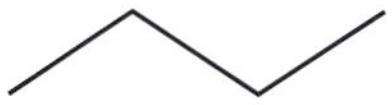
5	pentane	C_5H_{12}	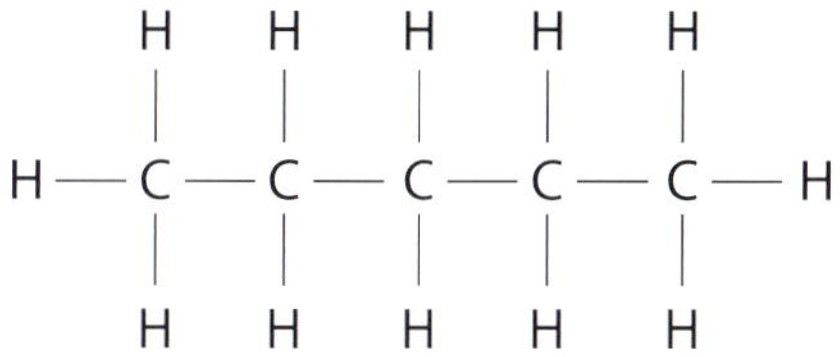	
6	hexane	C_6H_{14}	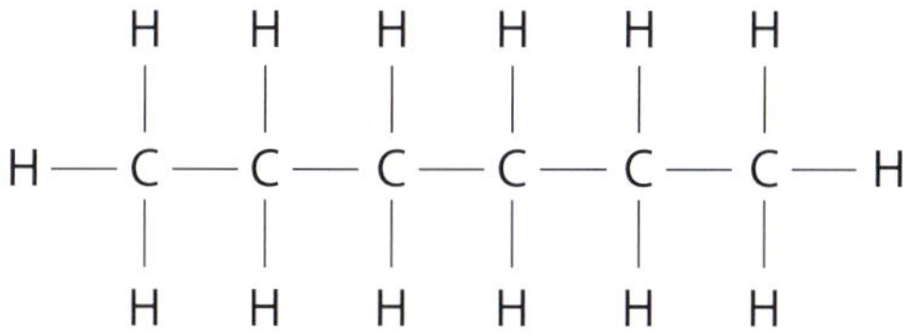	

Tip: Remember, you also need to be able to name and draw structural formulae for branched alkanes.

Cycloalkanes

Cycloalkanes are saturated and only contain carbon-carbon single bonds, but this time the carbon atoms are joined up in a ring. The smallest cycloalkane is cyclopropane.

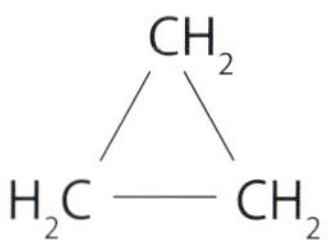

cyclopropane

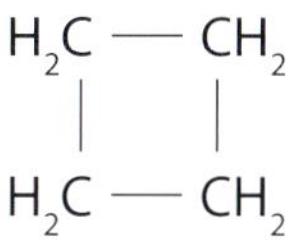

cyclobutane

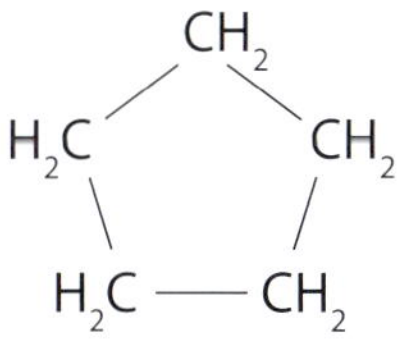

cyclopentane

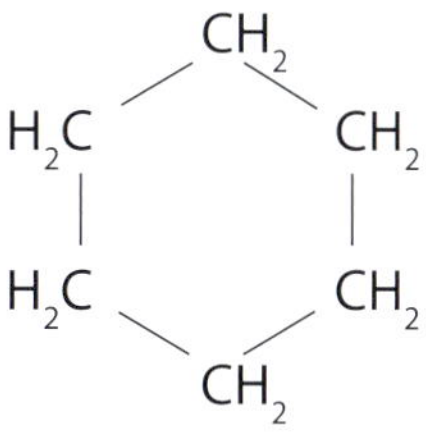

cyclohexane

The skeletal formulae are:

cyclopropane

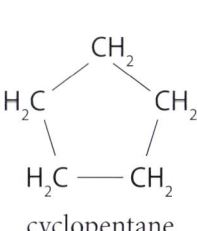

cyclobutane

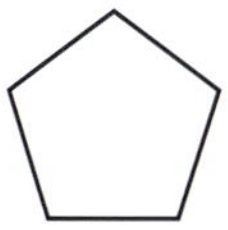

cyclopentane

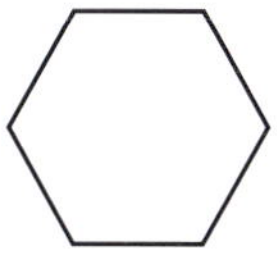

cyclohexane

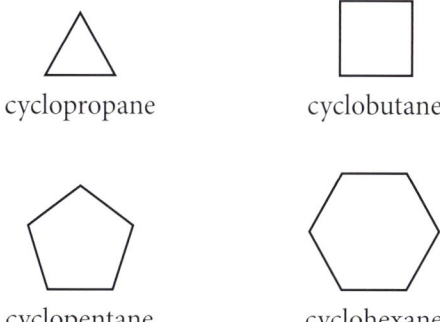

If you count the carbons and hydrogens, you will see that they **no longer fit the general formula** for alkanes C_nH_{2n+2}. By joining the carbon atoms in a ring, you have had to lose two hydrogen atoms. The general formula for a cycloalkane is C_nH_{2n} (the same as alkenes).

Isomers

Structural isomers are molecules which have the same molecular formula but a different structural formula.

You must be able to draw and name isomers for compounds with up to six carbons. The first alkane to have isomers is C_4H_{10}.

Worked example

Draw and name the isomers of C_4H_{10}.

Answer

First draw out the straight chain structure and name it:

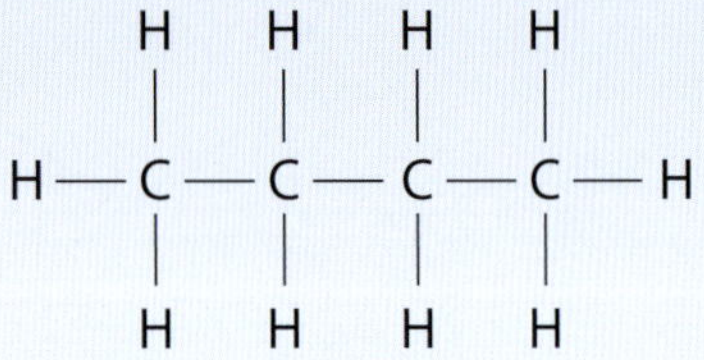

butane

Then shorten the carbon chain to three carbons and place a methyl group on the chain. It **cannot go on the end**, as this extends the chain length back to four carbons.

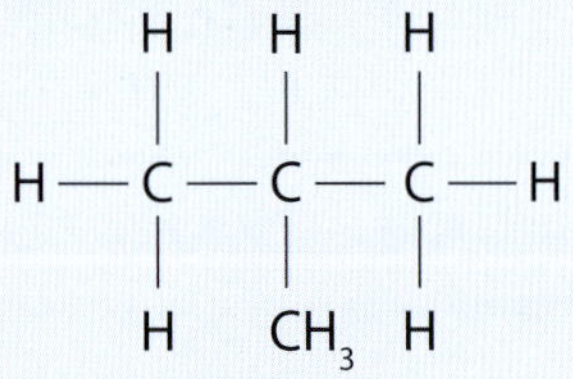

2-methylpropane

Butane and 2-methylpropane both have the **same molecular formula** C_4H_{10} but different structural formulae. Hence C_4H_{10} has two structural isomers.

Worked example

Draw and name the isomers of C_5H_{12}.

Answer

Draw out the straight chain structure and name it:

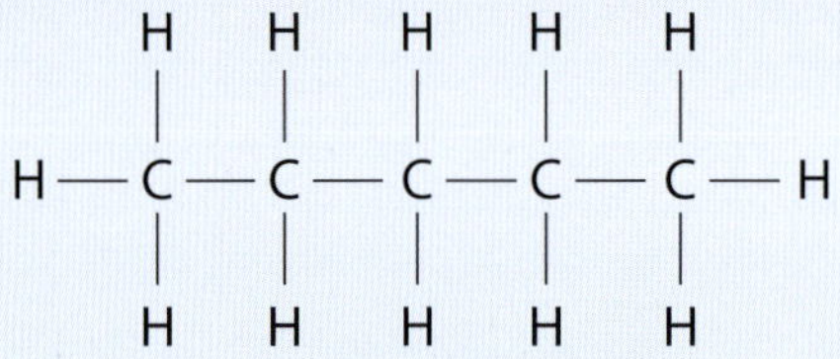

pentane

Then shorten the carbon chain to four carbons, and place a methyl group on the chain and name the isomer.

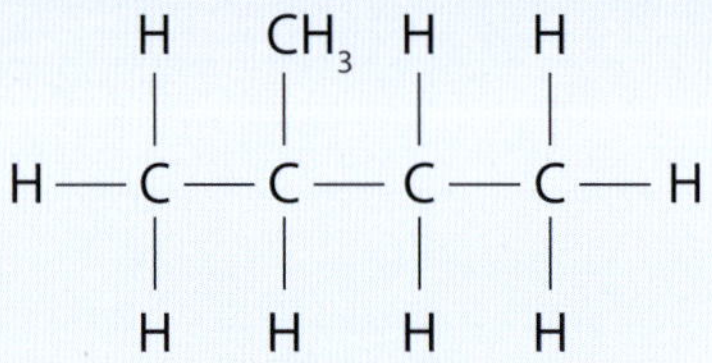

2-methylbutane

Consider whether you can change the position of the methyl to get another different structure. In this case you can't, because if you move it over one carbon then this is still position 2.

Shorten the carbon chain to three carbons, and place two methyl group on the chain. They cannot go on the end, so both must go on carbon 2.

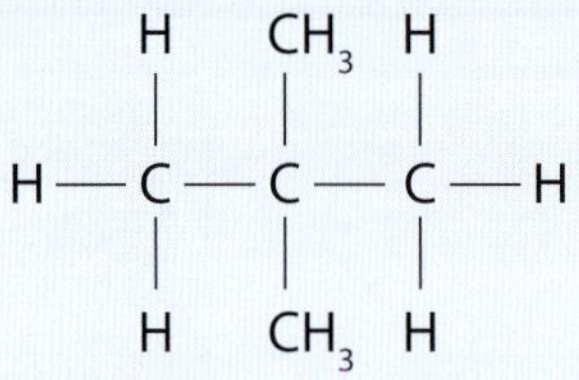

2,2-dimethylpropane

Hence C_5H_{12} has three isomers. All have the same molecular formula and a different structural formula.

Alkane fuels

Obtaining alkane fuels

1. Fractional distillation

Crude oil is a mixture consisting mostly of alkane hydrocarbons which have **different boiling points**. This difference in boiling points is used to separate them by **fractional distillation** at an oil refinery. This process separates the hydrocarbons into fractions.

A fraction is a mixture of molecules with similar boiling points.

Fractional distillation is the separating of a mixture of liquids of different boiling points by repeated evaporation and condensation.

The process of fractional distillation works in the following way:

1. Crude oil is **heated** and the vapour is passed into a **fractionating column** which is hot at the bottom and cooler at the top.
2. As the **vapour moves up** the column it **gets cooler**. Due to the **different chain lengths** and **boiling points** each fraction **condenses** at a different temperature.
3. The fractions are drawn off at different boiling points at different levels in the column.

The diagram below shows some of the fractions obtained during fractional distillation of crude oil.

Hydrocarbons with large molecules, such as bitumen, are collected near the bottom of the tower as they have a high boiling point, while those with small molecules and a lower boiling point are collected at the top.

Tip: The smaller hydrocarbons with lowest boiling points do not condense and exit the column at the top as gases.

Tip: The larger hydrocarbons present in crude oil do not vaporise because their boiling points are too high, and they are collected at the bottom of the column.

2. Cracking

Shorter chain alkanes are in very high demand as fuels or for synthesis of chemicals. However, longer chain alkanes are in less demand as they do not burn well and are less flammable. This means that there is a **surplus of the longer chain alkanes**, such as those in the bitumen fraction, from the fractional distillation of crude oil. These longer alkanes can be broken down into shorter, more useful alkanes by a process called **cracking**.

Cracking is the breakdown of larger saturated hydrocarbons (alkanes) into smaller more useful ones, some of which are unsaturated (alkenes).

Cracking is often carried out by heating, and

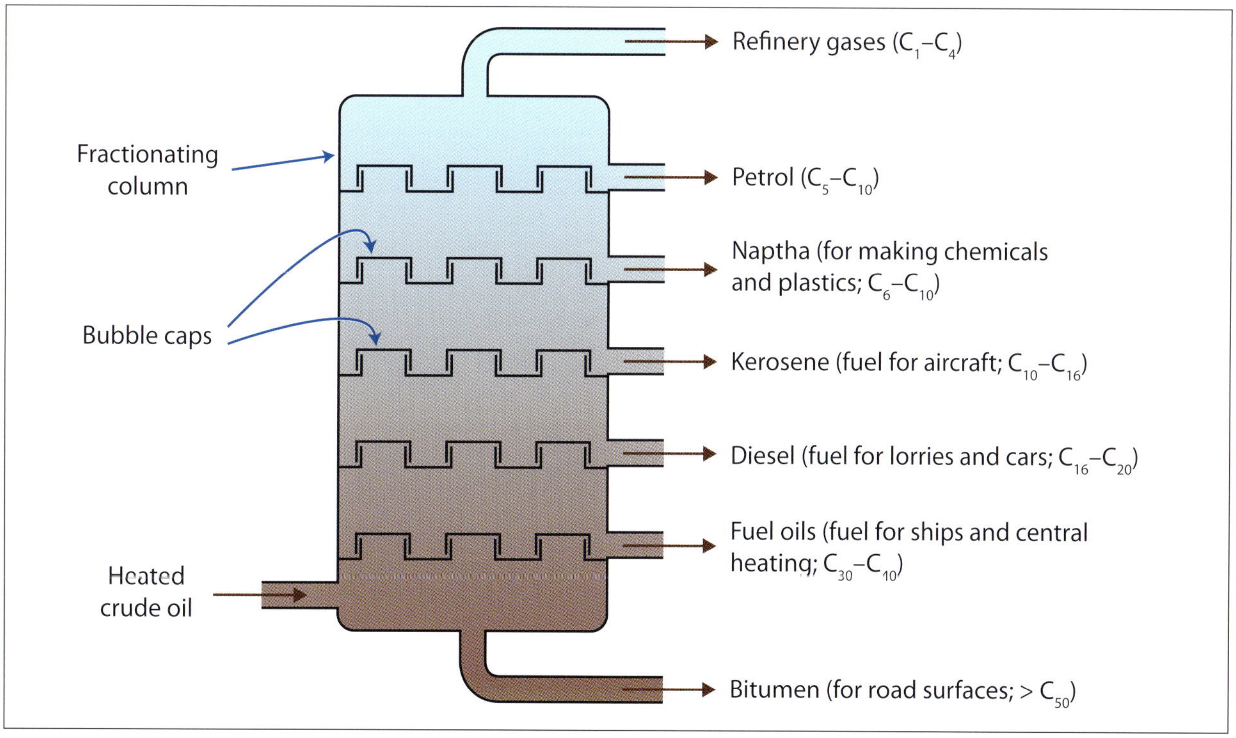

sometimes a catalyst is used. In this process, the large alkanes are thermally decomposed.

Tip: Thermal decomposition is the breakdown of a substance by heat.

The alkenes produced can be used as a starting material to make many other substances such as polymers (see chapter 5).

A **general equation** to describe cracking is:

$$C_xH_y \rightarrow C_aH_b + C_cH_d$$

where $x = a + c$ and $y = b + d$

The numbers of carbon and hydrogen atoms on the left- and right-hand sides of the equation have to balance. At least **one product** must be an **alkene** (unsaturated). For example,

$C_{18}H_{38}$	$\rightarrow$	$C_{10}H_{22}$	+	C_8H_{16}
saturated		saturated		unsaturated

Tip: You can tell whether a compound is unsaturated or not by the formula. If a formula follows C_nH_{2n+2} then the hydrocarbon is an alkane and is saturated. If the formula follows C_nH_{2n} then the hydrocarbon is an alkene and is unsaturated.

Worked example

Write an equation for the cracking of octane C_8H_{18}, to form ethene and one other hydrocarbon product. Name the other hydrocarbon product.

Answer

First write the formula of octane and ethene and represent the other product in the equation as C_xH_y.

$C_8H_{18} \rightarrow C_2H_4 + C_xH_y$

$8 = 2 + x$ so $x = 6$

$18 = 4 + y$ so $y = 14$

The other product is C_6H_{14}, hexane.

The equation is $C_8H_{18} \rightarrow C_2H_4 + C_6H_{14}$

Worked example

Write an equation for the thermal cracking of $C_{18}H_{38}$, to form butene and one other hydrocarbon product.

Answer

First write the formula of $C_{18}H_{38}$ and butene, and let the other hydrocarbon product in the equation be C_xH_y.

$C_{18}H_{38} \rightarrow C_4H_8 + C_xH_y$

$18 = 4 + x \quad x = 14$

$38 = 8 + y \quad y = 30$

The equation is $C_{18}H_{38} \rightarrow C_4H_8 + C_{14}H_{30}$

Worked example

One mole of a hydrocarbon is cracked to produce two moles of ethene, one mole of butene and one mole of octane C_8H_{18}. Write a balanced symbol equation for the reaction.

Answer

Allow C_xH_y to be the hydrocarbon and then write down the formula of the products using the information in the question.

Tip: Use the general formula of alkenes C_nH_{2n} to get the formula for ethene and butene.

$C_xH_y \rightarrow C_2H_4 + C_4H_8 + C_8H_{18}$

Then insert the number of moles given in the question.

$C_xH_y \rightarrow 2C_2H_4 + C_4H_8 + C_8H_{18}$

Remember that the equation must balance so the number of the carbons and hydrogens on both sides must be equal.

$x = (2 \times 2) + 4 + 8 = 16$

$y = (2 \times 4) + 8 + 18 = 34$

$C_{16}H_{34} \rightarrow 2C_2H_4 + C_4H_8 + C_8H_{18}$

3. Reforming

Reforming is a process in which the hydrocarbon molecules of petroleum are rearranged to improve their properties, usually with the loss of a small molecule such as hydrogen.

In reforming, a straight chain alkane is often converted into a branched alkane or cycloalkane with the same number of carbon atoms. Hydrogen is produced as a by-product of the reaction. A catalyst and a high temperature are needed. Reforming changes the shape of molecules rather than their size, unlike cracking which makes smaller molecules.

For example, hexane can be reformed into cyclohexane:

hexane	→	cyclohexane	+	hydrogen
C_6H_{14}	→	C_6H_{12}	+	H_2

This equation written structurally is:

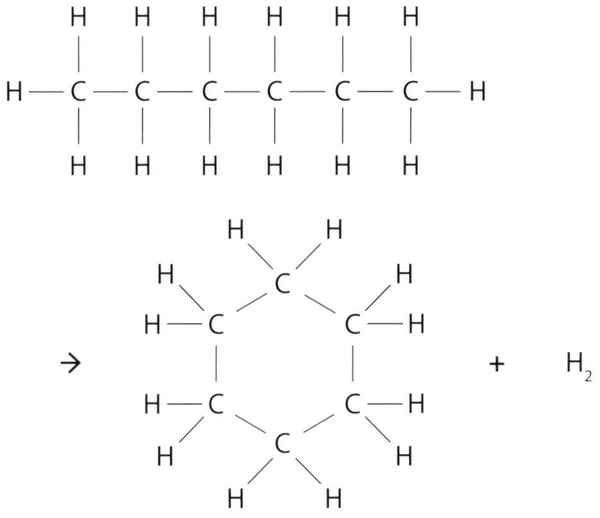

Benzene is a very useful compound made by reforming. It has the formula C_6H_6 and can be represented as:

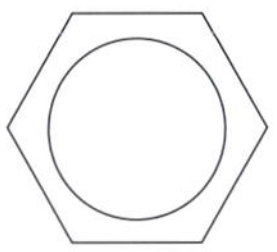

Tip: The circle represents delocalised electrons.

Hexane, C_6H_{14} can be reformed to form benzene, which can be used to make many different organic chemicals.

C_6H_{14}	→	C_6H_6	+	$4H_2$
hexane		benzene		hydrogen

This equation written structurally is:

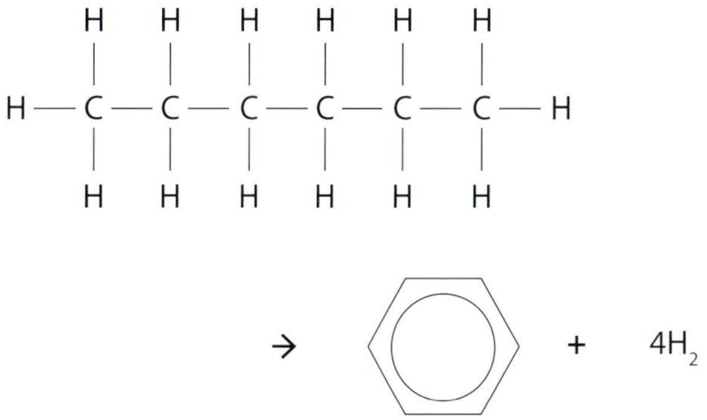

Combustion of alkanes

Combustion is the reaction of fuels with oxygen, forming oxides and releasing heat energy.

Alkanes undergo complete combustion in a plentiful supply of air and undergo incomplete combustion in a limited supply of air.

Combustion in a plentiful supply or air

Complete combustion occurs if there is a plentiful supply of oxygen from the air. The products are **carbon dioxide** and **water**, and energy is released. An orange flame is observed in the reaction (the higher the percentage of carbon present, the more orange the flame).

Worked example

Write a balanced equation for the complete combustion of methane, CH_4.

Answer

It is useful to first write the word equation and then put the correct formula underneath.

Word equation:

methane + oxygen → carbon dioxide + water

Unbalanced equation:

$$CH_4 + O_2 \rightarrow CO_2 + H_2O$$

We then balance the equation.

CO_2: there is 1 C atom in CH_4 so 1 CO_2 will be formed.

H_2O: there are 4 H atoms in CH_4 so 2 H_2O will be formed.

O_2: $CO_2 + 2H_2O$ contains 4 O atoms and so 2 O_2 will be formed.

The balanced equation is:

$$CH_4 + 2O_2 \rightarrow CO_2 + 2H_2O$$

Worked example

Write a balanced equation for the complete combustion of butane, C_4H_{10}.

Answer

Word equation:

butane + oxygen → carbon dioxide + water

Unbalanced equation:

$$C_4H_{10} + O_2 \rightarrow CO_2 + H_2O$$

We then balance the equation.

CO_2: there are 4 C atoms in C_4H_{10} so 4 CO_2 will be formed.

H_2O: there are 10 H atoms in C_4H_{10} so 5 H_2O will be formed.

O_2: 4 CO_2 + 5 H_2O contains 13 O atoms and so 6½ O_2 will be needed.

As there is a half in the balancing numbers of the equation, you can double all the balancing numbers.

The balanced equation is:

$$2C_4H_{10} + 13O_2 \rightarrow 8CO_2 + 10H_2O$$

Combustion in a limited supply of air

If limited oxygen is present, then alkanes undergo **incomplete** combustion to give **carbon monoxide** and **water**, and release energy. Sometimes **soot**, which is **particles of carbon**, is also produced, particularly with larger alkanes, but you do not need to include carbon in equations unless you are specifically asked to.

Worked example

Write an equation for the combustion of ethane in a limited supply of oxygen. Include state symbols.

Answer

Word equation:

ethane + oxygen → carbon monoxide + water

The alkanes are all gases, as is the oxygen and the carbon monoxide. Due to the heat energy given out the water is often formed as water vapour which is a gas.

Unbalanced equation:

$$C_2H_6(g) + O_2(g) \rightarrow CO(g) + H_2O(g)$$

Balanced equation:

$$C_2H_6(g) + 2\tfrac{1}{2}O_2(g) \rightarrow 2CO(g) + 3H_2O(g)$$

As there is a half in the balancing numbers in the equation it is usual to double all the values.

$$2C_2H_6(g) + 5O_2(g) \rightarrow 4CO(g) + 6H_2O(g)$$

Tip: Remember that in incomplete combustion carbon is also produced, but do not put it in equations unless you are asked to.

Carbon monoxide is a toxic gas which prevents haemoglobin in the blood carrying oxygen. Hence incomplete combustion is dangerous. Symptoms of carbon monoxide poisoning include headache, dizziness, nausea, and lack of concentration. Exposure to high concentrations can cause unconsciousness and death.

Environmental pollution due to combustion of alkane fuels

The combustion of fuels is a major source of atmospheric pollution. The table opposite shows some of the pollutants, how they are formed and the problems they cause.

Pollutant	How the pollutant is formed?	Environmental problems caused
carbon dioxide	Complete combustion of hydrocarbon fuels	Carbon dioxide is a greenhouse gas and leads to the greenhouse effect: it absorbs infra-red radiation given off by the Earth and causes the Earth's surface to warm. This leads to environmental problems such as: • sea level rises, • flooding, • climate change.
carbon monoxide	Incomplete combustion of fuels in limited oxygen	Carbon monoxide is a toxic gas as it combines with haemoglobin in the blood, preventing the blood from carrying oxygen, and can lead to death.
carbon particulates	Incomplete combustion of fuels in limited oxygen	The carbon particles pollute the air causing global dimming which stops the sun's rays reaching the Earth. They can cause respiratory problems and worsen asthma.
oxides of nitrogen (NO_x)	Nitrogen from the air reacts with oxygen at high temperature and pressure in engines. $N_2 + O_2 \rightarrow 2NO$ (nitrogen(II) oxide) $N_2 + 2O_2 \rightarrow 2NO_2$ (nitrogen(IV) oxide)	Oxides of nitrogen react with unburned hydrocarbons to produce photochemical smog. Oxides of nitrogen dissolve in water to form acid rain.
oxides of sulfur	Many fuels contain sulfur impurities which burn and produce acidic sulfur dioxide. $S + O_2 \rightarrow SO_2$. The sulfur dioxide reacts with water in the atmosphere to form sulfurous acid which falls as acid rain. $H_2O + SO_2 \rightarrow H_2SO_3$	Acid rain can: • react with and corrode/damage buildings, especially limestone buildings, • damage vegetation and defoiliate trees, • kill fish in lakes and rivers.
unburned hydrocarbons	Not all of the fuel burns, and some unburnt hydrocarbons leave the exhaust.	They react with nitrogen oxides (NO_x) to form ground level ozone (O_3) which is a component of smog. It irritates eyes, and causes respiratory problems.

Tip: You should say that acid rain **reacts** with limestone buildings. The term 'erodes' implies a physical process, which is incorrect.

Tip: Make sure you learn the equations below and both names of the product.

$N_2 + O_2 \rightarrow 2NO$

(nitrogen(II) oxide/nitrogen monoxide)

$N_2 + 2O_2 \rightarrow 2NO_2$

(nitrogen(IV) oxide/nitrogen dioxide)

Catalytic converters

The conversion of polluting and harmful emissions from car exhausts to **less polluting** or less harmful products is achieved by reactions on the surface of **catalytic converters**. A catalytic converter has a honeycomb ceramic structure coated with a metal catalyst such as **platinum** or **rhodium**. The use of a coating means that less metal is used, which keeps the cost down, and the **honeycomb structure** provides a **large surface area** for the reactions to take place which ensures a faster and more complete reaction.

The conversions which occur in a catalytic converter include:

1. Carbon monoxide is converted to carbon dioxide.

$CO + O_2 \rightarrow CO_2$

2. Unburned hydrocarbons are converted to carbon dioxide and water.

For example:

$C_8H_{18} + 25NO \rightarrow 8CO_2 + 9H_2O + 12½N_2$

or

$C_8H_{18} + 12½O_2 \rightarrow 8CO_2 + 9H_2O$

3. Oxides of nitrogen (NO_x: NO or NO_2) are reduced to N_2 and O_2.

nitrogen(II) oxide/nitrogen monoxide:

$2NO \rightarrow N_2 + O_2$

nitrogen(IV) oxide/nitrogen dioxide:

$2NO_2 \rightarrow N_2 + 2O_2$

Reduction is a reaction in which hydrogen is gained or oxygen is lost. In this case oxygen is lost.

Environmental problems associated with spillage of alkane fuels

Oil is carried from oil fields to refineries in oil tankers. If there is leakage from storage tanks or from the engine, some of the oil may enter waterways. If a ship sinks or runs aground in the ocean large amounts of oil can be spilled. Oil spills cause considerable damage to the environment. It does not dissolve and so it floats on the surface. Some of the environmental problems are as follows:

- Beaches are destroyed by oil and look ugly.
- Wildlife is harmed, for example by ingesting oil.
- Since most oils float, the creatures most affected by oil are animals like sea otters and seabirds that spend time at the ocean surface. Birds' feathers can become coated with oil, which prevents them from flying. It also destroys their natural waterproofing and insulation, leaving them vulnerable to either hypothermia or overheating.

Alternative fuels

A non-renewable resource is a resource that, once used, cannot be replaced in a human lifetime. Fossil fuels such as oil, coal and gas are non-renewable resources. Their supply is finite and will eventually run out. **A renewable resource is a resource that can be replaced as it is used.**

Alcohol and biodiesel are alternative fuels which are derived from renewable sources such as plants. Alcohol can be produced by fermenting sugar beet, a renewable resource. **Biodiesel is a fuel that is produced from renewable organic materials such as vegetable oils and animal fats.** Bioethanol and biodiesel are both biofuels. A biofuel is a fuel that is made from renewable plant or organic material.

The environmental impact of burning of biofuels is less than that of burning fossil fuels because

- they are derived from **renewable sources** rather than finite sources;
- they are **carbon neutral** as there are no net emissions of carbon dioxide to the atmosphere, since the carbon dioxide made when the fuel is manufactured and burnt is equal to the amount of carbon dioxide used when the raw plant material is grown;
- biofuels do not produce SO_2, so do not produce acid rain.

There are however also **disadvantages** to the use of crops for the production of alcohol and biodiesel. These include:

- our food supply may be depleted, as increasingly land is being used to grow crops for fuel – in some countries crops that could be used to feed people are instead used to provide the raw materials for biofuels (this is an **ethical** issue);
- production of crops is subject to the weather and climate;
- it takes a long time to grow the crops.

Substitution reactions of methane with halogens

The halogens are Group 7 in the Periodic Table. They are found as diatomic elements and have the formulae F_2, Cl_2, Br_2 and I_2.

Tip: Diatomic means there are 2 atoms bonded in the molecule.

A substitution reaction is one in which one group or atom is replaced by another group or atom.

For example, methane reacts with halogens in the presence of **ultraviolet light**. The light is needed to break the bond in chlorine and start the reaction. A **substitution reaction** occurs and a halogen atom replaces a hydrogen atom.

The reactions of halogens with alkanes produce a mixture of halogenoalkanes with varying numbers of halogen atoms. The reaction of methane with chlorine produces hydrogen chloride gas and a mixture of chloromethane (CH_3Cl), dichloromethane (CH_2Cl_2), trichloromethane ($CHCl_3$) and tetrachloromethane (CCl_4). A chain reaction may occur. Some of the reactions are as follows:

- methane + chlorine
  → chloromethane + hydrogen chloride

  $CH_4 + Cl_2 \rightarrow CH_3Cl + HCl$
- methane + chlorine
  → dichloromethane + hydrogen chloride

  $CH_4 + 2Cl_2 \rightarrow CH_2Cl_2 + 2HCl$
- methane + chlorine
  → trichloromethane + hydrogen chloride

  $CH_4 + 3Cl_2 \rightarrow CHCl_3 + 3HCl$
- methane + chlorine
  → tetrachloromethane + hydrogen chloride

  $CH_4 + 4Cl_2 \rightarrow CCl_4 + 4HCl$

Condition (in each of the four examples):

- ultraviolet light

You must be able to apply your knowledge of these equations to the reactions of methane with bromine, fluorine or iodine.

Worked example

Write an equation for the reaction between bromine and methane to produce tribromomethane.

Answer

First write down the correct formula.

$CH_4 + Br_2 \rightarrow CHBr_3 + HBr$

Tip: Remember bromine is diatomic.

Then balance the equation.

$CH_4 + 3Br_2 \rightarrow CHBr_3 + 3HBr$

Tip: In an exam when you are asked to write an equation, you are expected to write a balanced symbol equation.

Questions

1. Hexane C_6H_{14} is a saturated hydrocarbon. It has several branched chain structural isomers.
   (a) Explain the meaning of the term saturated hydrocarbon. [2]
   (b) Write the skeletal formula of hexane. [1]
   (c) Define the term structural isomers. [2]
   (d) Draw the skeletal formula and name two branched chain isomers of C_6H_{14}. [4]
   (e) Write a balanced symbol equation for the combustion of hexane in a plentiful supply of air. [2]
   (f) Name two combustion products, formed from the combustion of hexane in a limited supply of air, which are different to those in 1(e). [2]
   (g) Write the skeletal, structural and molecular formula of cyclohexane. [3]

2. Name two structural isomers of
   (a) C_4H_9Cl [2]
   (b) C_5H_{12} [2]
   (c) C_3H_8O, which are alcohols [2]

3. Crude oil is a mixture of hydrocarbons which is separated by fractional distillation.
   (a) Explain the process of fractional distillation. [3]

(b) Suggest why fractions such as lubricating oils are not as useful as petrol or gas fractions. [1]
(c) Why is cracking necessary? [1]
(d) What is reforming? [1]
(e) Write an equation for reforming of hexane to form C_6H_6 [1]
(f) Write equations for cracking of
(i) C_7H_{16} to form ethene and one other product [1]
(ii) $C_{10}H_{22}$ to form propene and one other product [1]
(iii) $C_{16}H_{34}$ to form two molecules of ethene and one molecule of butene and one other product. [1]

4. Liquified petroleum gas (LPG) contains liquefied propane and butane. It undergoes combustion and is used in gas fires.
(a) What is meant by the term combustion? [2]
(b) Name all the products when propane burns in a plentiful supply of air. [2]
(c) Name all the products when butane burns in a limited supply of air. [2]
(d) Write a balanced equation for the incomplete combustion of propane to form two gaseous products. [2]

5 (a) When some alkane fuels burn in an internal combustion engine, nitrogen(II) oxide and carbon monoxide are often released. Explain how these pollutants form. [3]
(b) State the problems caused by the pollutants nitrogen(II) oxide and carbon monoxide. [2]
(c) Write balanced symbol equations for the conversion of nitrogen(II) oxide and carbon monoxide into less harmful substances in a catalytic converter. [2]
(d) State two environmental problems associated with the spillage of alkane fuels. [2]

6. Different pollutant gases are produced from petrol fuel in cars. Catalytic converters are used to convert the pollutants to less harmful products.
(a) Write equations for the formation of the following in cars.
(i) Nitrogen(II) oxide
(ii) Nitrogen(IV) oxide
(iii) Nitrogen dioxide
(b) Name a metal catalyst used in a catalytic converter and give the symbol for the element. [2]
(c) Name the substance(s) which each of the following are converted to in a catalytic converter.
(i) Unburned hydrocarbons [1]
(ii) Carbon monoxide [1]
(iii) Nitrogen(II) oxide [1]
(iv) Nitrogen(IV) oxide [1]
(d) Oxides of nitrogen can be reduced in a catalytic converter.
(i) What is reduction? [1]
(ii) Write a balanced symbol equation for the reduction of nitrogen monoxide. [1]
(e) Explain why petrol is considered a non-renewable resource. [1]
(f) Name two alternative fuels which are renewable. [2]
(g) State two reasons why burning biofuels has less of an impact on the environment than burning fossil fuels. [2]

7. Methane undergoes a substitution reaction with chlorine to form chloromethane.
(a) Why is UV light needed in this reaction? [1]
(b) Write a word equation for the reaction to form chloromethane. [1]
(c) Write a balanced symbol equation for the reaction to form chloromethane. [1]
(d) Explain why this reaction is a substitution reaction. [1]

8. Write balanced symbol equations for the reaction of
   (a) methane and chlorine to form dichloromethane [1]
   (b) methane and chlorine to form tetrachloromethane [1]
   (c) bromine and methane to form bromomethane [1]
   (d) fluorine and fluoromethane to form tetrafluromethane [1]

9. Methane is fully substituted by chlorine in a reaction.
   (a) Give the condition for this reaction. [1]
   (b) Write a balanced symbol equation for this reaction. [1]
   (c) Name the two products. [1]

3: ALKENES

Students should be able to:

- **8.3.1** write the general formulae for alkenes as C_nH_{2n};
- **8.3.2** demonstrate an understanding and explain that alkenes and cycloalkenes are unsaturated compounds and that they decolourise bromine water (qualitative test required);
- **8.3.3** recall the structural and molecular formulae for alkenes with up to six carbon atoms;
- **8.3.4** apply IUPAC rules to name alkenes with up to six carbon atoms;
- **8.3.5** demonstrate an understanding of the bonding in alkenes in terms of sigma and pi bonds;
- **8.3.6** recall that the C=C bond is a centre of high electron density and use this to explain the difference in reactivity of alkanes and alkenes;
- **8.3.7** define the terms electrophile and heterolytic fission;
- **8.1.10** demonstrate understanding that geometrical isomers result from restricted rotation due to an energy barrier about the carbon-carbon double bond and exist and E and Z forms;
- **8.1.11** draw and identify the structural formula of E and Z isomers;
- **8.3.8** demonstrate an understanding of and write appropriate balanced symbol equations for:
  - the addition reactions of alkenes with hydrogen in the presence of a nickel catalyst, to form an alkane (knowledge of the application of catalytic hydrogenation to the manufacture of margarine is expected; however, detailed structure of the oil molecule is not expected);
  - the reaction of symmetrical alkenes with hydrogen halides to produce monohalogenoalkanes and alkenes with halogens to produce dihalogenoalkanes (electrophilic addition mechanism required including the use of curly arrows);
  - the hydration of alkenes using steam in the presence of a catalyst to produce alcohols; and
  - the addition polymerisation of alkenes, including ethene and propene; [this is discussed in chapter 5 Polymers]

Introduction to alkenes

The general formula of alkenes is C_nH_{2n}, and they have a double carbon carbon bond C=C. The **functional group** of the alkenes is **C=C**, a carbon carbon double bond. The simplest alkene is ethene. Some examples of alkenes are given in the table below. You should be able to name and write the formulae for different alkenes.

Tip: You must give the position of the double bond for alkenes above propene.

Name	*n*	Molecular formula	Structural formula	Skeletal formula
ethene	2	C_2H_4	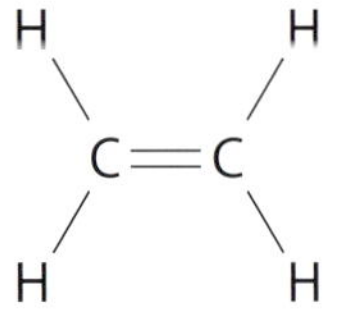 or CH_2CH_2	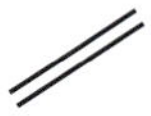
propene	3	C_3H_6	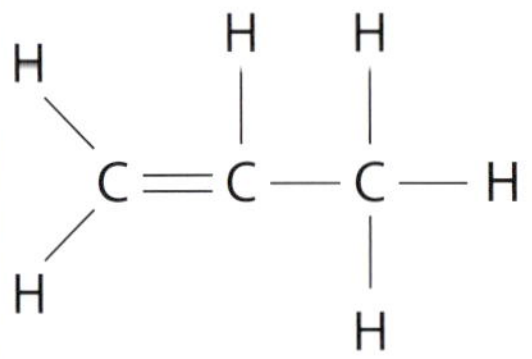 or CH_2CHCH_3	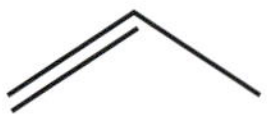

Name	*n*	Molecular formula	Structural formula	Skeletal formula
but-1-ene	4	C_4H_8	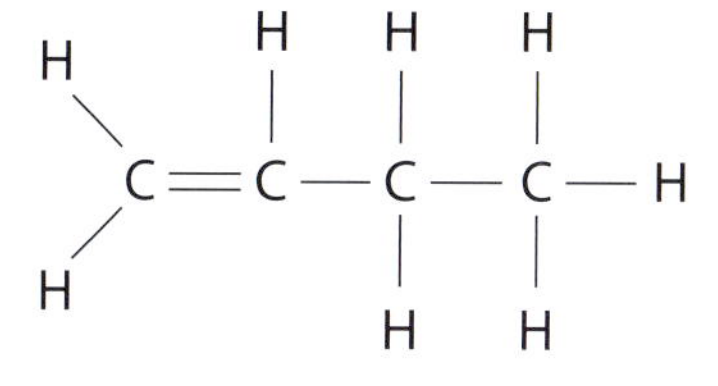 or $CH_2CHCH_2CH_3$	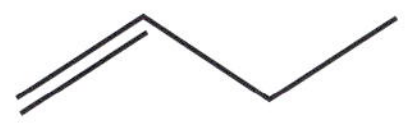
but-2-ene	4	C_4H_8	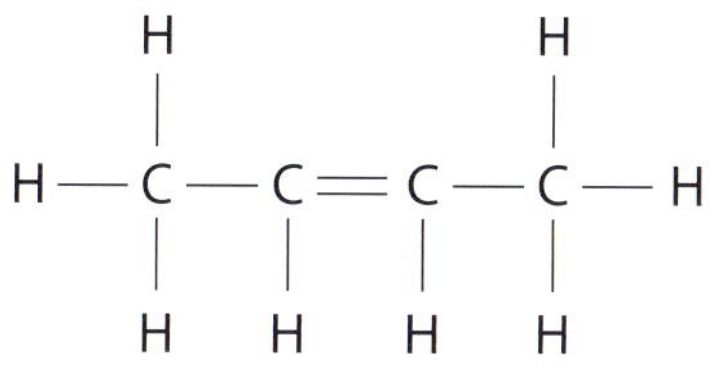 or $CH_3CHCHCH_3$	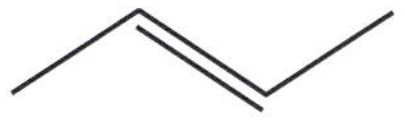
pent-2-ene	5	C_5H_{10}	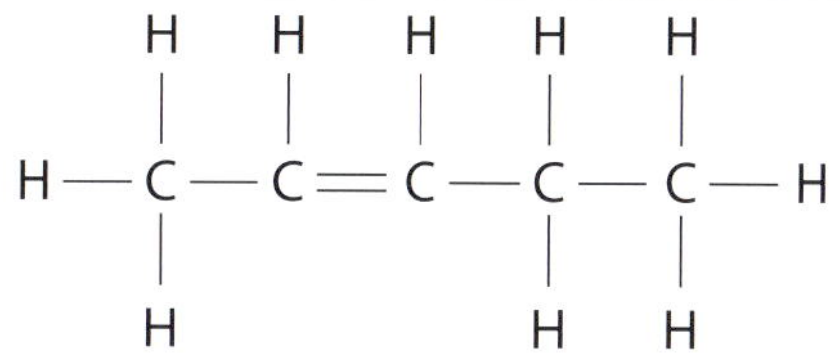 or $CH_3CHCHCH_2CH_3$	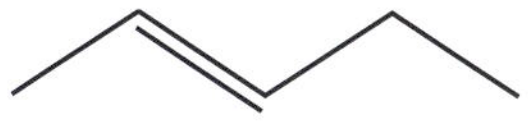

Tip: In a structural formula without bonds shown, it is possible to find the position of a carbon carbon double bond by looking for CHCH.

A **diene** is an alkene with two C=C bonds in the main carbon chain. Examples include:

- CH_2=C=CH–CH_3 buta-1,2-diene
- CH_2=CH–CH=CH_2 buta-1,3-diene
- CH_2=CH–CH_2–CH=CH_2 penta-1,4-diene

The bonding in alkenes

An atomic orbital is the space where electrons are found (shell). They have different shapes – they may be spherical (s) orbitals or dumbbell shaped (p) orbitals as shown on the following axes.

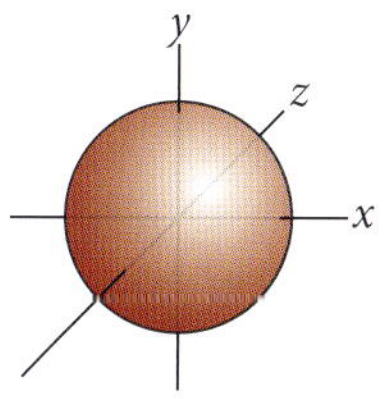

An s orbital (spherical)

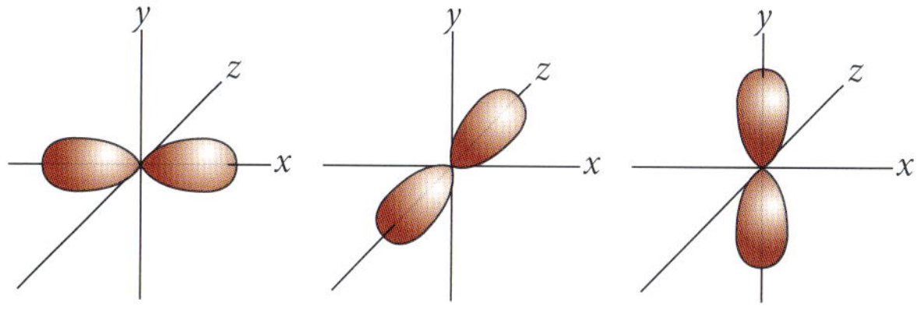

Three p orbitals (dumbbell) along different axes

Sigma bonds, σ

A sigma bond is a covalent bond formed by the linear overlap of atomic orbitals.

A sigma bond is formed by the overlap of two orbitals that are pointing directly towards one another. If two atoms are connected by a sigma bond, rotating one of the atoms around the bond axis doesn't break the overlap, and so doesn't break the bond, as shown in the diagram that follows.

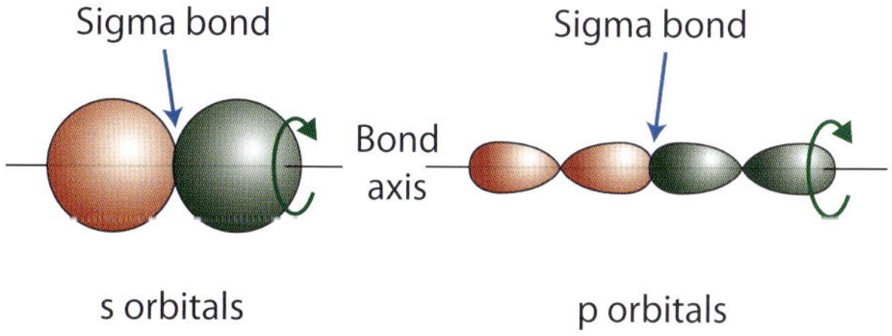

Rotating one atom around the bond axis does not break the bond

Pi bonds, π

A pi bond is a covalent bond formed by the sideways overlap of p orbitals.

The following diagram shows the formation of a pi bond. Each carbon atom contributes one electron from a p orbital to the electron pair in a pi bond. The pi bond is formed from the sideways overlap of parallel p orbitals on adjacent atoms.

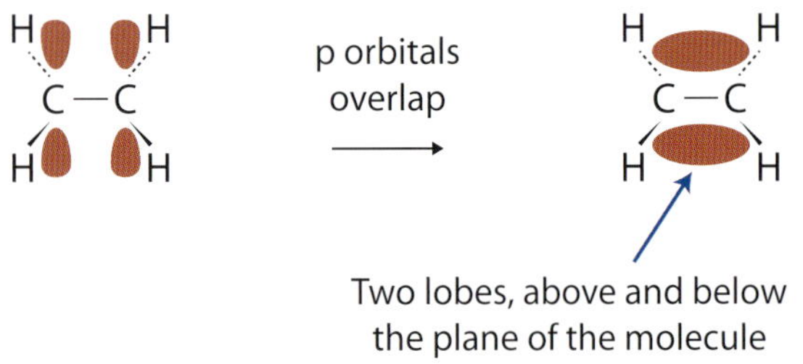

A pi bond cannot be rotated as the overlap breaks, as shown in the following diagram.

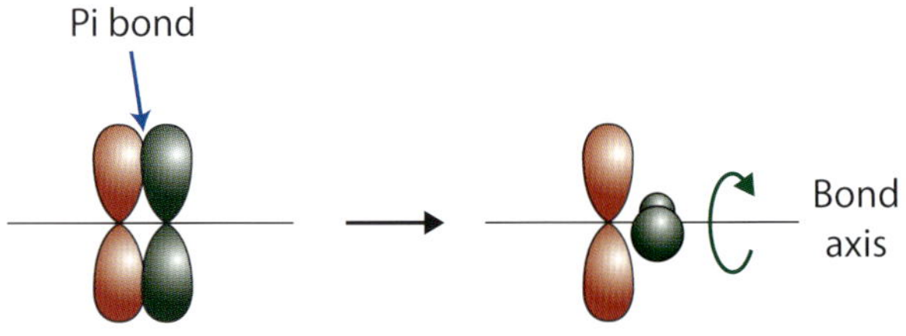

Rotating one atom around the bond axis breaks the bond

The carbon carbon double bond in alkenes

Alkenes have a **carbon carbon double bond** which is made up of two parts:

- a sigma bond,
- a pi bond.

A **carbon carbon single bond** is a sigma bond (as indeed are all single bonds).

For example, as shown in the structural formulae below, ethene has five sigma bonds and one pi bond, whereas ethane has seven bonds, all of which are sigma bonds.

Ethene

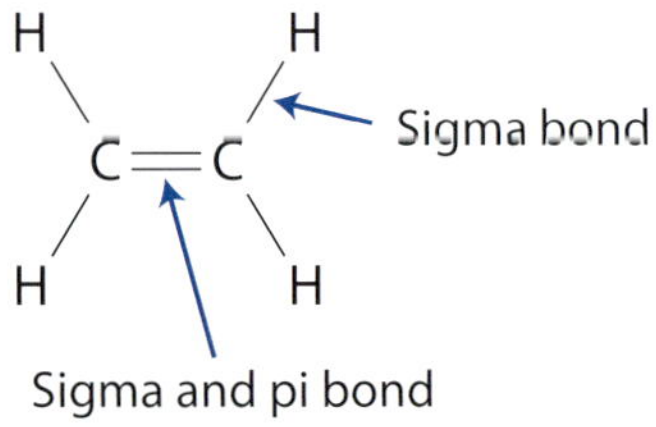

Ethane

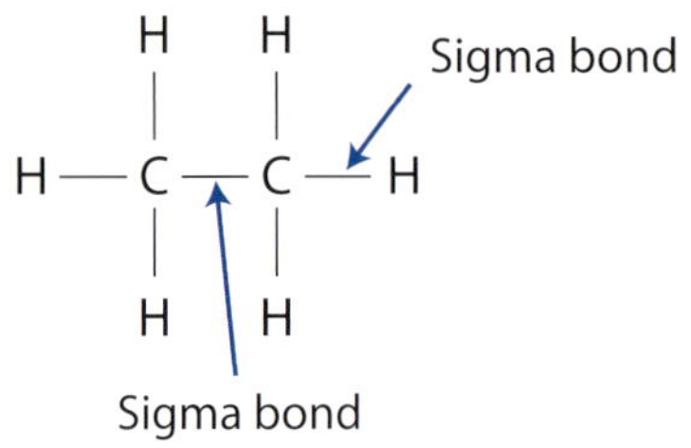

Carbon has four electrons in its outer shell which are used in bonding. Each carbon in the double bond of an alkene uses three of its electrons in the formation of three sigma bonds, and one electron in the formation of a pi bond.

The two electrons in the pi bond are not situated directly between the carbon atoms, and so they are not 'on average' as close to the nuclei as the sigma bond electrons. This means that they attract the nuclei less and are not as strong as a sigma bond. However pi and sigma together are stronger together so a double bond is stronger than a single bond.

Therefore:

- a pi bond is weaker than a sigma bond;
- a double bond is stronger and shorter than a single bond.

Later in this chapter you will study the addition reactions of alkenes. Alkenes undergo addition reactions because the C=C is a centre of high electron density, and because the pi bond in alkenes is weak and projects out of the molecule making it more open to attack by electrophiles. Alkanes do not undergo addition reactions because all the bonds in alkanes are sigma.

Stereoisomers

Alkenes have structural isomers and special types of isomers called geometric isomers, which are a type of stereoisomer.

Stereoisomers are molecules which have the same molecular formula but a different arrangement of atoms in 3D space.

> **Tip:** Structural isomers and stereoisomers are both molecules which have the same molecular formula but structural isomers have different structural formula whereas stereoisomers are molecules have a different arrangement of atoms in 3D space. Geometric isomers are stereoisomers.

Geometric isomers are molecules with the same structural formula, but a different arrangement of atoms due to the presence of one or more C=C bonds.

Why do geometric isomers occur?

If an alkene is rotated about the double bond, then the pi bond breaks as the sideways overlap of the p orbitals is broken. We say there is **restricted rotation due to an energy barrier** about the double bond at room temperature. This leads to two different structures, which are geometric isomers. Geometric isomers will occur if:

- there is a C=C bond (which has an energy barrier to rotation), and
- each carbon in the double bond must be attached to two different atoms or groups.

Consider but-1-ene, shown below. The two atoms on the first carbon (circled) are the **same** – they are both **H**. Hence but-1-ene will not have E-Z isomers. However but-2-ene, shown below, will have E-Z isomers because each carbon in the double bond is attached to two different atoms/groups – an **H** and a **CH_3**.

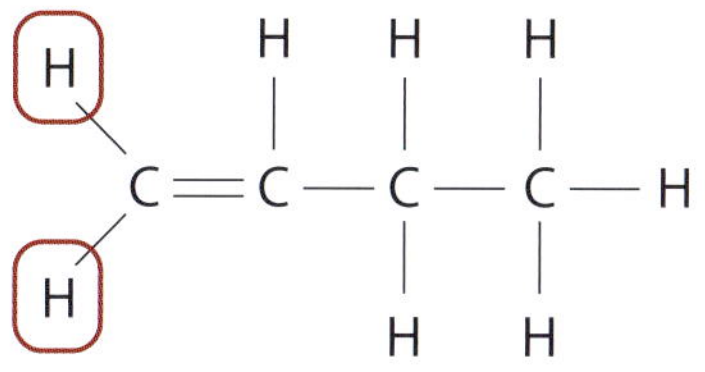

but-1-ene has no E-Z isomers

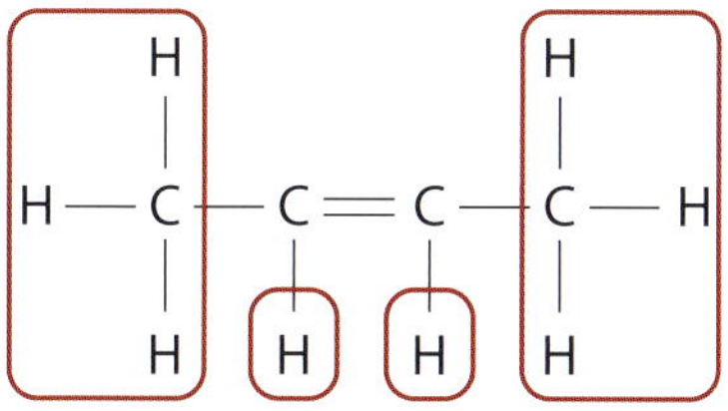

but-2-ene has E-Z isomers

Identifying E-Z isomers

Geometic isomers exist in **E** and **Z** forms.

Z means the highest priority atoms/groups are on the SAME side of the double bond.

> **Tip:** The Z comes from the German word *zusammen* meaning 'together'.

E means the highest priority atoms/groups are on the OPPOSITE side of the double bond.

To identify E-Z isomers, look at the first carbon in the double bond and decide on the priority of the groups attached to it. This is done using priority rules: the **higher the atomic number** of **the atom attached directly to the carbon of the C=C** then the **higher the priority**. If two atoms are the same, consider the total atomic number of the atoms bonded directly to them. Remember that atoms attached by double bonds have their atomic number counted twice.

Then, if both of the substituents of higher priority are on the **same** side of the plane of the C=C bond, the arrangement is **Z**; if they are on **opposite** sides, the arrangement is **E**.

Drawing E-Z isomers

The procedure for drawing E-Z isomers is as follows:

1. Draw out the general structure of an alkene.
2. Place the groups of highest priority on the **same** side – this is the Z arrangement. Add the other groups/atoms.
3. To draw the E arrangement, simply swap around **one** of the atoms/groups on the first or second carbon.

The E-Z isomers of but-2-ene are shown below. On each carbon the two atoms attached to the carbon of the double bond are H (atomic number 1) and C (atomic number 6). Carbon has the higher atomic number and higher priority and so in the Z isomer, both methyl groups are on the same side of the carbon–carbon double bond, but in the E isomer they are on opposite sides.

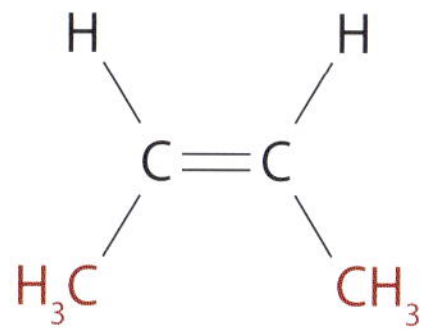

Z-but-2-ene

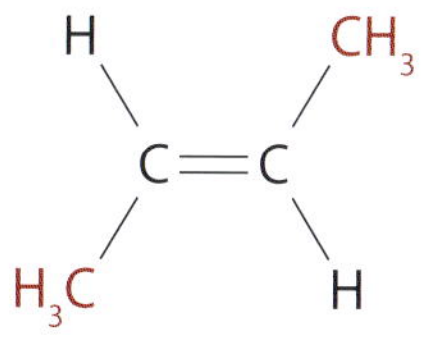

E-but-2-ene

> **Tip:** If you have drawn Z, then to draw the E simply swap around one of the atoms/groups on the second carbon.

Worked example

Draw and label the E-Z isomers of 1-bromo-1-fluoro-2-iodoethene.

Answer

First draw the structural formula. Then consider the priority of the atoms bonded to the left carbon and then to the right carbon of the C=C. Then draw the two isomers.

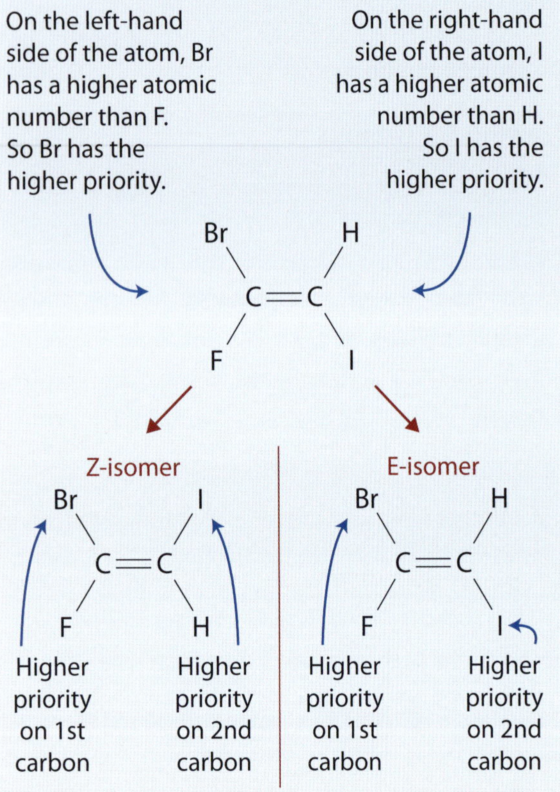

Tip: The isomers are named by placing a capital E or Z followed by a dash and then the name, for example, E-1-bromo-1-fluoro-2-iodoethene.

Worked example

Classify the isomer shown below as E or Z.

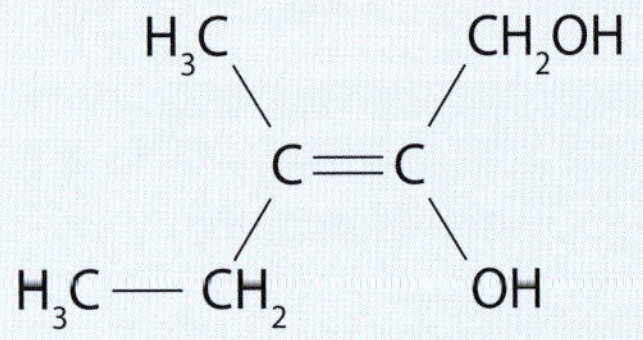

Answer

When the molecule contains groups rather than single atoms, the procedure works in a similar way. First, look at the atoms that are bonded directly to each carbon in the double bond. Then, move one atom away from the double bond and look at the atoms bonded there.

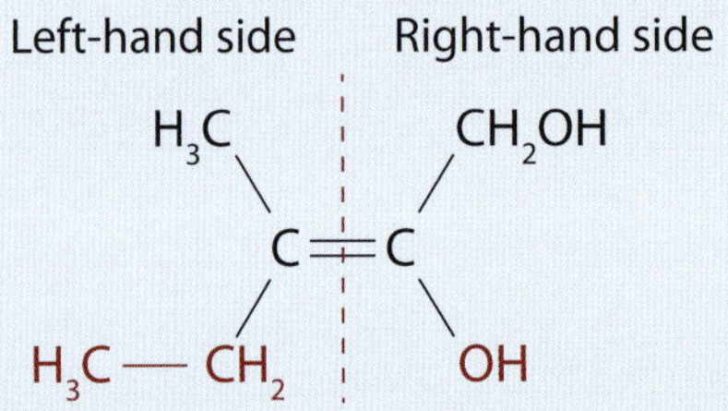

Considering the left-hand side:
CH_3 has the C atom bonded directly to the C=C, atomic number 6. CH_2CH_3 also has a carbon directly bonded to the C=C. This is the same priority.

Now look at all the atoms bonded directly to these carbons.

CH_3 has three H atoms. This is a total atomic number of 3. CH_2CH_3 has two H atoms and a C atom directly attached to the carbon of the double bond. The total atomic number is 8. So the bottom group, CH_2CH_3, has the higher priority.

Considering the right-hand side:
CH_2OH has a carbon directly bonded to the C=C, atomic number 6. OH has the O directly bonded to C=C, atomic number 8. So the bottom group, OH, has the higher priority.

Since both of the substituents of higher priority are on the same side of the plane of the C=C bond, the arrangement is Z.

Structural isomers

Alkenes also have **structural isomers** due to the position of the double bond and because cycloalkanes have the same general formula to the alkenes. For example, C_3H_6 has the isomers propene and cyclopropane, shown below.

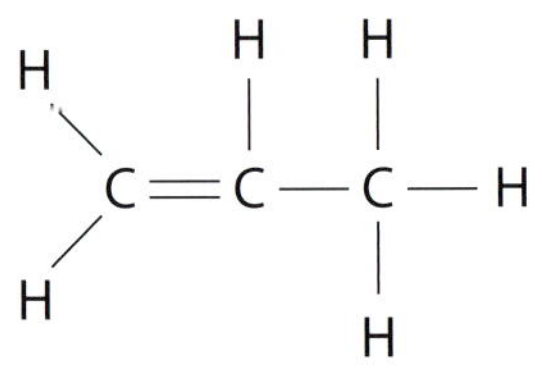

propene

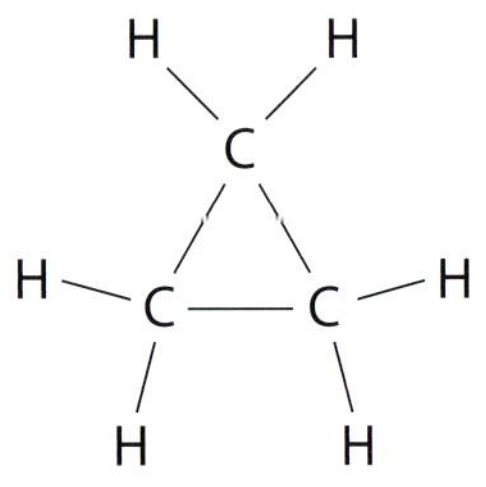

cyclopropane

C_4H_8 has geometric and structural isomers. In total it has five isomers, as shown below.

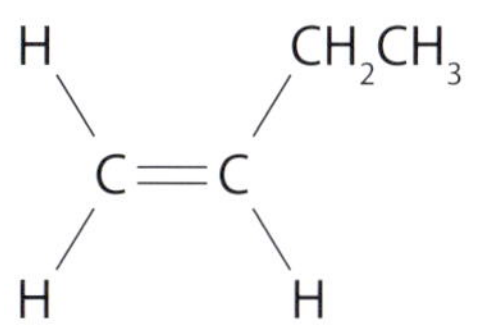
but-1-ene

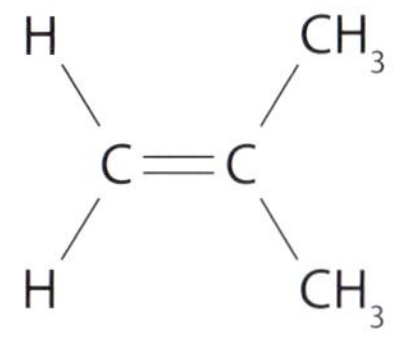
2-methylpropene

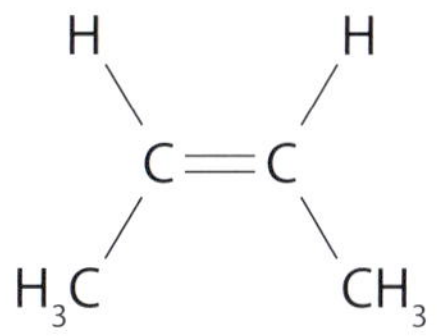
Z- but-2-ene

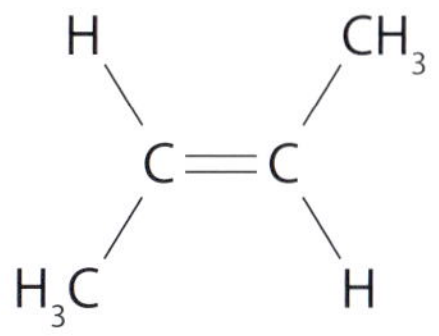
E-but-2-ene

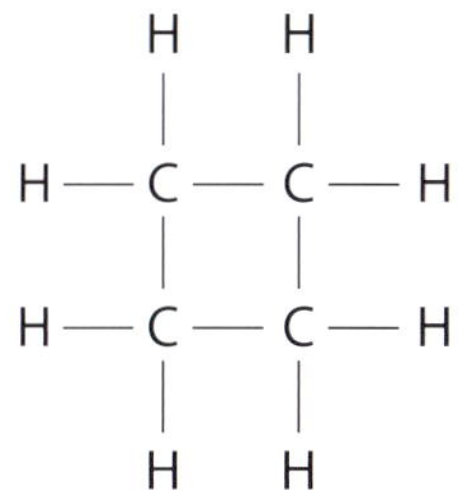
cyclobutane

Addition reactions

An addition reaction is when two or more molecules combine to form a larger one.

The reactant added 'adds across' the double bond, this means that one atom from the reactant joins to one carbon and the other atom from the reactant joins to the other carbon. There is only **one product**.

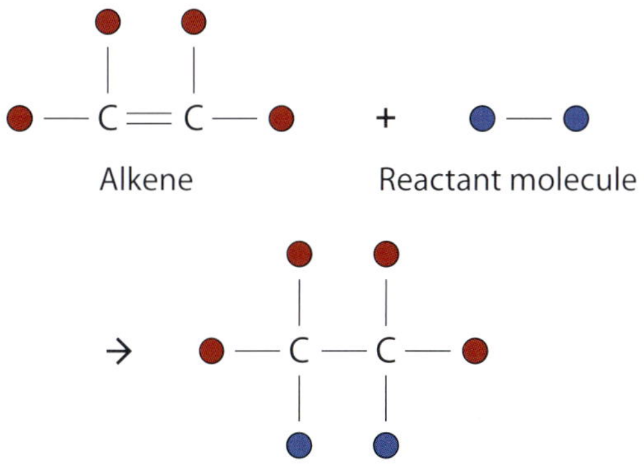

Double bond breaks and one atom of the reactant molecule joins on to each of the carbons of the double bond

You need to understand and write equations for the addition reactions of alkenes with:

1. hydrogen,
2. steam,
3. halogens, and
4. hydrogen halides.

1. Addition of hydrogen

Alkenes react with hydrogen to form **alkanes**.

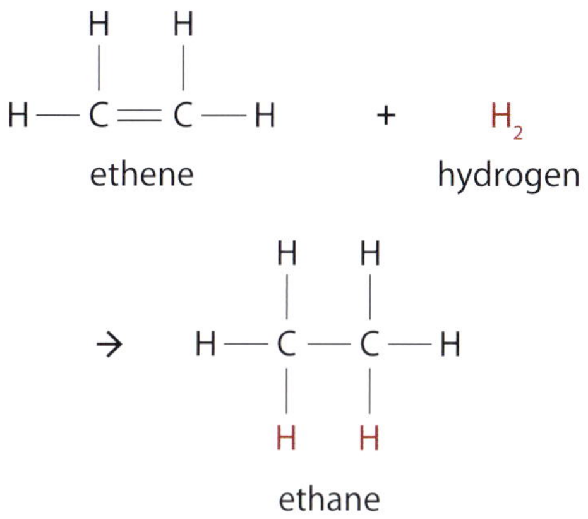

Molecular equation:
$C_2H_4 + H_2 \rightarrow C_2H_6$

Conditions:

- catalyst of finely divided nickel
- temperature of 140–160°C

This is an industrial reaction and is called **catalytic hydrogenation**.

Hydrogenation is the addition of a hydrogen molecule across a C=C.

> **Tip:** Remember that a catalyst is a substance which alters the speed of a chemical reaction but does not get used up. In this case, it is **heterogeneous catalysis** – the catalyst is in a different phase from the reactants.

This reaction is used in industry to 'harden' oils, which means that the melting point of the oil is raised and it is changed into solid fat. Vegetable oils undergo catalytic hydrogenation to form solid margarine. The double bonds of the oil have hydrogen added on and the unsaturated oil becomes a saturated fat. The conditions are:

- bubble hydrogen through the vegetable oil
- at 140–160°C
- using a finely divided nickel catalyst.

> **Tip:** You do not need to recall the structure of an oil molecule.

Worked example

Write a structural equation for the reaction of but-2-ene and hydrogen. Name the organic product.

Answer

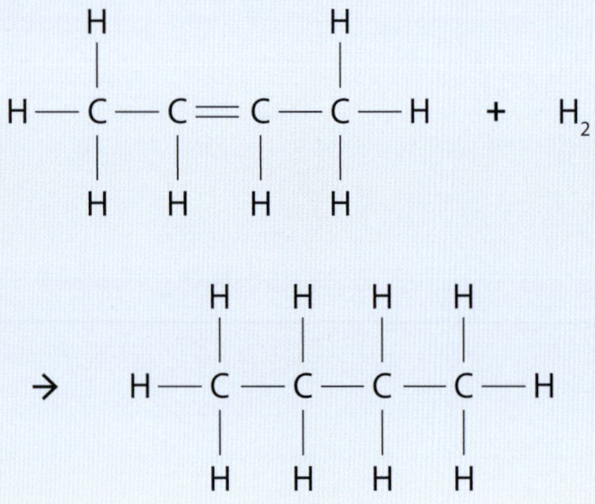

The organic product is butane.

2. Addition of steam – hydration

In this reaction steam is added on to alkenes to form **alcohols**.

Hydration is the addition of water to a molecule.

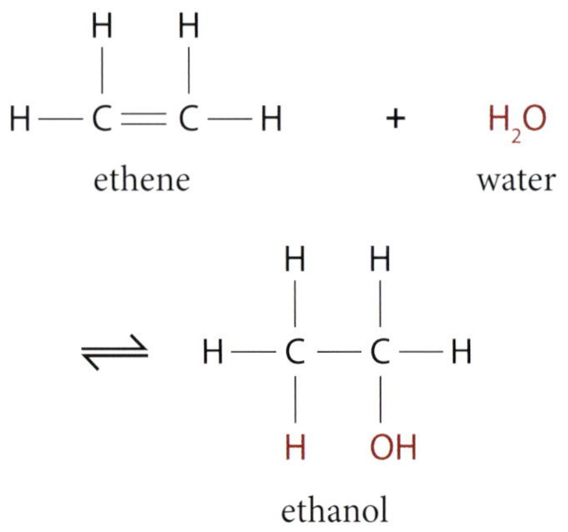

Molecular equation:

$C_2H_4\ (g) + H_2O\ (g) \rightleftharpoons C_2H_5OH\ (l)$

> **Tip:** Remember to include equilibrium arrows in this reaction.

Conditions:

- catalyst of concentrated phosphoric acid
- 60 atm pressure
- temperature of 300°C

This reaction is used in industry to produce ethanol.

3. Addition of halogens (halogenation)

Halogens react with alkenes to form **dihalogenoalkanes**.

ethene + bromine → 1,2-dibromoethane

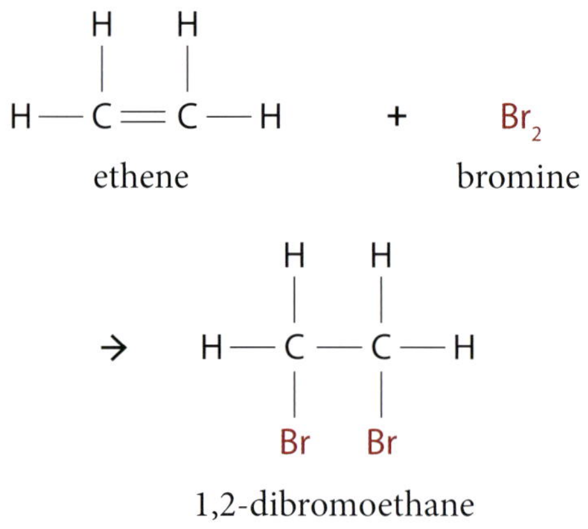

Molecular equation:

$C_2H_4 + Br_2 \rightarrow C_2H_4Br_2$

Condition:

- use a solution of bromine water

> **Tip:** Note that the bromine adds across the double bond so when bromine reacts with but-2-ene the product is 2,3-dibromobutane:
>
> but-2-ene + Br_2 → 2,3-dibromobutane
>
> 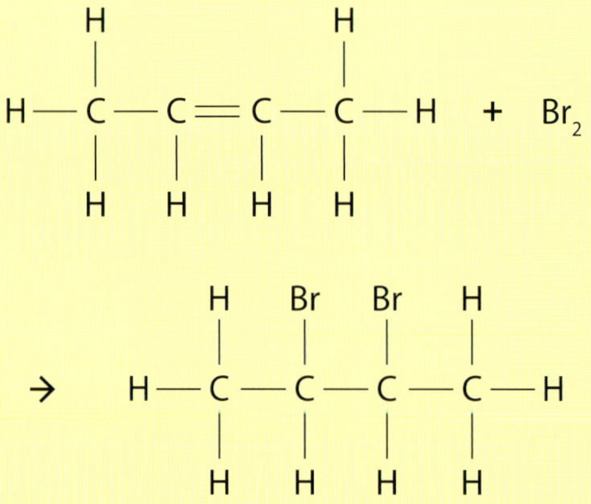
>
> Molecular equation:
>
> $C_4H_8 + Br_2 \rightarrow C_4H_8Br_2$

The reaction using bromine water is **a test for the presence of a C=C** or a test for unsaturation. The steps to test to determine if a sample is unsaturated are as follows:

- Shake the unknown sample with a few cm^3 of **bromine water**.
- If the bromine water changes from **orange to colourless**, i.e the bromine water is decolourised, then the sample is **unsaturated** and contains a C=C. Two layers are observed.
- If the bromine water does not change colour the unknown sample is saturated.

Alkenes and cycloalkenes are both unsaturated and will have a positive test with bromine water.

An addition reaction also occurs between ethene and chlorine.

ethene + chlorine → 1,2-dichloroethane

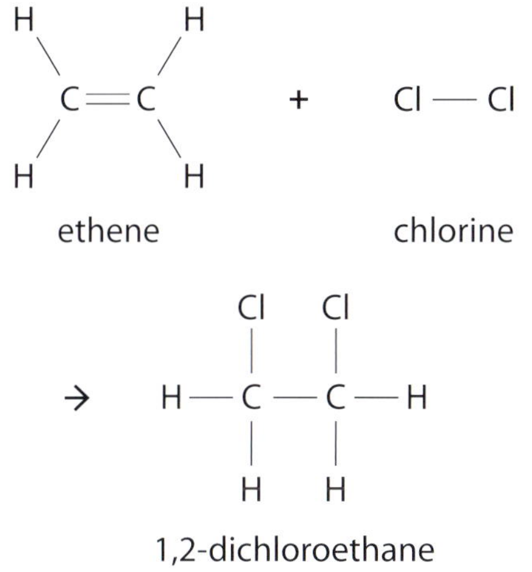

Molecular equation:
$C_2H_4 + Cl_2 \rightarrow C_2H_4Cl_2$

Tip: Chlorine water is virtually colourless so this is not a valid test for unsaturation because it is too difficult to detect the colour change.

4. Addition of hydrogen halides to symmetrical alkenes

A symmetrical alkene is one which has identical atoms or groups attached to each end of the carbon carbon double bond. Ethene and but-2-ene are symmetrical alkenes.

Tip: You do not need to study the reaction of unsymmetrical alkenes such as propene or but-1-ene as these may have different products.

Hydrogen halides include hydrogen chloride, hydrogen bromide, hydrogen fluoride and hydrogen iodide. The hydrogen halide adds across the double bond of an alkene and produces a **monohalogenoalkane**, a product which has one halogen atom.

ethene + HBr → bromoethane

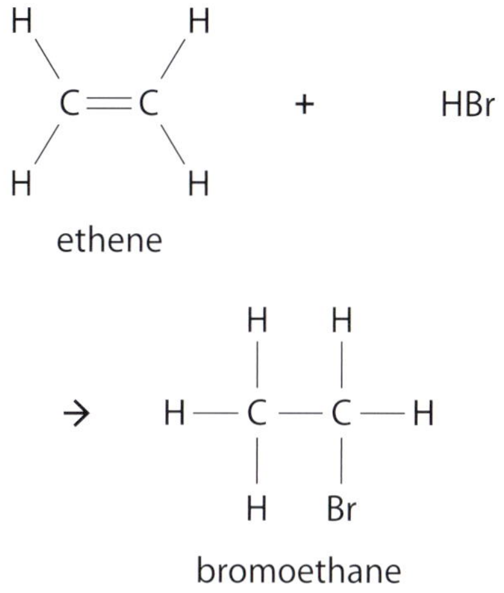

Molecular equation:
$C_2H_4 + HBr \rightarrow C_2H_5Br$

Condition:

- HBr is unstable and must be made from concentrated sulfuric acid and sodium bromide.

Mechanism

A mechanism is a series of steps which shows how a reaction takes place step by step. A mechanism shows how the electrons move by using **curly arrows**. A curly arrow shows **movement of an electron pair**. The arrow must start from touching the middle of a bond or from a lone pair.

The name of the mechanism you will study is **electrophilic addition**. The reactions of halogens with ethene and the reaction of hydrogen bromide with ethene both have an electrophilic addition mechanism.

An electrophile is an ion or molecule that accepts a pair of electrons.

Mechanism for the reaction of hydrogen bromide with ethene

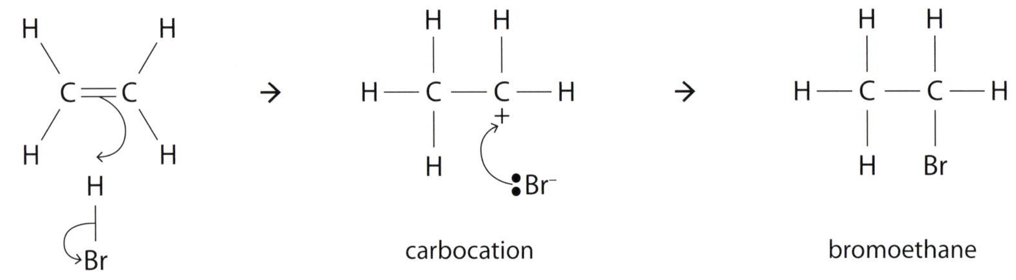

Heterolytic fission is bond breaking in which both shared electrons go to one single atom. Heterolytic fission produces two ions. For example:

$HBr \rightarrow H^+ + :Br^-$

Here the Br^- takes both electrons. This bond fission produces the electrophile H^+.

In this mechanism the electrophile attacks the high centre of electron density in the double bond.

Mechanism for hydrogen bromide reacting with ethene

The mechanism of the reaction of hydrogen bromide with ethene is electrophilic addition (see diagram below).

In this mechanism the electrons in the pi bond are attracted to the slightly positive hydrogen atom of the hydrogen bromide, which acts as an electrophile. The HBr bond breaks heterolytically and the shared pair of electrons from the bond go to the Br and it becomes Br^-. The pi bond of the double bond breaks and a new bond forms between a carbon and the hydrogen. This forms a carbocation, which is unstable and reacts with bromide quickly to form bromoethane.

A carbocation is a positive ion where the positive charge is on a carbon atom.

Tip: In an exam if asked to draw a mechanism you simply need to draw a flow scheme with curly arrows, similar to that above.

Tip: Note how the curly arrows start by touching the centre of the bond or from the middle of a lone pair.

Mechanism for bromine reacting with ethene

The reaction of bromine with ethene is also an electrophilic addition (see diagram below).

Tip: Note that the bromine molecule becomes polarised (charged) as it approaches the carbon carbon double bond and then it splits heterolytically, $Br_2 \rightarrow Br^+ + :Br^-$, and both electrons go to one bromine forming the Br^+ electrophile.

Why are alkanes more reactive than alkenes?

Alkanes are more reactive than alkenes. This is because a double bond is a centre of **high electron density**. The pi bond, caused by the overlap of p orbitals, **projects out of the plane** of the molecule and so the electrons in the bond are easily attacked by electrophiles.

Alkanes which have **lower electron density**, and the **electrons are in the plane** of the molecule are not as easily attacked by electrophiles. Hence alkanes are less reactive than alkenes.

Mechanism for the reaction of bromine with ethene

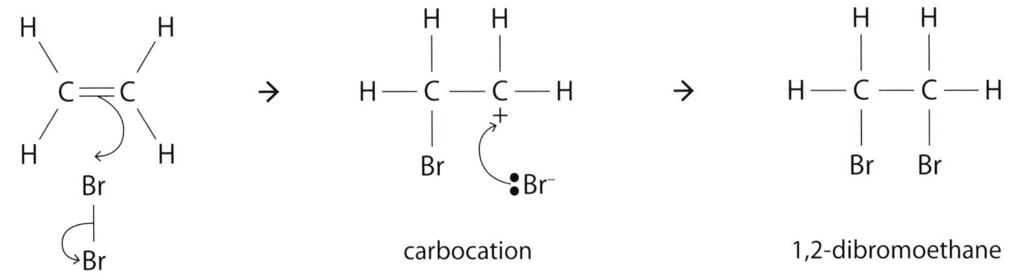

Questions

1. Give the IUPAC name for
(a) $CH_3CHCHCH_2CH_2CH_3$
(b) $CH_3C(CH_3)CHCH_2CH_2CH_3$
(c) $CH_3CClCHCH_2CH_3$
(d) $CH_2CHCH(CH_3)CH_3$
(e) $CH_2CClCH_2CH_2CH_3$
(f) CH_2CCHCH_3 [7]

2. Alkenes contain a functional group which is made of a sigma bond and a pi bond. They are more reactive than alkanes.
(a) What is meant by the term sigma bond? [1]
(b) What is meant by the term pi bond? [1]
(c) Name the functional group in an alkene. [1]
(d) Draw a diagram to show an ethene molecule before and after formation of a pi bond. [2]
(e) Explain why ethene is referred to as an unsaturated hydrocarbon. [2]
(f) Explain why the bond between carbon atoms in ethene is stronger than the bond between carbon atoms in ethane. [2]
(g) Copy and complete the table below. [1]
(h) Explain why the pi bond in ethene makes it more reactive than ethane. [2]

Compound	Structural formula	Number of pi bonds present in compound	Number of sigma bonds present in compound
ethene			
ethane			

3. Which one of the following molecules could exist as E-Z isomers? [1]
A $CH_3CH{=}CH_2$
B $CH_3CH{=}CHCH_3$
C $CH_3CH_2CH{=}CH_2$
D $(CH_3)_2C{=}CHCH_3$

4 (a) Draw and name an isomer of C_4H_8 which is a cycloalkane. [1]
(b) Draw and name a branched chain isomer of C_4H_{10}. [1]

5. The compound X, $CH_3CHCHCH_2CH_3$, exists as E-Z isomers.
(a) Give two reasons why X exists as E-Z isomers. [2]
(b) Draw the E isomer of X. [1]

6. The compound shown below has two functional groups.

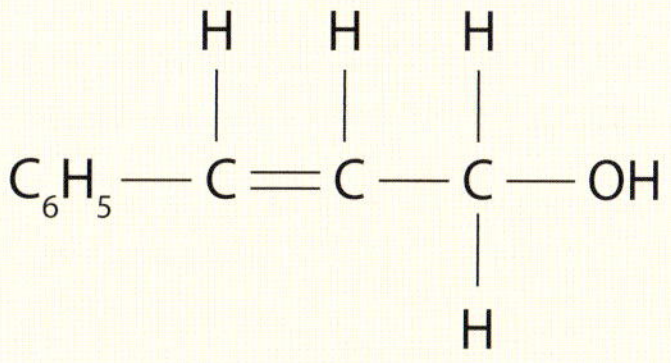

(a) Name the two functional groups present in this compound. [2]
(b) Draw the structure of the E isomer of this compound. [1]

7. Write equations for the reactions below and name the products.
(a) hydrogenation of 2-methylbut-2-ene [2]
(b) reaction of ethene and hydrogen bromide [2]
(c) reaction of ethene and chlorine [2]
(d) hydration of ethene [2]
(e) propene + chlorine [2]

8. Suggest a balanced symbol equation for
(a) the combustion of ethene in a plentiful supply of air [2]
(b) the combustion of butene in a limited supply of air [2]

9. Suggest the name and structure for the product of the reaction of
(a) but-1-ene and chlorine [2]
(b) pent-2-ene and chlorine [2]
(c) hydrogen and 2-chloropent-2-ene [2]

10. Alkenes undergo hydrogenation reactions.
(a) State what is meant by hydrogenation. [1]
(b) State the conditions needed for hydrogenation. [2]
(c) Write an equation for the hydrogenation of pentene and name the organic product. [2]
(d) Oleic acid, $CH_3(CH_2)_7CH{=}CH(CH_2)_7COOH$, is found in olive oil. Write an equation for the hydrogenation of oleic acid. [1]

11. Compare the reaction of bromine with ethane to the reaction of bromine with ethene. Include in your answer the type of reaction, names of the products, and the conditions required for each reaction to take place. **Your quality of written communication will be assessed in this answer. [6]**

12. The reaction below occurs at room temperature.

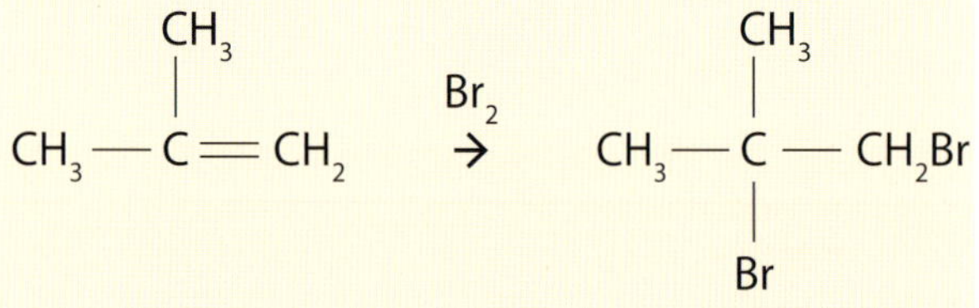

A B

(a) Give the IUPAC name for A and for B. [2]
(b) Explain if A can form E-Z isomers. [1]
(c) State the colour change observed in this reaction. [1]
(d) Give the name for the mechanism of this reaction. [1]
(e) Draw a flow scheme to show the mechanism of the reaction of chlorine and ethene. [3]
(f) Draw the structure and name the product when $CH_3CH{=}CHCH{=}CHCl$ is reacted with an excess of hydrogen. [2]

13. The compound 3-methylpent-2-ene reacts with hydrogen bromide in an electrophilic addition reaction.
(a) What is an electrophile? [2]
(b) Name the functional group present in 3-methylpent-2-ene. [1]
(c) Name the product when 3-methylpent-2-ene reacts with hydrogen. [1]
(d) Suggest the structure of the product when $CH_3CH{=}CHCH{=}CHCl$ is reacted with an excess of chlorine. [1]
(e) Explain if the structure below is the E or Z isomer. [3]

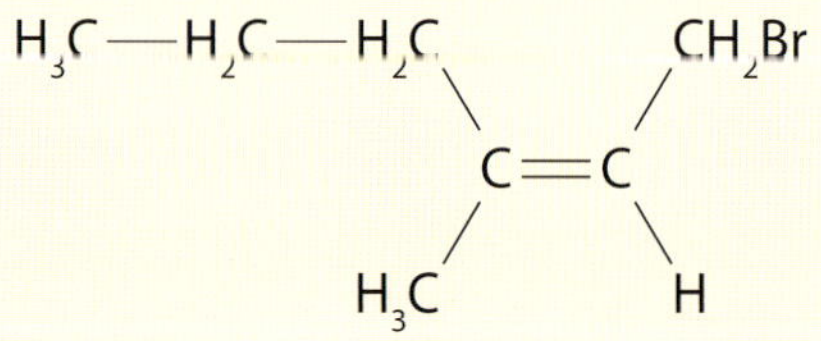

4: POLYMERS

Students should be able to:

- **8.4.1** demonstrate an understanding that addition polymers are made from molecules containing C=C bonds;
- **8.4.2** demonstrate an understanding that polythene is chemically inert and this leads to a need for waste management strategies, including:
  - incineration to release energy;
  - recycling; and
  - using it as feedstock for cracking;
- **8.4.3** evaluate how chemists can limit the problems linked to polymer disposal by:
  - removing toxic waste gases caused by the incineration of plastics; and
  - continuing to develop biodegradable polymers;
- **8.8.1** describe the process of condensation polymerisation to produce nylon 6,6.

Addition polymerisation

When alkene molecules react with other alkene molecules a **polymer** is formed.

A polymer is a large molecule formed when monomers join together.

Monomers are the many small molecules that join together to form a polymer.

The word 'poly' means 'many', referring to the many monomers that join together. The name of a polymer is formed from the word 'poly' followed by the name of the polymer, in brackets. For example, lots of ethene molecules join together to make the polymer poly(ethene), better known as polythene. Similarly, many propene molecules join together to make poly(propene).

In the reaction between monomers the C=C double bonds open up and the molecules join onto each other to make a long chain molecule. The exact number of molecules that join together varies, but is likely to be several hundred. When drawing the polymer structure the bonds on either end are left 'open' as shown in the example of polythene below.

Addition polymerisation is the process of joining many small molecules (monomers) together to form a large molecule.

Tip: Remember that alkenes undergo **addition** polymerisation **not** additional polymerisation.

An addition polymer **does not** have a carbon **carbon double bond** and as a result it is unreactive (inert). Polythene, for example, is chemically inert and as a result it is difficult to dispose of.

Tip: Only monomers with a double bond (i.e. alkenes) can form addition polymers.

Drawing structures

The **repeating unit** is the part of the structure that repeats many times. We show this by drawing 'open' bonds on the end of the structure. For example, the repeating unit of the polymer polythene is shown in the following way:

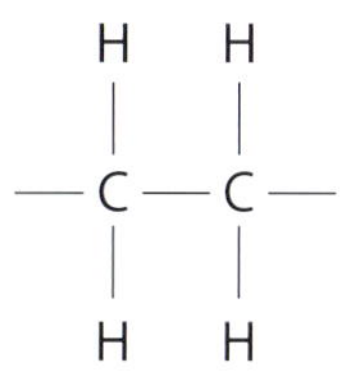

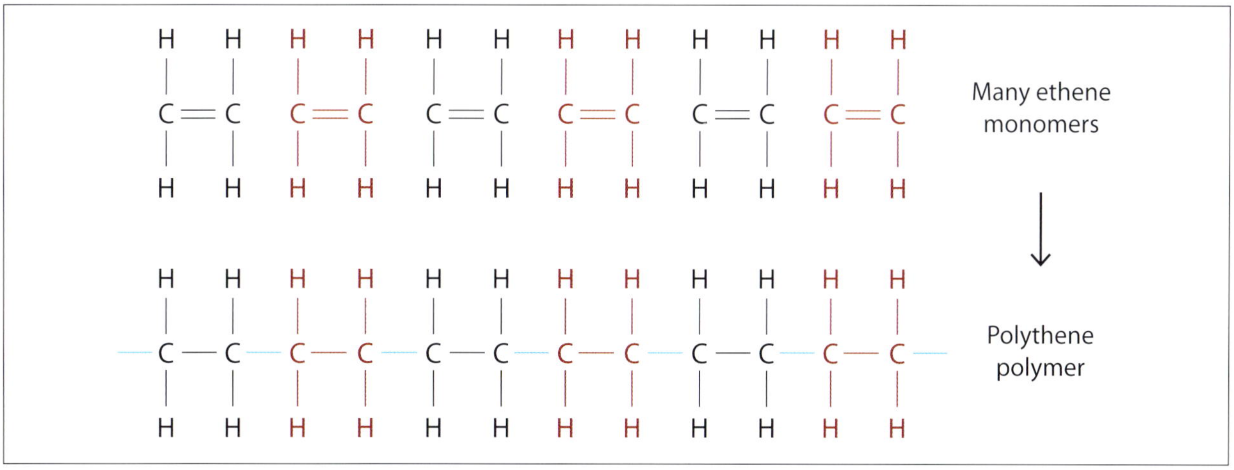

A **polymer** is made up of many (*n*) repeats of the repeating unit. The structure of a polymer is drawn with brackets and an *n* to show that it is made up of many repeating units. For example, the polymer polyethene is represented as follows:

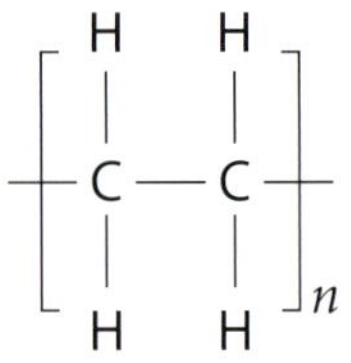

You may be asked to draw a polymer showing several repeating units. To do this simply link together the required number of repeating units.

Worked example
Draw the structure of polythene, showing 3 repeating units.

Answer

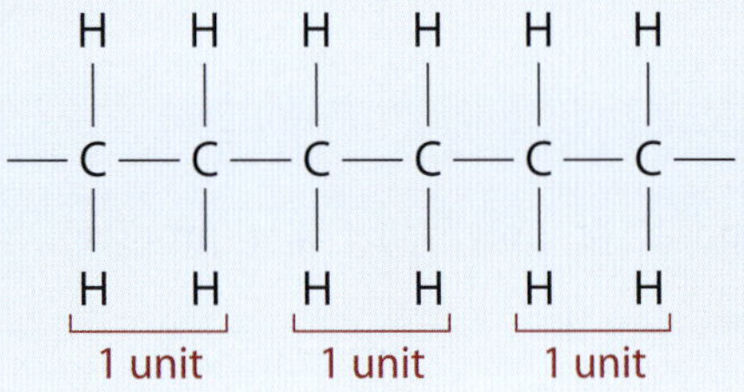

You may also be asked to write an equation for polymerisation. The chemical **equation** for polymerisation of ethene is:

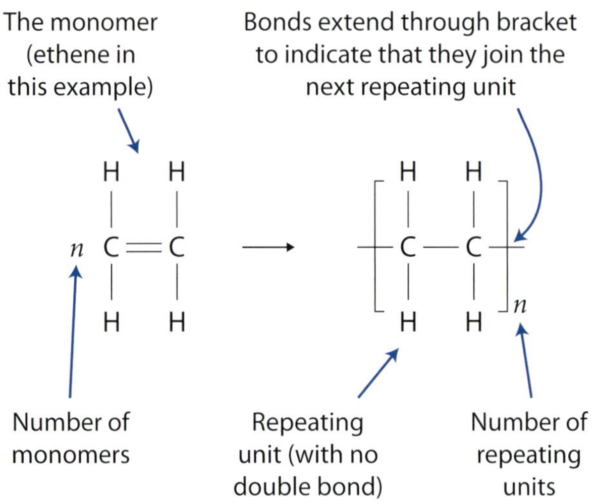

Some examples of polymers and repeating units are shown in the table below.

Monomer	Repeating unit of polymer	Polymer	Equation for formation of polymer
ethene 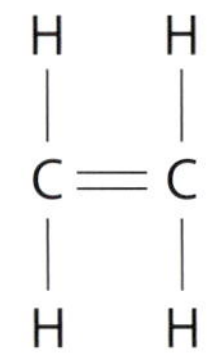	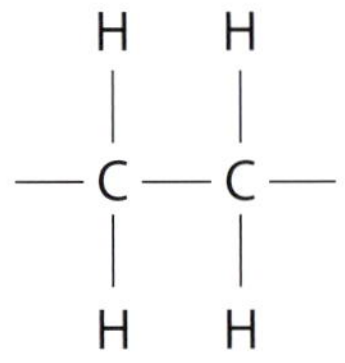	poly(ethene) *common name polythene*	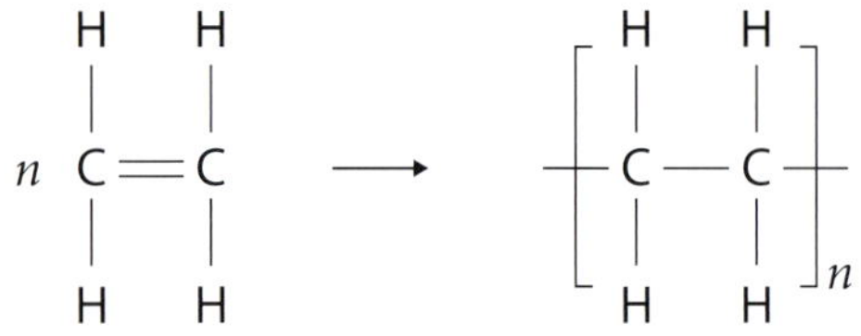
propene 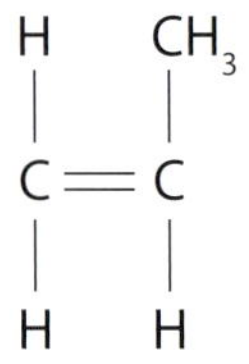	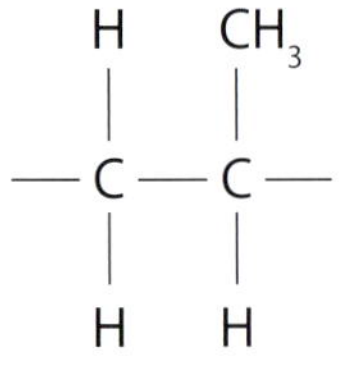	poly(propene) *common name polypropene*	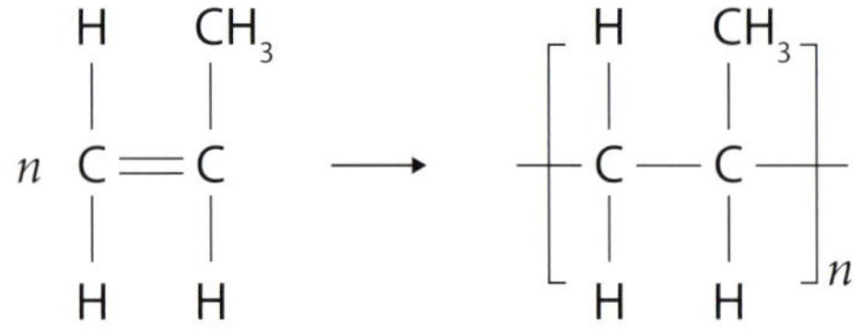

Worked example
Write an equation for the polymer formed from the monomer shown.

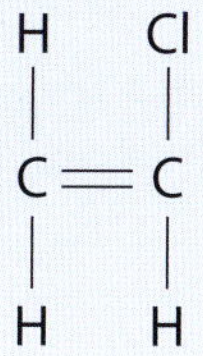

Answer
First write the general polymerisation equation.

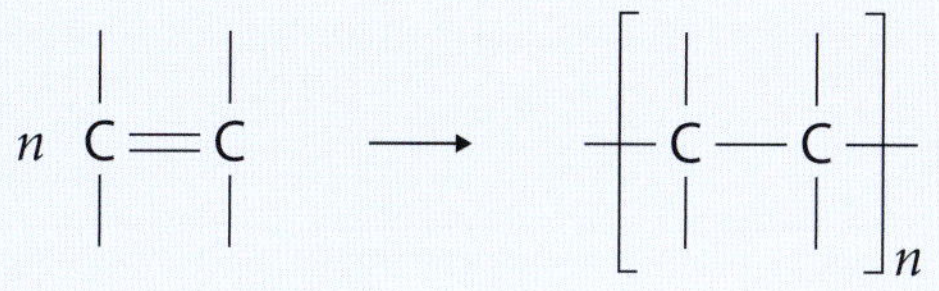

Then add in the different atoms or groups from the monomer, H and Cl in this case.

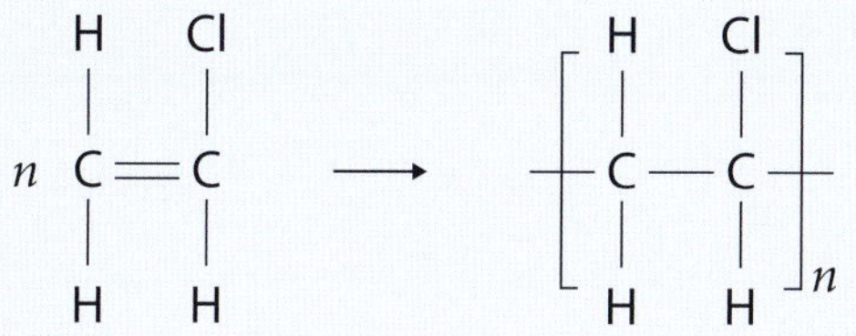

You must also be able to deduce the structure of a monomer from the given structure of a polymer.

Worked example
The structure below shows part of a polymer chain. Draw the repeating unit of the polymer and the monomer.

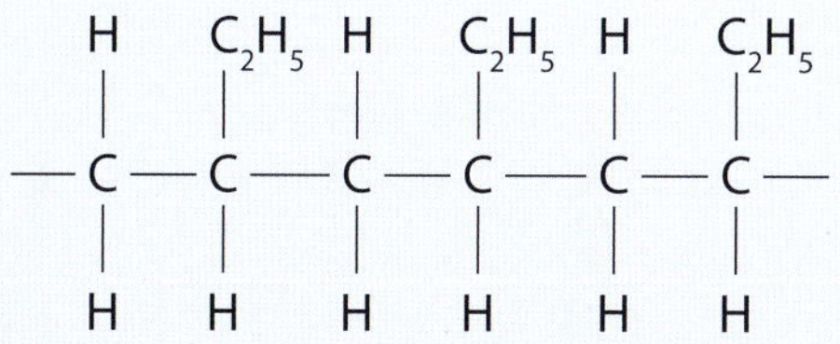

Answer
It is important to be able to identify the **repeating unit** from the polymer. It is circled below.

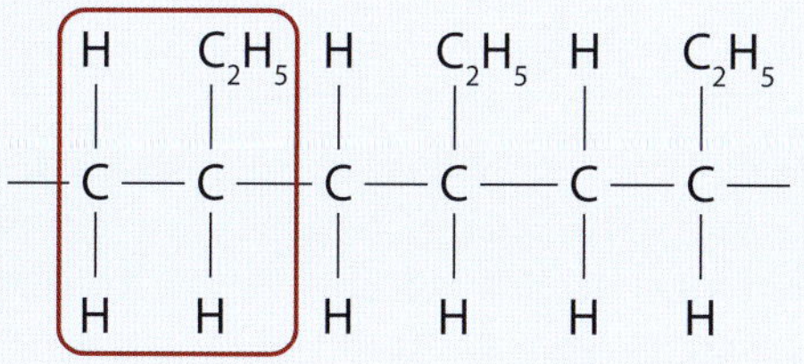

So the repeating unit is:

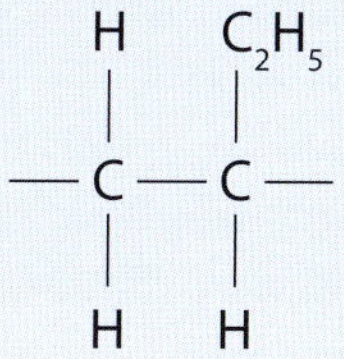

Tip: When asked to draw the structure of a repeating unit of a molecule you should not draw brackets around it and you should not put an *n* beside it – it is not the polymer.

To draw the monomer, add a double bond and remove the open bonds at the ends:

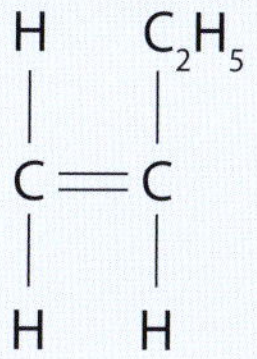

Disposal of polythene

The disposal of polythene is a problem for two reasons:

- Polythene is **non-biodegradeable**. A non-biodegradeable material is one which is not decomposed by microorganisms in the environment.
- Polythene is **chemically inert** and does not react with alkalis or acid (apart from concentrated nitric acid).

Tip: Inert means that a substance does not react with others.

Addition polymers such as polythene are often disposed of by burying them in landfill sites where, due to their inertness and non-biodegradability, they last for a long time. Landfill sites are an eyesore, and they waste land which could otherwise be used for building or agriculture.

Waste management strategies

More sustainable **waste management strategies** can be used to dispose of polymers. These include:

- **Incineration to release energy**. This involves combustion of the polymers at very high temperatures. The advantage of incineration is that it **releases a lot of energy** which can be used to heat homes or to generate electricity. However, toxic waste gases are also released: for example, hydrogen chloride is released when PVC is burned. Chemists need to ensure that these toxic waste gases are removed before they pass into the atmosphere. This can be achieved by placing a base or carbonate in the incineration chimney to react with acidic gases, neutralising them before they are released to the environment. Polluting gases, such as carbon dioxide which can cause global warming, are also released.

- **Recycling**. Recycling involves melting the waste polymer and forming it into a new product. It has the advantage that it reduces the volume of crude oil used to make more plastics, so it conserves resources. However, it can be an expensive process as the different polymers must be separated from each other first.
- **Using it as a feedstock (raw material)** for cracking. Polymers can be cracked to break them into smaller molecules, which can then be used to make other materials or more plastics. This process also conserves crude oil resources.

Limiting the problems of polymer disposal

Chemists can limit the problems linked to polymer disposal in two ways:

- **Removing toxic waste gases** caused by the incineration of plastics, as detailed above.
- Continuing to **develop biodegradable polymers** which can be broken down in the environment by microorganisms.

Condensation polymerisation

Condensation polymers are polymers formed by the elimination of small molecules, such as hydrogen chloride or water, when monomers bond together.

Nylon is a type of condensation polymer known as a **polyamide**. Polyamides are condensation polymers where the repeating units are held together by amide links. An amide link has the structure:

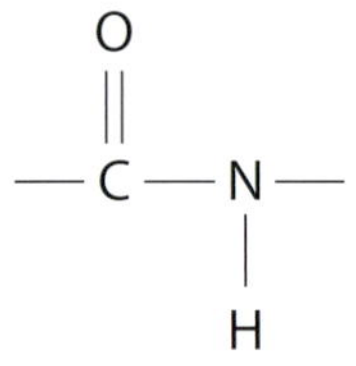

Nylon-6,6 is made in industry by reacting two monomers, each of which contain six carbon atoms – hence its name. One of the monomers is a six-carbon acid with a -COOH group at each end called **hexanedioic acid** ($HOOC(CH_2)_4COOH$).

The other monomer is a six-carbon chain with an amino group, $-NH_2$, at each end. This monomer is called **1,6-diaminohexane/hexane-1,6-diamine** ($H_2N(CH_2)_6NH_2$).

A condensation reaction occurs, as shown below, between the two monomers and water is removed.

> **Tip:** It is a good idea to write out the monomers and surround the elements of water to help you get the correct structure of the polymer.

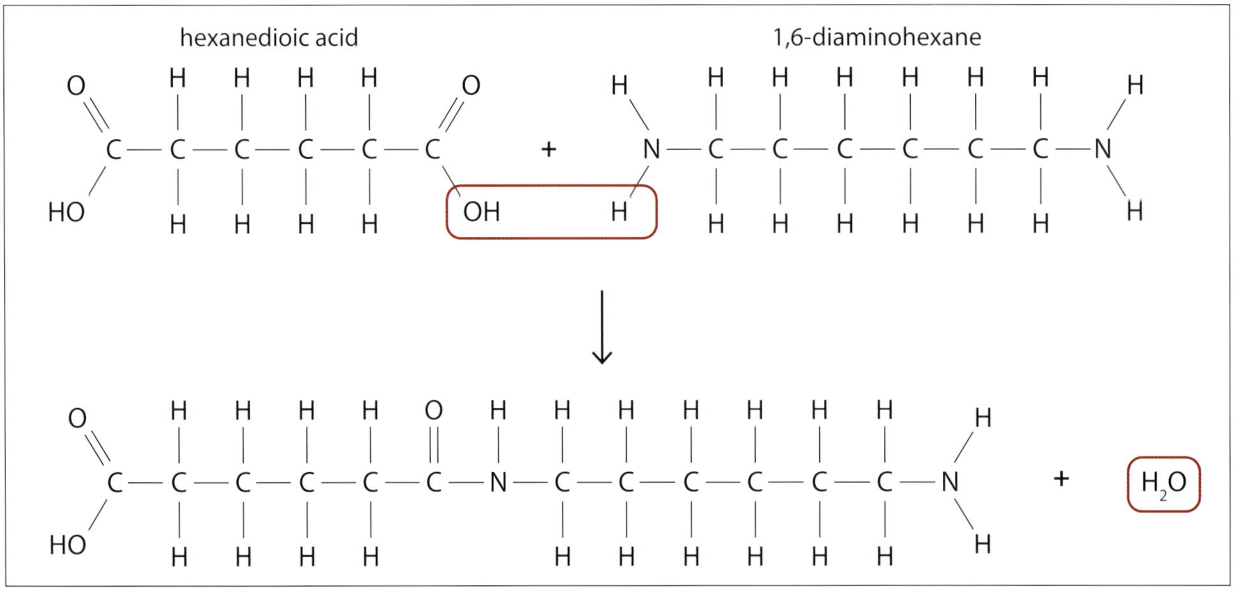

This keeps on happening, and so you get a chain which looks like this:

$$-\underset{\substack{\|\\O}}{C}-(CH_2)_4-\underset{\substack{\|\\O}}{C}-\underset{\substack{|\\H}}{N}-(CH_2)_6-\boxed{\underset{\substack{|\\H}}{N}-\underset{\substack{\|\\O}}{C}}-(CH_2)_4-\underset{\substack{\|\\O}}{C}-\underset{\substack{|\\H}}{N}-(CH_2)_6-\underset{\substack{|\\H}}{N}-\underset{\substack{\|\\O}}{C}-(CH_2)_4-\underset{\substack{\|\\O}}{C}-$$

Amide link

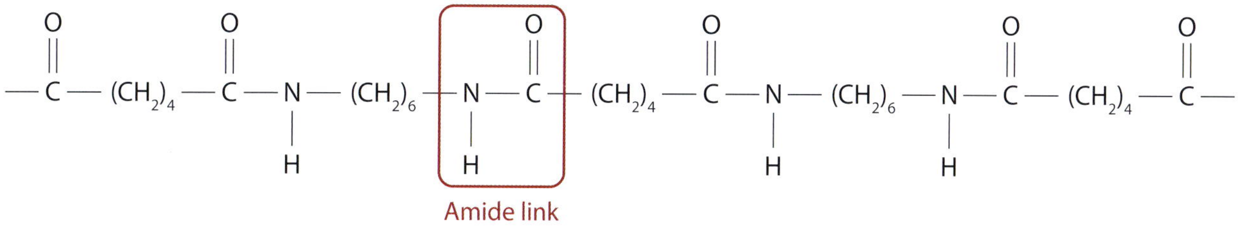

The polyamide contains many amide links. One is circled above. The repeating unit of nylon 6,6 is:

$$-\underset{\substack{\|\\O}}{C}-(CH_2)_4-\underset{\substack{\|\\O}}{C}-\underset{\substack{|\\H}}{N}-(CH_2)_6-\underset{\substack{|\\H}}{N}-$$

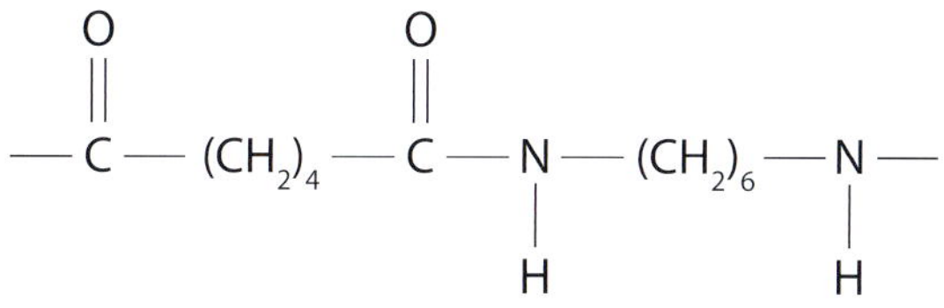

Polyamides can be hydrolysed because the amide link reacts with water and they are broken up into the acid and amine starting materials. As a result they are **biodegradeable**.

A biodegradeable polymer is a polymer which can be hydrolysed by the action of microorganisms.

> **Tip:** Remember hydrolysis is breaking up molecules by reaction with water.

Instead of using the hexanedioic acid, a molecule containing two **acyl chloride** groups (**COCl**) such as hexanedioyl dichloride can be used. In this case hydrogen chloride is removed instead of water:

Note that when using **condensation polymerisation** to make nylon **two different** monomers are used (an acid/acyl chloride and 1,6-diaminohexane) and, as well as the polymer, **water or hydrogen chloride is produced**. By contrast, in **addition polymerisation**, only **one monomer** is used (the alkene) and there is only **one product**.

Laboratory preparation of nylon

To produce nylon in the laboratory, a solution of **decanedioyl dichloride** (an **acyl chloride**) **in cyclohexane** is floated on an aqueous solution of **1,6-diaminohexane** at room temperature. Nylon forms at the interface and can be pulled out as fast as it is produced forming a long thread often referred to as the 'nylon rope trick'. The nylon formed is called **nylon 6,10** because of the lengths of the carbon chains of the monomers. The method is as follows:

1. Dissolve 1,6-diaminohexane in distilled water in a beaker.

2. Dissolve decanedioyl dichloride in cyclohexane in another beaker.

hexanedioyl dichloride

$$Cl-\underset{\substack{\|\\O}}{C}-CH_2CH_2CH_2CH_2-\underset{\substack{\|\\O}}{C}-Cl$$

hexane-1,6-diamine

$$\underset{\substack{|\\H}}{\overset{H}{N}}-CH_2CH_2CH_2CH_2CH_2CH_2-\underset{\substack{|\\H}}{\overset{H}{N}}$$

↓

$$\left[-\underset{\substack{\|\\O}}{C}-CH_2CH_2CH_2CH_2-\boxed{\underset{\substack{\|\\O}}{C}-\underset{\substack{|\\H}}{N}}-CH_2CH_2CH_2CH_2CH_2CH_2-\underset{\substack{|\\H}}{\overset{H}{N}}-\right] + HCl$$

Amide link

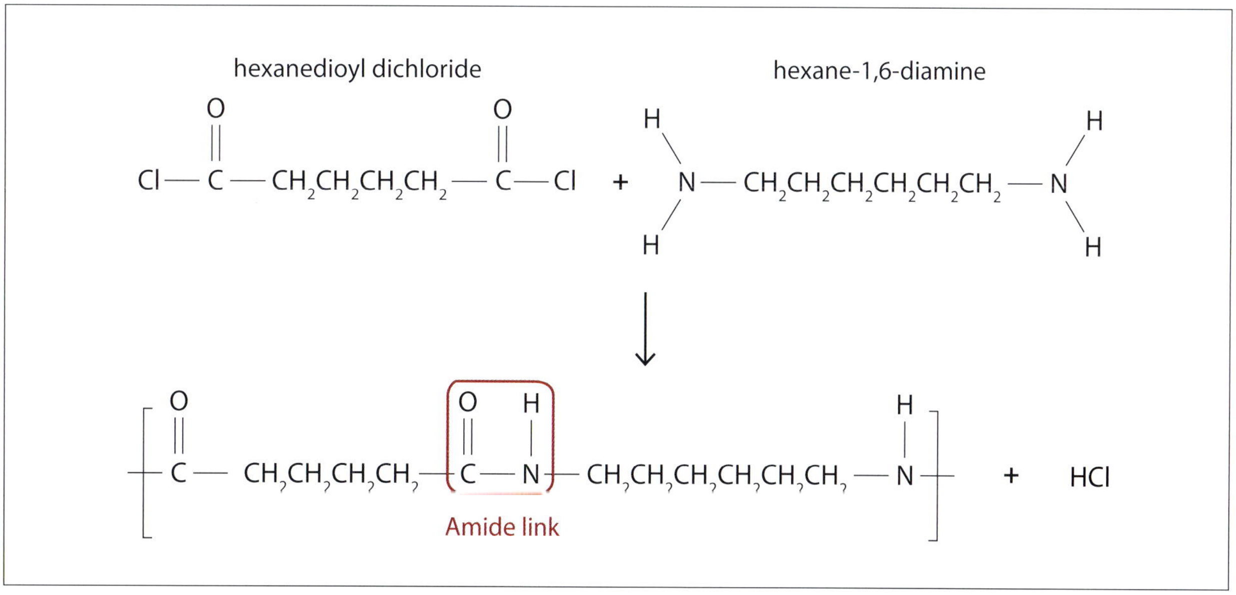

3. Carefully pour the decanedioyl dichloride solution onto the solution of 1,6-diaminohexane, ensuring that mixing of solutions is minimised by pouring down the wall of the beaker or down a glass rod. The decanedioyl dichloride should float on top.

4. A greyish film of nylon will form at the interface. Use tweezers to pull out the nylon formed. It should pull out as a thread which you can wind around a glass rod as shown below.

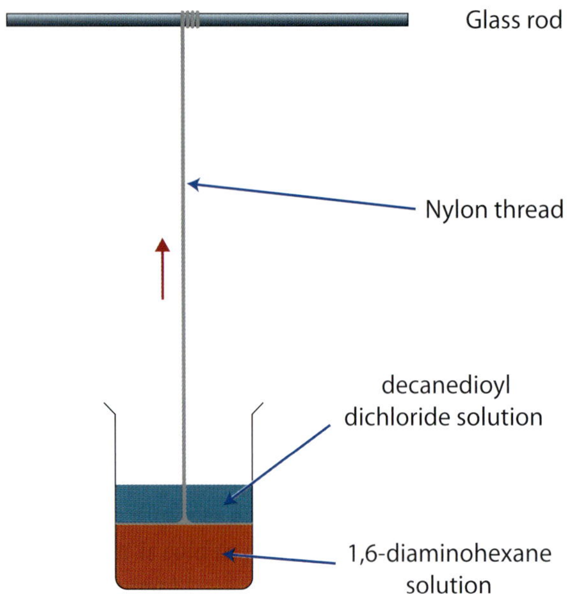

The equation for the reaction taking place is:

$H_2N(CH_2)_6NH_2$ + $Cl-\underset{\underset{O}{\|}}{C}-(CH_2)_8-\underset{\underset{O}{\|}}{C}-Cl$

$\rightarrow -\underset{\underset{H}{|}}{N}-(CH_2)_6-\underset{\underset{H}{|}}{N}-\underset{\underset{O}{\|}}{C}-(CH_2)_8-\underset{\underset{O}{\|}}{C}-$ + HCl

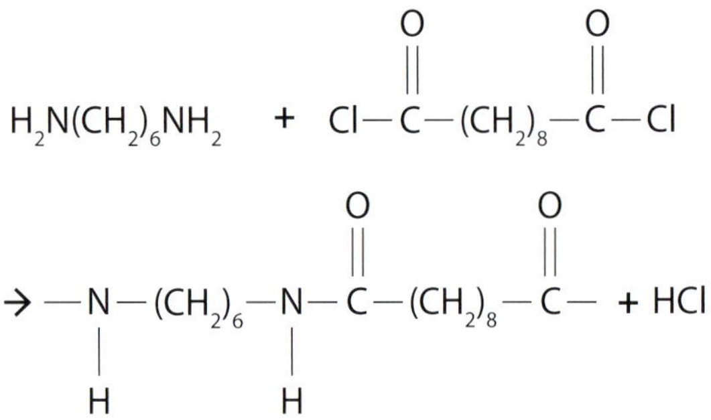

This reaction repeats to make a polymer. The **repeating unit** of nylon 6,10 is:

$-\underset{\underset{H}{|}}{N}-(CH_2)_6-\underset{\underset{H}{|}}{N}-\underset{\underset{O}{\|}}{C}-(CH_2)_8-\underset{\underset{O}{\|}}{C}-$

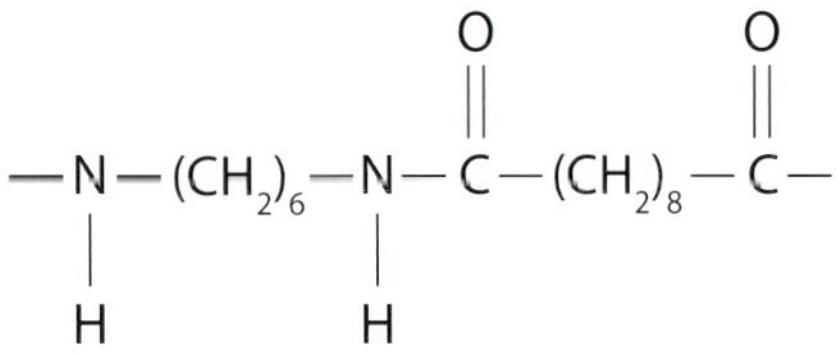

When carrying out this procedure, observe the following safety precautions:

- Keep away from naked flames as cyclohexane is flammable.
- Wear goggles and gloves as the acyl chloride is corrosive and cyclohexane is toxic if ingested.
- Use a fume cupboard to remove the fumes of the organic chemicals as cyclohexane is toxic if inhaled.

Questions

1. (a) What is a polymer? [1]
   (b) What is a monomer? [1]
   (c) What functional group do monomers that form addition polymers contain? [1]
   (d) Write an equation for the polymerisation of ethene. [3]
   (e) Suggest the name of the addition polymer formed from the monomer styrene. [1]
   (f) Suggest the name and draw the skeletal formula of the monomer used to make poly(bromoethene). [2]

2. Write an equation for the polymerisation of the following monomers:
   (a)

   $\begin{array}{cc} H & C_6H_5 \\ | & | \\ C=C \\ | & | \\ H & H \end{array}$ [3]

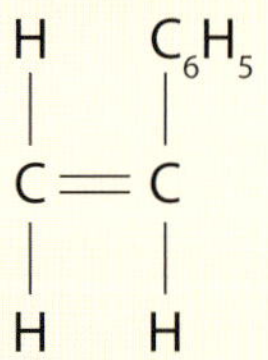

   (b)

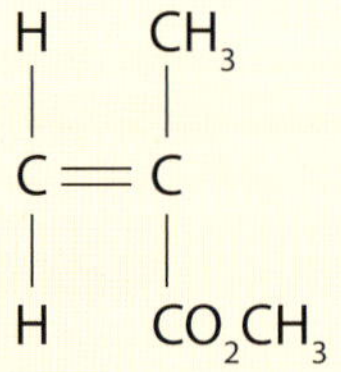

   $\begin{array}{cc} H & CH_3 \\ | & | \\ C=C \\ | & | \\ H & CO_2CH_3 \end{array}$ [3]

3. Draw three repeating units of the polymer made from the monomer shown:

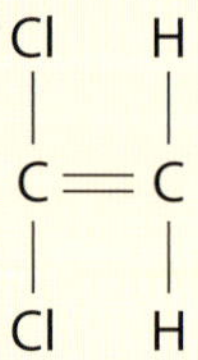

   $\begin{array}{cc} Cl & H \\ | & | \\ C=C \\ | & | \\ Cl & H \end{array}$ [2]

4. For each of the monomers A and B shown below write
(a) the structure of the repeating unit, [2]
(b) the structure of the polymer. [2]

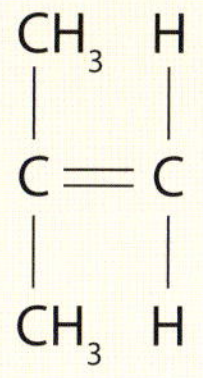

A

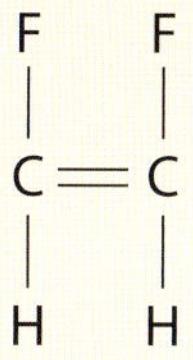

B

5. Part of the structure of a polymer is shown below.

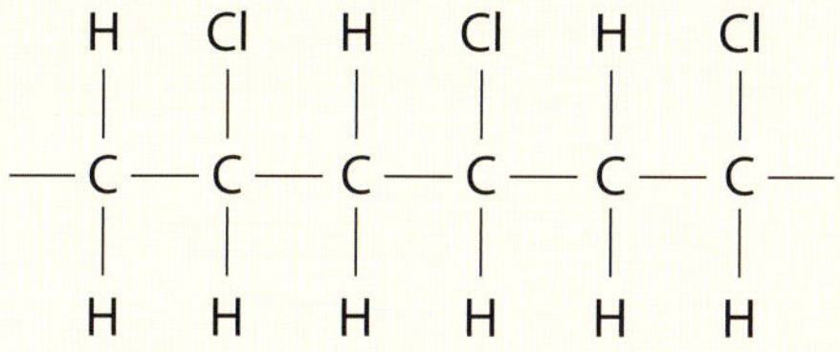

(a) Draw the repeating unit of this polymer. [1]
(b) Draw the skeletal formula of the monomer used to make this polymer. [1]
(c) Explain if this polymer is a hydrocarbon. [1]
(d) Explain why disposing of this polymer using incineration can lead to environmental problems. [1]
(e) State two ways chemists can limit the problems linked to polymer disposal. [2]

6. Ethene is used in many industrial reactions, such as the one represented below.

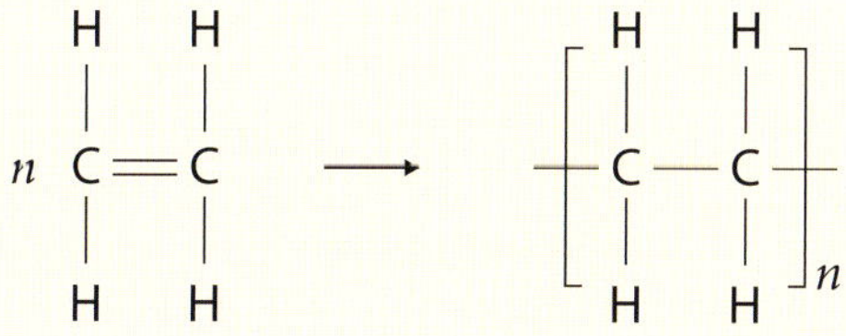

(a) State fully the type of chemical reaction shown above. [2]
(b) Name the product formed in this reaction. [1]
(c) What does ***n*** represent in the equation above? [1]
(d) Describe two waste management strategies which could be used to dispose of the polymer above, detailing how they are beneficial to the environment. [4]

7. Compare the polymerisation reaction used to make nylon with the polymerisation reaction used to produce ethene. You do not need to give equations. **Your quality of written communication will be assessed in this answer.** [6]

8. Polyamides such as nylon have many uses.
(a) Suggest why nylon is easier to dispose of than polythene. [2]
(b) The polyamide nylon-6,6 is made by a condensation reaction between 1,6-diaminohexane and hexanedioic acid. Draw a section of the polymer showing two repeating units. [2]
(c) Define condensation polymerisation.

9. Poly(propene) and nylon are both polymers.
(a) Draw two repeating units of poly(propene). [1]
(b) What type of polymer is nylon? [1]
(c) Nylon-6,10 can be made in the laboratory from solutions of decanedioyl dichloride and 1,6-diaminohexane at room temperature. Describe the preparation. [5]
(d) Why is the nylon prepared in (c) called nylon-6,10? [1]

5: ALCOHOLS

Students should be able to:

8.5.1 explain that alcohols can be classified as primary, secondary or tertiary;

8.5.2 write the general formula of alcohols as $C_nH_{2n+1}OH$;

8.5.3 recall molecular and structural formulae with up to six carbons (referring to primary, secondary and tertiary alcohols);

8.5.4 apply IUPAC rules to name alcohols with one hydroxyl group and up to six carbon atoms;

8.5.5 describe the preparation of alcohols from halogenoalkanes;

8.5.6 describe the industrial preparation of ethanol from:

- the reaction of steam with ethene in the presence of phosphoric acid; and
- the fermentation of sugars to make ethanol;

8.5.7 discuss the use of ethanol in alcoholic beverages and its use as a recreational drug which can have beneficial and harmful effects; and

8.5.8 use balanced symbol equations for the reactions of alcohols with:

- concentrated phosphoric acid to form alkenes by elimination (mechanism not required); and
- potassium dichromate(VI) in dilute sulfuric acid to oxidise primary alcohols to aldehydes and carboxylic acids, and secondary alcohols to ketones (using Benedict's or Fehling's solution to distinguish an aldehyde from the other products).

Introduction to alcohols

Alcohols contain the hydroxyl functional group (-OH). The general formula is $C_nH_{2n+1}OH$.

Tip: Note that the hydroxyl functional group is OH. This is different to the hydroxide ion OH^-.

Classification of alcohols

Alcohols are classified as primary, secondary or tertiary.

A **primary alcohol** is an alcohol which has one carbon atom directly bonded to the carbon atom that is bonded to the -OH group (exception is methanol).

Tip: Methanol only has one carbon atom, but is still referred to as a primary alcohol.

A **secondary alcohol** is an alcohol which has two carbon atoms directly bonded to the carbon atom that is bonded to the -OH group.

A **tertiary alcohol** is an alcohol which has three carbons atoms directly bonded to the carbon atom that is bonded to the -OH group.

Examples of primary, secondary and tertiary alcohols are shown below.

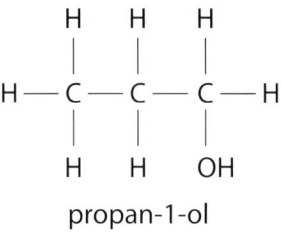

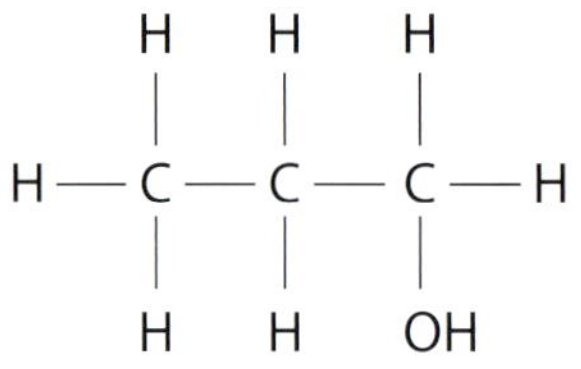

propan-1-ol

Primary

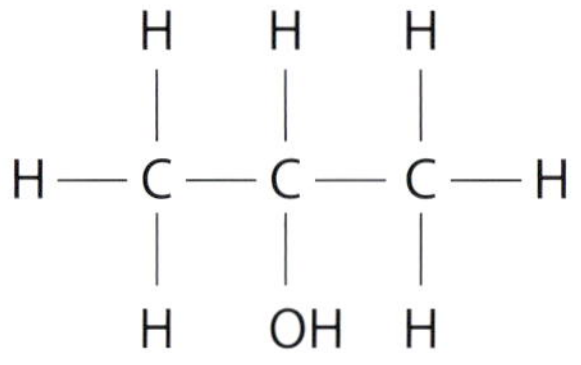

propan-2-ol

Secondary

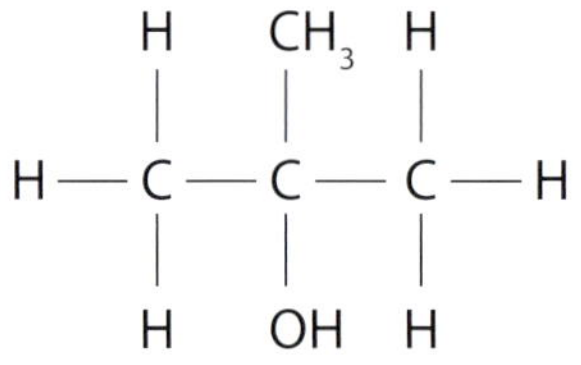

2-methylpropan-2-ol

Tertiary

Isomers

Some alcohols have isomers. For example both propan-1-ol and propan-2-ol (shown above) are isomers of C_3H_7OH. They have the same molecular formula but different structural formulae, as the OH is in a different position in each case.

Reactions of alcohols

1. Oxidation

Oxidation is a reaction in which oxygen is gained or hydrogen is lost.

Acidified potassium dichromate(VI) is an oxidising agent. It is made by adding a few drops of dilute sulfuric acid to potassium dichromate(VI) solution ($K_2Cr_2O_7$). Primary, secondary and tertiary alcohols react differently when warmed with potassium dichromate(VI):

- **Primary** alcohols are oxidised to **aldehydes** which can be oxidised further to **carboxylic acids**.
- **Secondary alcohols** are oxidised to **ketones**.
- **Tertiary alcohols cannot** be oxidised.

If there is a reaction, the acidified potassium dichromate(VI) changes in colour from **orange to green**.

Naming aldehydes, ketones and carboxylic acids

It is useful to know how to name aldehydes, ketones and carboxylic acids for this reaction. Aldehydes and ketones both contain the carbonyl functional group, C=O, but differ in the position of the carbonyl group.

For an **aldehyde** the **carbonyl group** is at the **end** of the chain. Methanal is the simplest aldehyde and has formula HCHO. Propanal is CH_3CH_2CHO:

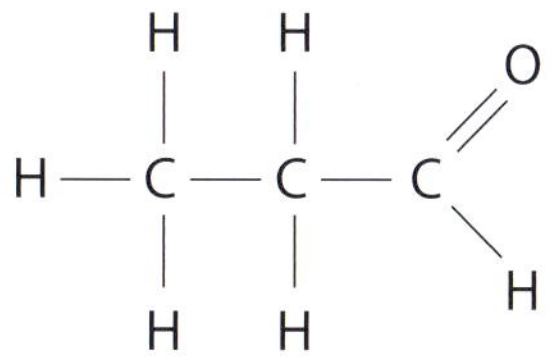

Tip: For an aldehyde, always write CHO. It is not COH.

For a **ketone** the **carbonyl group** is **in** the chain. Propanone is the simplest ketone and has the formula CH_3COCH_3:

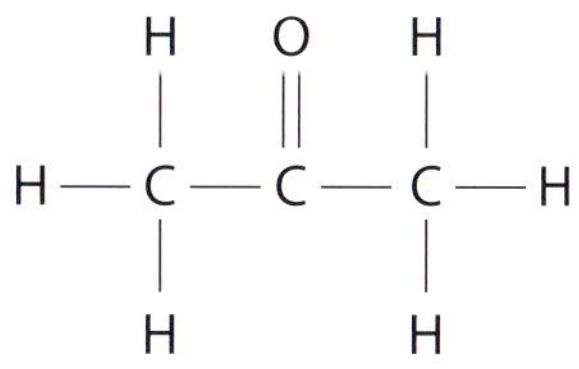

For ketones with five or more carbons, the position of the carbonyl group must be given.

A **carboxylic acid** has a carboxyl functional group, COOH. The carbon of the functional group is included in the longest carbon chain. Methanoic acid, HCOOH is the simplest carboxylic acid. Propanoic acid is CH_3CH_2COOH:

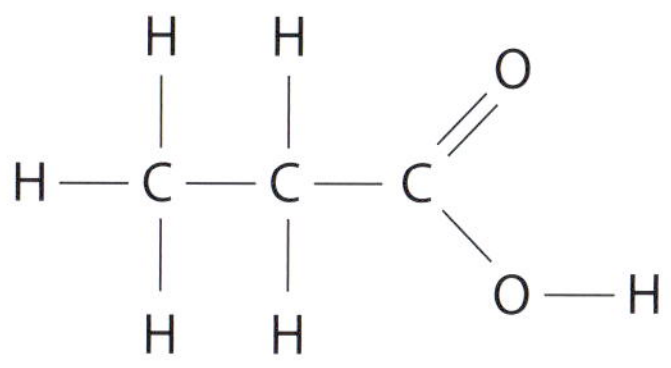

Writing equations for oxidation reactions

In an equation an oxidising agent such as acidified potassium dichromate(VI) can be represented as [O].

Mild oxidation of a primary alcohol produces an aldehyde

$C_2H_5OH + [O] \rightarrow CH_3CHO + H_2O$
ethanol ethanal

Conditions:

- [O] is acidified potassium dichromate(VI)
- warm in a hot water bath

Observation:
Solution changes from **orange to green** and **change in smell** (from alcohol smell to apple smell of aldehyde).

If this reaction is used to prepare an aldehyde, distillation apparatus should be used, so that the aldehyde can be distilled off as soon as it is formed, removing it from contact with the oxidising agent and preventing it oxidising further to the carboxylic acid.

Strong oxidation of primary alcohol produces a carboxylic acid

$C_2H_5OH + 2[O] \rightarrow CH_3COOH + H_2O$
ethanol ethanoic acid

Conditions:

- [O] is acidified potassium dichromate(VI)
- warm in a hot water bath

Observation:
Solution changes from **orange to green** and **change in smell**.

If this reaction is used to prepare a carboxylic acid, reflux apparatus should be used (see next page) so that the aldehyde is in contact with the oxidising agent and fully oxidised.

Oxidation of a secondary alcohol to a ketone

$CH_3CH(OH)CH_3 + [O] \rightarrow CH_3COCH_3 + H_2O$
propan-2-ol propanone

Conditions:

- [O] is acidified potassium dichromate(VI)
- warm in a hot water bath

Observation:
Solution changes from **orange to green** and **change in smell**.

Distinguishing between alcohols using oxidation

To distinguish between primary, secondary and tertiary alcohol first **warm** the samples in separate test tubes **with acidified potassium dichromate(VI)** in a hot water bath. If the colour:

- changes from orange to green – it is a primary/secondary alcohol;
- remains orange – it is a tertiary alcohol.

The primary alcohol produces an aldehyde and the secondary alcohol a ketone. To distinguish between an aldehyde and a ketone, use the test in the table below. The ketone does not react.

Fehling's solution and **Benedict's** solution are variants of essentially the same thing. Both contain copper(II) ions in an alkaline solution and are **blue solutions**.

Worked example
Describe how you could use simple test tube reactions to distinguish between butan-2-ol and 2-methyl propan-2-ol. Your answer should include reagents, conditions, observations and an explanation of the chemistry involved.

Answer
Take separate test tubes of butan-2-ol and 2-methyl propan-2-ol and add a few drops of acidified potassium dichromate(VI). Warm in a hot water bath.

There is a colour change from orange to green with the butan-2-ol. This is because it is a secondary alcohol and can be oxidised.

The acidified potassium dichromate(VI) stays orange in the 2-methyl propan-2-ol. This is because it is a tertiary alcohol and cannot be oxidised.

2. Elimination

An elimination reaction is one where a small molecule is removed from a larger molecule.

Alkenes can be produced from alcohols by acid-catalysed elimination reactions. A molecule of water is removed. This reaction can also be termed **dehydration**.

Conditions:

- concentrated sulfuric/phosphoric acid catalyst
- temperature of 170°C

Test	Observation with aldehyde	Observation with ketone	Equation for positive test
Warm with Benedict's or Fehling's solution	Red precipitate forms	No reaction; solution remains blue	$Cu^{2+} + e^- \rightarrow Cu^+$ copper(II) ions are reduced to a red precipitate of copper(I) oxide, Cu_2O, The aldehyde is oxidised to the acid $RCHO + [O] \rightarrow RCOOH$

Test to distinguish between an aldehyde and a ketone.

The equation for the dehydration of propan-1-ol is shown below.

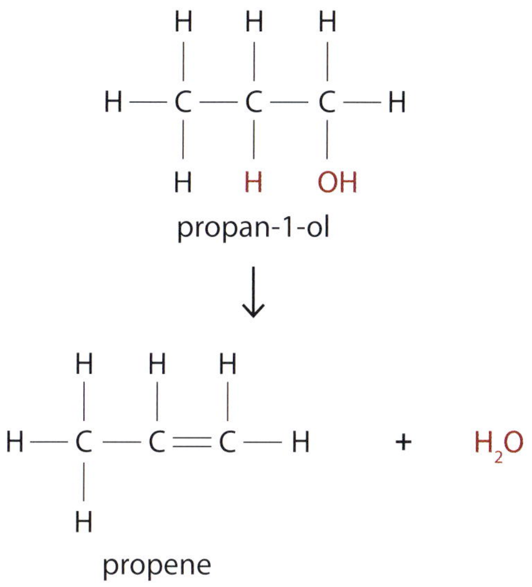

$CH_3CH_2CH_2OH \rightarrow CH_3CHCH_2 + H_2O$

or $C_3H_7OH \rightarrow C_3H_6 + H_2O$

Laboratory preparation of a liquid organic compound

A liquid organic compound can be prepared in the laboratory using the following general method:

1. Add reactants and **reflux** for 30 minutes.
2. Distill and collect the crude product over a boiling point (bpt) range.
3. Dry by adding drying agent (anhydrous sodium sulfate) and swirling until it changes from cloudy to clear.
4. Filter to remove drying agent.
5. Redistill and collect at sharp bpt (1–2 degrees either side of bpt).

What is reflux?

You will note that this general method uses a process called **reflux**.

Reflux is the repeated boiling and condensing of a reaction mixture.

It ensures that organic compounds can be heated for a long time without loss of vapour – organic compounds are volatile and evaporate readily. A condenser in the upright position is used during heating, to condense any vapour.

Reflux and distillation diagrams

You may be asked to draw diagrams of the apparatus set up for reflux or for distillation. When you do so, make sure you include all the items listed below.

Tip: It is important that you draw these diagrams as cross sections.

Refluxing

A labelled diagram should include:

- the condenser in the upright position,
- a flask,
- a heat source,
- the water flowing correctly through the condenser,
- anti-bumping granules for smooth boiling.

Tip: Diagrams with gaps at the joints or showing a closed apparatus will be penalised.

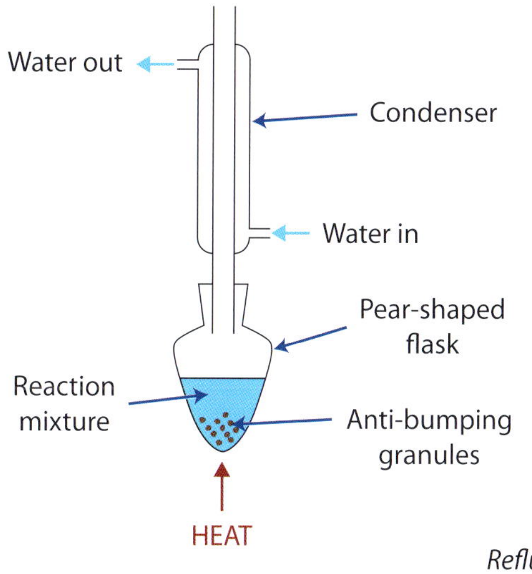

Refluxing

Distillation

A labelled diagram, such as the one shown overleaf, should include:

- the condenser in the sideways position,
- a flask,
- a side-arm connection/still head,
- a thermometer (with the bulb opposite the exit to the condenser),
- a heat source,
- the water flowing correctly through the condenser,
- an appropriate collecting vessel,
- anti-bumping granules.

Tip: As before, diagrams with gaps at the joints or showing a closed apparatus will be penalised.

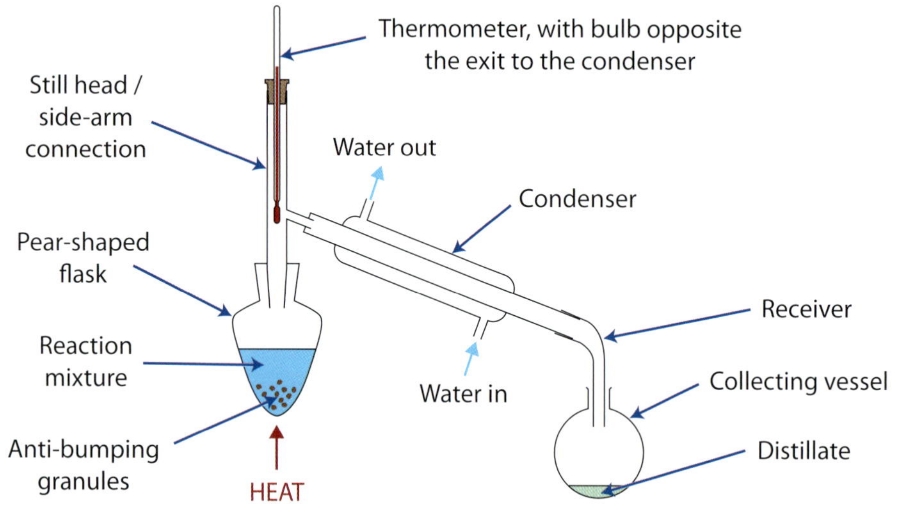

Distillation

Most organic compounds are flammable. Therefore, instead of using a Bunsen burner as the heat source, a water bath, sand bath or electric heating mantle can be used.

When separating the crude product from the reaction mixture, several distillations will be carried out. For the first distillation collect the crude product distillate **over a range**. For the final distillation, if the product is pure, it should distil over a **narrow range** at the expected boiling point.

Drying

Sometimes organic liquids may be dried by the following method:

1. Place the product in a beaker or conical flask.
2. Add a spatula of a drying agent, for example anhydrous magnesium sulfate/anhydrous sodium sulfate/anhydrous calcium chloride, and swirl.
3. Add more drying agent until the liquid is clear/no longer cloudy.
4. Decant/filter off the drying agent

Laboratory preparation of an alcohol from a halogenoalkane

An alcohol can be prepared from a halogenoalkane in the laboratory using the following method:

1. Place the halogenoalkane in a pear shaped/ round bottomed flask.
2. Add dilute sodium hydroxide solution. (The solution is made in ethanol/water so that everything will dissolve and the solutions will mix and react.)
3. Add some **anti-bumping granules**. These make the **boiling even and smooth** by preventing the production of large bubbles of gas which can cause 'bumping'.
4. Heat under reflux.
5. Distil off the alcohol.

The reaction that is occurring is a **substitution** reaction. If a halogenoalkane is heated under reflux with a solution of sodium or potassium hydroxide, the halogen is replaced by -OH and an alcohol is produced.

Worked example

Write an equation for the preparation of propan-1-ol from 1-bromopropane.

Answer

This is a subsitution reaction. The bromine (or other halogen) in the halogenoalkane is simply replaced by an -OH group:

$$CH_3CH_2CH_2Br + NaOH \rightarrow CH_3CH_2CH_2OH + NaBr$$

The yield of the reaction is not 100% for different practical and theoretical reasons. For example:

- Practical reason: some of the product is lost in distillation;
- Theoretical reason: side reactions occur, producing different products.

Industrial production of ethanol

Ethanol can be produced industrially by two methods: fermentation and the reaction of steam with ethene.

1. By fermentation

Fermentation is the breakdown of sugars to produce ethanol and carbon dioxide, using yeast. The yeast produces an enzyme which converts glucose to ethanol and carbon dioxide.

Conditions:

- **temperature of 35°C**, as the enzyme in yeast works best around this temperature: above this temperature the enzyme is denatured; below this temperature the reaction is too slow.
- **absence of air** to prevent the oxidation of the ethanol formed to ethanoic acid (vinegar).
- the sugars are **in solution**.
- use **yeast** as the enzyme.

An equation for the fermentation of the sugar glucose is:

$$\underset{\text{glucose}}{C_6H_{12}O_6(aq)} \rightarrow \underset{\text{ethanol}}{2C_2H_5OH(aq)} + 2CO_2(g)$$

> **Tip:** Ethanol can be written CH_3CH_2OH or C_2H_5OH. It is best not to use a molecular formula (C_2H_6O) unless asked for in a question.

Once the fermentation solution reaches about 15% ethanol the yeast can no longer function and fermentation stops. Ethanol produced industrially by fermentation is separated by fractional distillation. Fermentation is a slow reaction.

2. By the reaction of steam with ethene

In this method, ethene is hydrated using steam and a catalyst of concentrated phosphoric acid to produce ethanol (see page 40). **Hydration is the addition of water to a molecule**. For example:

$$CH_2{=}CH_2 + H_2O(g) \rightleftharpoons C_2H_5OH$$

> **Tip:** Remember to include equilibrium arrows in this reaction.

Conditions:

- catalyst of concentrated phosphoric acid
- pressure of 60 atm
- temperature of 300°C

The unreacted ethene and steam is passed back over the catalyst to increase the yield. This is a fast reaction. The ethanol produced in this process is very pure, but the main disadvantage of the method is that it requires ethene which comes from crude oil, a finite resource.

Uses of ethanol

Ethanol is used in **alcoholic beverages as a recreational drug**.

There are some **beneficial effects** of consuming alcohol in moderation:

- It may reduce the risk of cardiovascular disease.
- It may reduce the risk of dementia.
- It causes relaxation and may have social benefits for those who find shyness a difficulty.

However the consumption of alcohol can also have **harmful effects**:

- Excessive drinking can lead to liver damage.
- Excessive drinking can lead to brain damage.
- It reduces inhibitions, leads to a lack of coordination and impairs driving. This can result in accidents and injuries.

Questions

1. Give the IUPAC name for each of the following alcohols.

(a) 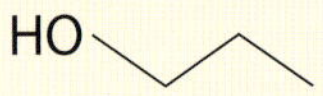

(b) 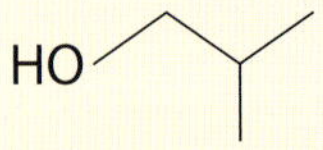

(c) 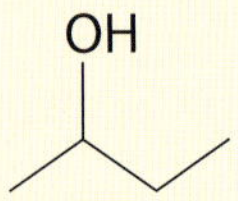

(d) 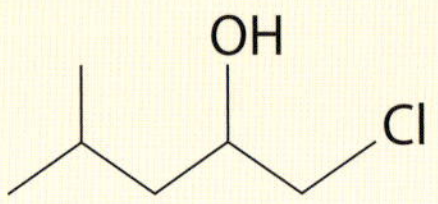

(e) 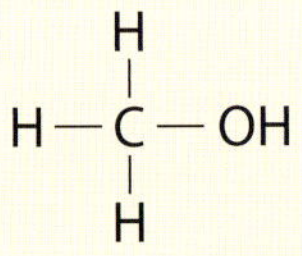

(f) 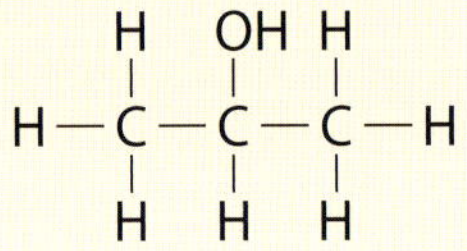

(g) 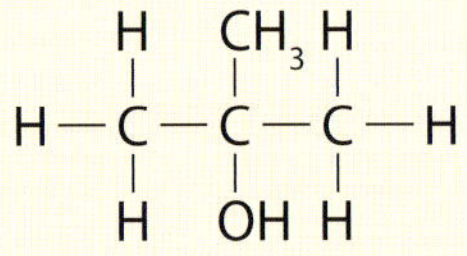

(h) 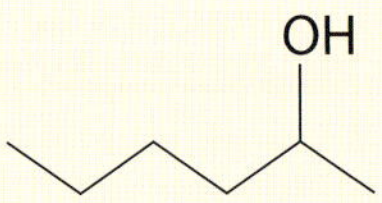

(i) $(CH_3)_2CHCH_2OH$

2. Classify each alcohol in question 1 as primary, secondary or tertiary. [9]

3. Classify the following alcohols as primary, secondary or tertiary.
(a) ethanol
(b) 2-methylpropan-1-ol
(c) 2,3-dimethylbutan-2-ol
(d) 2-methylbutan-2-ol
(e) 2-methylpropan-2-ol
(f) butan-1-ol
(g) 2-methylpentan-1-ol
(h) propan-2-ol [8]

4. Alcohols are a homologous series. They have a general formula and a functional group.
(a) What is meant by the term functional group? [1]
(b) Name the functional group in propan-1-ol. [1]
(c) Explain if ethanol is a hydrocarbon. [1]
(d) What is the general formula of the alcohols? [1]
(e) State three other features of the homologous series of alcohols. [3]
(f) Suggest a balanced symbol equation for the combustion of ethanol in a plentiful supply of air. [2]
(g) Suggest the names of the products formed when ethanol undergoes combustion in a limited supply of air. [2]
(h) Explain why 2-methylbutan-2-ol is a tertiary alcohol. [1]

5. (a) What is meant by the term structural isomer? [2]
(b) Draw the skeletal formula and name two alcohol isomers of C_3H_8O. [2]

6. The following alcohols are oxidised using acidified potassium dichromate(VI) solution. The conditions of the oxidation are also given.

A	pentan-3-ol	reflux
B	butan-1-ol	distillation
C	hexan-1-ol	reflux

Name and give the structure of the organic product in each of the oxidation reactions for A, B and C. [3]

7. Four structural isomers exist with formula $C_4H_{10}O$.

(a) Copy and complete the table to give the names, structure and classification of each isomer of $C_4H_{10}O$.

Name	Structure	Classification – primary, secondary or tertiary
butan-1-ol		
	$CH_3C(OH)(CH_3)CH_3$	
		primary

(b) Name any of the alcohols from the table which do not react with acidified potassium dichromate(VI). [1]

(c) What is observed when butan-1-ol is warmed with acidified potassium dichromate(VI)? [1]

(d) Write an equation for the complete oxidation of butan-1-ol using [O] to represent the oxidising agent and name the organic product. [2]

8 Which one of the following statements is **not** correct about the alcohol shown below?

$CH_3CH_2CH(OH)CH_3$

A It has the molecular formula $C_4H_{10}O$.
B It is butan-2-ol.
C It can be oxidised to an aldehyde.
D It is a secondary alcohol.

[1]

9. Propan-1-ol is refluxed with an oxidising agent to produce propanoic acid.

(a) Explain what is meant by the term reflux and why it is necessary in this experiment. [2]

(b) Write an equation for the overall oxidation of propan-1-ol into propanoic acid. [1]

(c) Name a suitable oxidising agent and state the colour change which would occur in the reaction mixture. [2]

(d) Suggest how you would change the experimental setup to produce propanal rather than propanoic acid. [3]

(e) Name the starting material which you could oxidise to prepare a sample of propanone by oxidation. [1]

(f) What is observed when Fehling's solution is warmed with (i) propanone (ii) propanal? [2]

10. Describe how you could use simple test tube reactions to distinguish between 2-methylbutan-2-ol and pentan-1-ol. In your answer give reagents, conditions, observations and an explanation of the chemistry involved.

In this question you will be assessed on using your written communication skills including the use of specialist scientific terms. [6]

11. Propan-1-ol can undergo an elimination reaction.

(a) Define elimination. [1]

(b) Write an equation for elimination of water from propan-1-ol and state the catalyst and temperature. [3]

(c) State what is observed if some bromine water is added to the products from the reaction in (b). [1]

12. Ethanol can be produced in the laboratory by refluxing bromoethane with an alkali or in industry from ethene.

(a) Write an equation for the reaction of bromoethane with sodium hydroxide. [1]

(b) Name the type of reaction in (a). [1]

(c) This reaction is carried out using reflux. State why anti-bumping granules are added. [1]

(d) State how the condenser is set up for reflux. [1]

(e) Suggest why electrical heating is preferred over using a Bunsen flame when preparing an alcohol from a halogenoalkane. [1]

(f) Describe how an impure sample of an organic liquid can be dried. [3]

(g) Why is the yield not 100%? Give a practical reason and a theoretical reason. [2]

(h) Write an equation for the production of ethanol from ethene, and name the catalyst used. [2]

6: SPECTROSCOPIC TECHNIQUES

Students should be able to:

8.6.1 interpret and read a combination and of infrared (IR) spectroscopy and mass spectrometry to identify organic compounds, and:

- explain that the absorption of infrared radiation arises from molecular vibrations;
- demonstrate understanding that groups of atoms within a molecule absorb infrared radiation at characteristic frequencies;
- use infrared spectra to deduce functional groups present in organic compounds given wavenumber data;
- recall the meaning of and identify the base peak, molecular ion peak, M+1 peak and fragmentation ions in a mass spectrum; and
- suggest formulae for the fragment ions in a given mass spectrum.

Infrared spectroscopy

If a range of infrared frequencies are passed, one at a time, through a sample of an organic compound, it will be observed that some frequencies get absorbed by the compound:

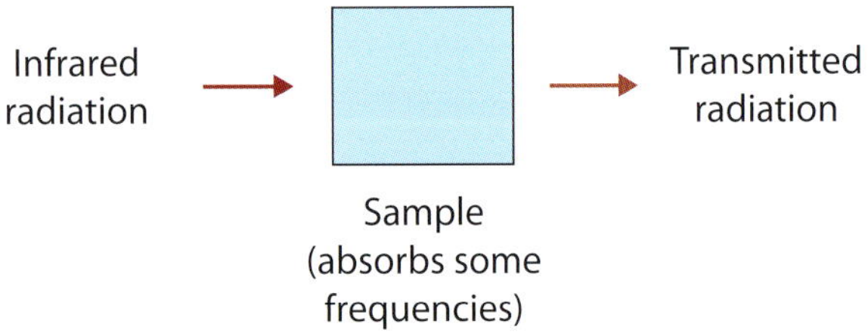

Infrared spectra

The frequency of the wavelengths absorbed depends on the bonds present and their environment. An **infrared spectrum** is a graph showing how the percentage transmittance varies with the frequency of the infrared radiation. If the transmittance is low it means that much of that frequency has been absorbed. An example of an infrared spectrum is shown next.

Tip: Notice that an unusual measure of frequency is used on the horizontal axis.

$$\text{wave number} = \frac{1}{\text{wavelength in cm}} \ \text{cm}^{-1}$$

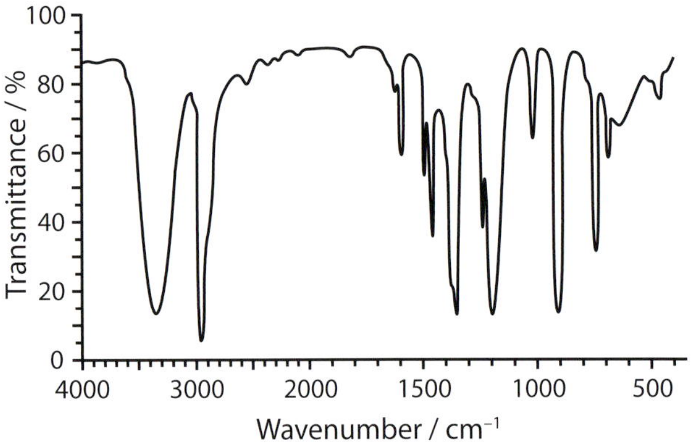

Deducing the functional groups present in organic compounds

When infrared radiation passes through a compound, **different groups of atoms** in the molecule **absorb the infrared** radiation at certain **characteristic frequencies**, causing the **bonds to vibrate**. The wavelength of the infrared radiation absorbed depends on the bond and its environment. As a result, the absorption of infrared radiation with a particular frequency can be used to detect specific bonds or groups of atoms in a molecule.

For example the -OH bond in an alcohol absorbs at 3200–3500 cm^{-1} and a peak at this point on the infrared spectra can be used to identify an alcohol. You can see an absorbance in this range in the example spectrum given above, showing that it is a spectrum for an alcohol.

By using infrared spectra, with tables of wavenumbers, it is possible to identify the functional groups present in a molecule. Tables of characteristic absorptions in infrared spectroscopy, similar to that below, will be given to you if you need to do this.

Wavenumber / cm^{-1}	Bond	Compound
750–1100	C-C	Alkanes, alkyl groups
1000–1300	C-O	Alcohols, carboxylic acids
1600–1700	C=C	Alkenes
1650–1800	C=O	Carboxylic acids, aldehydes, ketones
2500–3200	O-H	Carboxylic acids
2850–3000	C-H	Alkanes, alkyl groups, alkenes
3200–3500	O-H	Alcohols

For example, the structure of propan-1-ol is shown below.

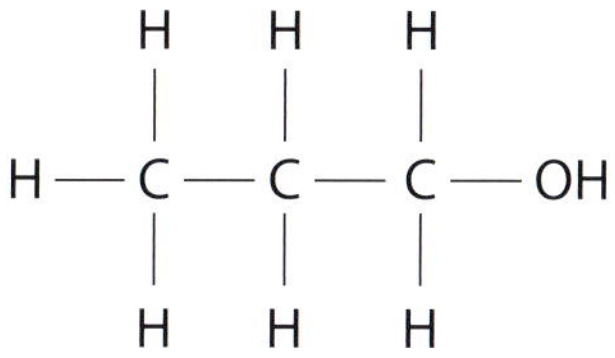

We can predict that, in the infrared spectrum for propan-1-ol:

- there will be an absorbance at 3200–3500 due to the -OH bond.
- there will be an absorbance at 2800–3000 due to C-H of the alkyl group.
- there will be an absorbance at 1000–1300 due to C-O.

Worked example
Explain if the spectrum below belongs to an alcohol, aldehyde or carboxylic acid. Use the characteristic absorptions from the table above.

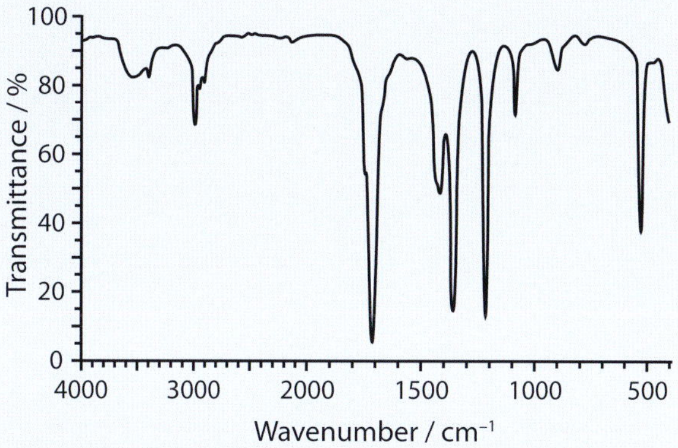

Answer
There is no OH absorption at 3200–3500 therefore it is not an alcohol.
There is no OH at 2500–3200 therefore it is not a carboxylic acid.
There is a C=O absorption at 1650–1800 so could be an aldehyde.

Other uses of infrared spectrometry

Infrared spectroscopy can also be used to **monitor the progress** of a reaction. For example, in the reaction oxidising ethanol to ethanoic acid the infrared absorbances will change as one functional group is converted to another. The absorbance for the -OH bond of an alcohol at 3200–3500 will decrease, while the absorbances for the C=O for an acid at 1650–1800 and -OH at 2500–3200 will appear. The reaction is finished when the -OH alcohol absorbance disappears.

The infrared spectrum of a compound is unique and can be used to **identify an unknown substance** by **matching** the infrared spectrum of the unknown substance with the infrared spectrum of a pure compound.

It is also possible to determine whether or not a prepared molecule is pure by generating an infrared spectrum and comparing it to a database of spectra.

Worked example
Propenenitrile is manufactured from propene, ammonia and oxygen. Suggest how you would show using infrared spectroscopy that no propene was present in the product.

Answer
The infrared spectrum for a compound is unique. If the product is pure no propene will be present and the infrared spectrum of the product will exactly match that of a pure sample of propenenitrile.

Mass spectrometry

In a mass spectrometer a molecule (M) is bombarded by electrons and positive ions are formed. A molecular ion (M^+) is formed by loss of one electron:

$M \rightarrow M^+ + e$

Tip: A molecular ion is an ion formed by the removal of an electron from a molecule.

This ion is detected in the recorder of the mass spectrometer and a peak is printed on a graph called a **mass spectrum**. The *x*-axis of the mass spectrum is labelled with the mass/charge ratio, or **m/z**, or even m/e. The *y*-axis is labelled with the **abundance** (usually given as a percentage). The more common a particular mass of a particle, the higher the abundance, and the higher the peak.

The **molecular ion peak** (**M**$^+$) has the **highest value of m/z** and it gives the **relative formula mass** of the molecule.

A molecular ion peak is the peak produced by an ion formed by the removal of one electron from a molecule.

Sometimes there is a small peak one unit to the right of the molecular ion peak – this is called the M+1 peak. It has very low abundance and is due to one carbon atom in the molecule having mass number 13 instead of mass number 12.

An M+1 peak is a peak produced by a molecular ion with an increased mass due to the presence of one carbon-13 atom.

The base peak is the peak of greatest abundance in a mass spectrum (that is, the tallest peak).

The spectrum of ethanol is shown below.

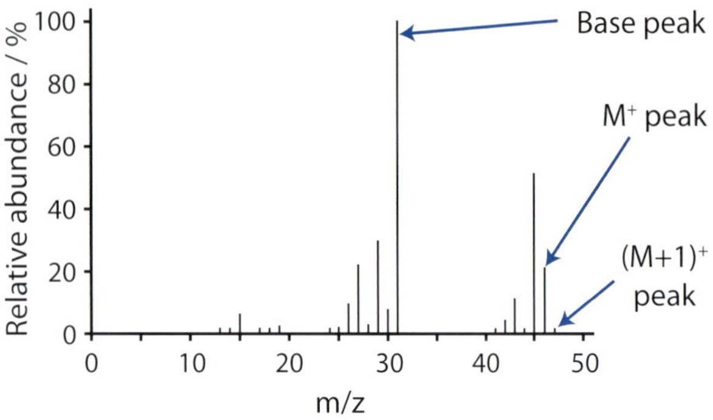

The base peak in this spectrum is at 31. The molecular ion peak is at 46, and this is the relative formula mass of ethanol. There is a peak with very small abundance at 47, which is the M+1 peak, due to the presence of one carbon-13 atom in a molecule of ethanol.

Fragmentation ion peaks

Other peaks are also present in a mass spectrum. These are due to bonds breaking in the molecule and the molecule breaking up. These events form positively-charged **fragmentation ions** (sometimes called fragment ions) which have different masses and hence different peaks, called **fragmentation ion peaks**.

A fragmentation ion is a positively charged ion produced when the molecular ion breaks apart.

The m/z of some common fragmentation ion peaks are shown in the following table.

Peak	m/z
CH_3^+	15
$C_2H_5^+$ / CHO^+	29
OH^+	17
CH_3CO^+ / $C_3H_7^+$	43
CO^+	28

For example ethanol may break at some of the positions below and form fragmentation ions with the masses shown.

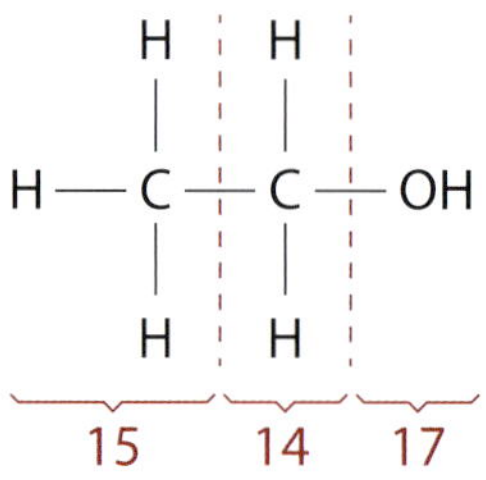

- The peak at m/z 47 is the M+1 peak. It is caused by $C_2H_5OH^+$ with one of the carbon atoms of mass 13:
  $(13 + 12 + (5 \times 1) + 16 + 1) = 47$
- The peak at m/z 46 is the molecular ion peak. It is caused by $C_2H_5OH^+$
- The peak at m/z 45 is caused by the ion $C_2H_5O^+$
- The peak at m/z 31 is the base peak. It is caused by the ion CH_2OH^+
- The peak at m/z 29 is caused by the ion $CH_3CH_2^+$
- The peak at m/z 15 is caused by the ion CH_3^+
- The peak at m/z 14 is caused by the ion CH_2^+
- The peak at m/z 17 is caused by the ion OH^+

The mass spectrum of pentan-2-one $CH_3COCH_2CH_2CH_3$ is shown below. The numbers above each peak shows the m/z value.

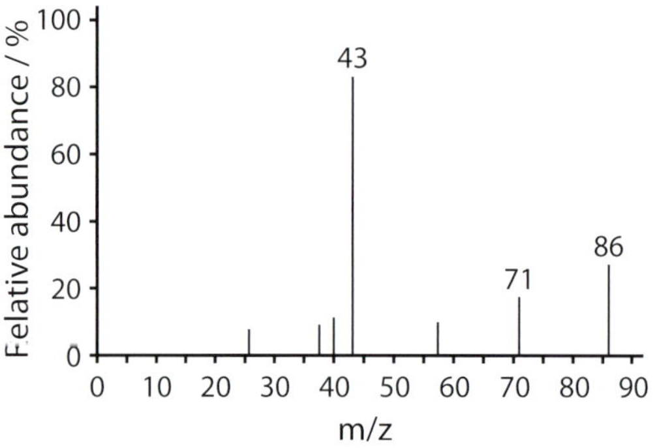

The molecular ion peak with the highest m/z value is at 86 and has formula $CH_3COCH_2CH_2CH_3^+$. This peak gives the relative formula mass of the compound. The other peaks are for fragmentation ions. The peak at 71 could be due to $CH_3COCH_2CH_2^+$ and the peak at 43 could be due to $C_3H_7^+$ or CH_3CO^+.

Questions

For these questions use the table of bond absorptions found on page 60.

1. The infrared spectrum of a compound is shown below.

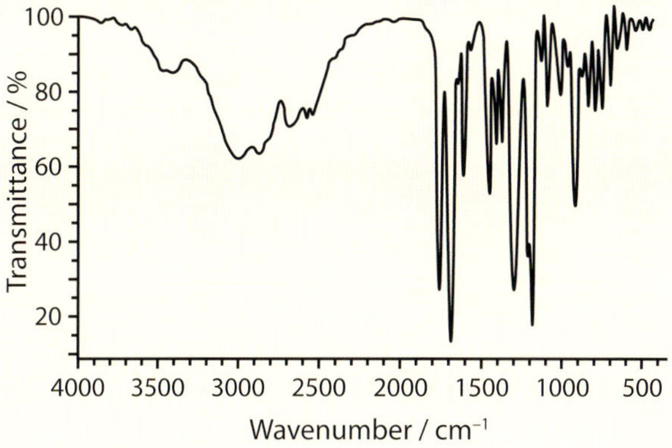

(a) What evidence is there in the spectrum that the compound is not an alcohol or an aldehyde or ketone? [2]

(b) What evidence is there in the spectrum that the compound may be a hydrocarbon? [1]

2. There are two functional groups in propen-2-ol. Each of these functional groups contains a bond with a characteristic absorption range in the infrared spectrum.

(a) Copy and complete the structure of propen-2-ol showing all bonds. [1]

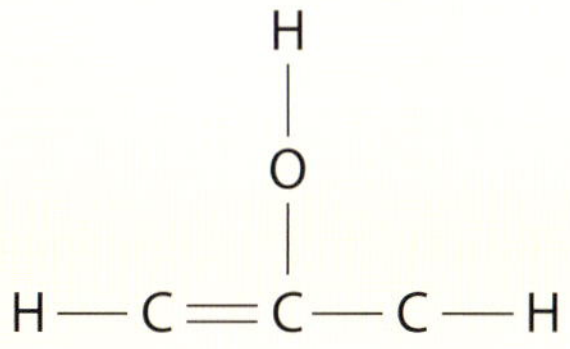

(b) Suggest a bond and its absorption range for each of the two functional groups present in propen-2-ol. [2]

3. Compounds A, B, C and D are isomers with the molecular formula $C_4H_{10}O$. They all have a broad absorption in their infrared spectra in the range 3230–3500 cm^{-1}.

(a) Identify the bond responsible for this absorption. [1]

(b) Compounds A and B are both straight chain compounds. A can be oxidised to form butanal and B can be oxidised to form butanone. Give the IUPAC name for A and B. [2]

(c) Isomer C is resistant to oxidation. Draw and name the structure of C. [2]

(d) Isomer D is a branched chain isomer that can be oxidised to form compounds E and F. Compound E is obtained by distilling it off as it forms during the oxidation. Compound F is formed when the oxidation takes place under reflux.

(i) Draw the structure and name isomer D. [2]

(ii) Identify the functional groups in E and F. [2]

(iii) A student attempted to oxidise D and the infrared spectrum of the product obtained by the student is shown below.

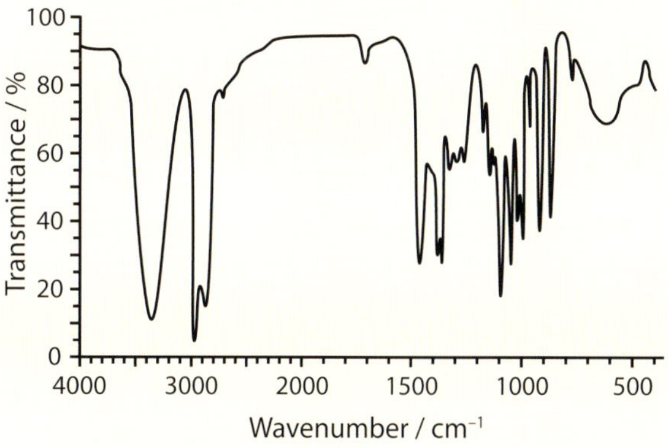

Suggest two ways in which the spectrum shows that compound D has not been oxidised. [2]

4. The infrared spectrum of an alcohol is shown below.

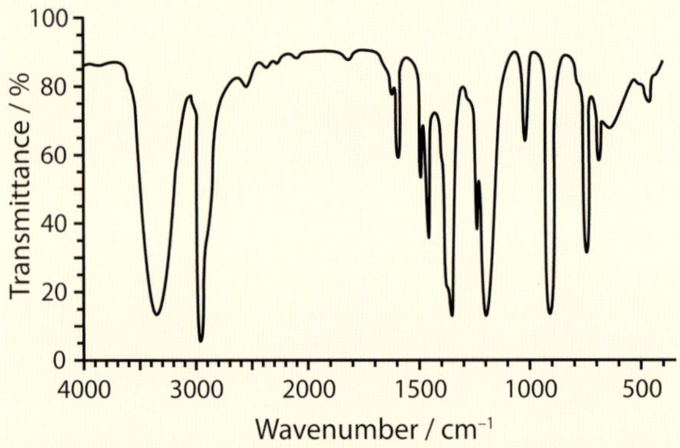

(a) Explain why this infrared spectrum of this compound supports the fact that it is an alcohol. [2]

(b) Explain how infrared spectroscopy can be used to exactly identify this alcohol. [1]

(c) How would mass spectrometry help identify the alcohol? [1]

(d) This alcohol can be oxidised. How could infrared spectroscopy be used to show when the oxidation is complete? [2]

(e) State a reagent and condition used to oxidise the alcohol. [2]

(f) Suggest why it is difficult to determine the distinguish between spectrums of the isomers butan-1-ol and butan-2-ol using infrared spectroscopy? [1]

5. A simple mass spectrum of ethanol is shown below. The numbers above the peaks are the m/z values.

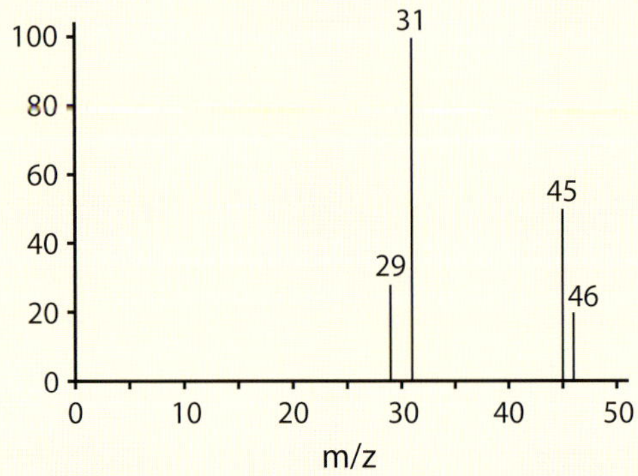

(a) What label should be placed on the *y*-axis? [1]

(b) What is meant by the term m/z? [1]

(c) State how the relative formula mass of ethanol can be determined from the mass spectrum. [1]

(d) Suggest formulae for the fragmentation ions found at m/z 29, 31 and 45. [3]

(e) State the m/z value for the base peak. [1]

6. The mass spectrum for a compound is shown below. Which peak gives the relative formula mass of the compound? [1]

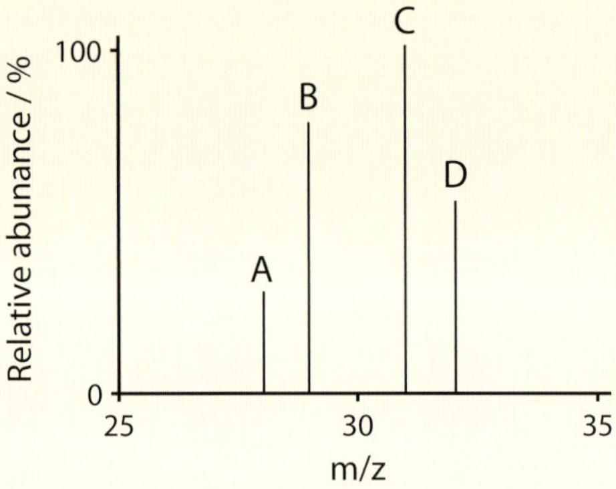

7: MAKING AND PURIFYING ORGANIC COMPOUNDS – THE PREPARATION OF ASPIRIN

Students should be able to:

8.7.1 investigate the main steps in the production and recrystallisation of laboratory grade aspirin;

8.7.2 determine the purity of laboratory synthesised aspirin using ferric chloride;

8.7.3 determine the theoretical and actual percentage yield from a laboratory prepared sample of aspirin;

8.7.4 determine the melting point of laboratory synthesised aspirin compared to industrially prepared aspirin;

8.7.5 suggest and explain any modifications they would make to their method and/or the product to improve its quality and/or yield.

Preparation of an organic solid

The exact method to prepare an organic solid depends on the actual solid being prepared, but in general the method is as follows:

1. **Preparation** – react suitable quantities of the reactants to produce the product.
2. **Separation of the crude (impure) product** – the solid is separated from the reaction mixture by **suction filtration** using a Büchner funnel.
3. **Purification of the product** – this removes impurities and is carried out by **recrystallistion**.
4. **Drying the product** – this is carried out by sucking air over the solid in the Büchner funnel, and drying in a low temperature oven.
5. **Checking the purity** – by carrying out a melting point determination.

Suction filtration

Suction filtration is often called Büchner filtration or vaccum filtration. It is used in a preparation to separate the solid product from the reactants as it is **faster** than normal gravity filtration and the solid is left quite **dry**. The apparatus for suction filtration is shown below. The method is as follows:

1. Place filter paper in a Büchner funnel.
2. Place the Büchner funnel in a Büchner flask.
3. Attach the flask to a suction pump and suck air through the flask. The suction draws the liquid through the filter paper into the Büchner flask and leaves the crude product in the filter paper.

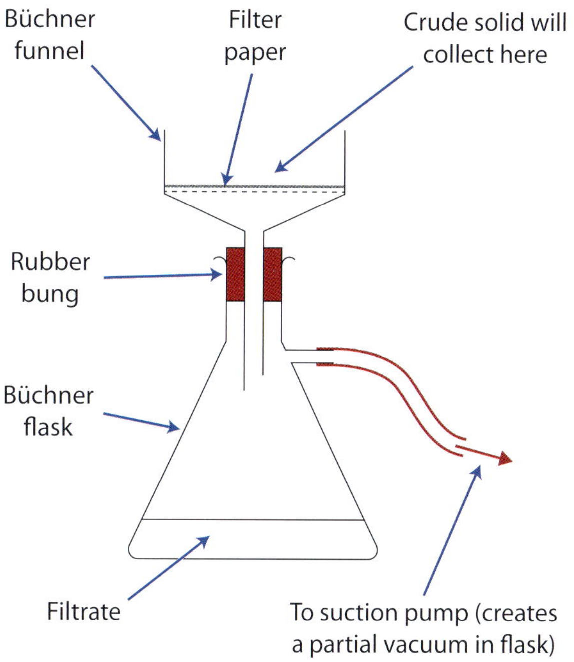

Tip: Make sure you can draw this diagram showing suction filtration.

Purification by recrystallisation

Recrystallisation is a method of purifying a solid by dissolving the impure crystals in the minimum volume of hot solvent, filtering whilst hot and cooling the filtrate to crystallise.

The general method of recrystallisation is to find a solvent that dissolves the product **more readily** at a **high temperature** than at a low temperature, make a hot solution, and allow it to crystallise on cooling. Any insoluble impurities can be removed by gravity filtration and other impurities remain dissolved in the solvent.

Tip: Remember, the material to be recrystallised should be sparingly soluble in the solvent at room temperature and very soluble near the boiling point.

The method to recrystallise and dry a solid is as follows:

1. Dissolve the impure solid in the **minimum volume of hot solvent.** *(A minimum volume of hot solvent is used to ensure that as much of the solute is obtained as possible.)*
2. Filter when **hot** by **gravity filtration**, using a hot funnel, or fluted filter paper, to remove insoluble impurities. *(Filtering through a hot filter funnel and using fluted paper prevents precipitation of the solid.)*
3. Allow the filtrate to cool and crystallise. The impurities will remain in solution.
4. Filter off the crystals using **suction** filtration.
5. **Wash** by pouring over some **ice cold solvent** which removes any aqueous impurities. *(The solvent is cold to prevent the crystals from dissolving.)*
6. **Dry** by sucking air over the crystals in the Büchner funnel and then in a low temperature oven. An alternative method of drying is to place the solid in a **desiccator** with a drying agent.

Several recrystallisations could be carried out to **improve** the purity and quality of the product. However, the disadvantage of several recrystallisations is that the yield will be reduced.

Checking the purity of an organic solid using melting point

The melting point of a substance is not the exact point at which it melts but rather the **range of temperatures** from when the sample starts to melt until it has completely melted. The greater the range the more impurities are present. A **pure** substance melts over a **narrow** range of temperatures. An **impure** substance melts over a **wide range** of temperatures and the melting point is lower than that of the pure product.

The method to find a melting point is as follows:

1. Place some solid in a capillary tube/melting point tube, sealed at one end.
2. Heat slowly using melting point apparatus.
3. Record the temperatures at which the solid starts and finishes melting.
4. Repeat and average the temperatures.
5. Compare the temperatures with known values in a data book.

Aspirin

Aspirin (acetylsalicylic acid) is a painkiller. It is manufactured by acylating **2-hydrobenzoic acid** (salicylic acid) using **ethanoic anhydride** (acetyl anhydride). It is also possible to use ethanoyl chloride, but this is very reactive, hydrolyses easily and gives off corrosive fumes of hydrogen chloride. Ethanoic anhydride, by contrast, is less corrosive, less easily hydrolysed, and gives a less violent reaction with no corrosive fumes of hydrogen chloride.

Acylation is the process of replacing a hydrogen atom in certain molecules by an acyl group (RCO-).

The equation for the preparation of aspirin is shown below and also shown structurally in the box:

$$C_6H_4(OH)COOH + (CH_3CO)_2O \rightarrow HOOCC_6H_4OCOCH_3 + CH_3COOH$$

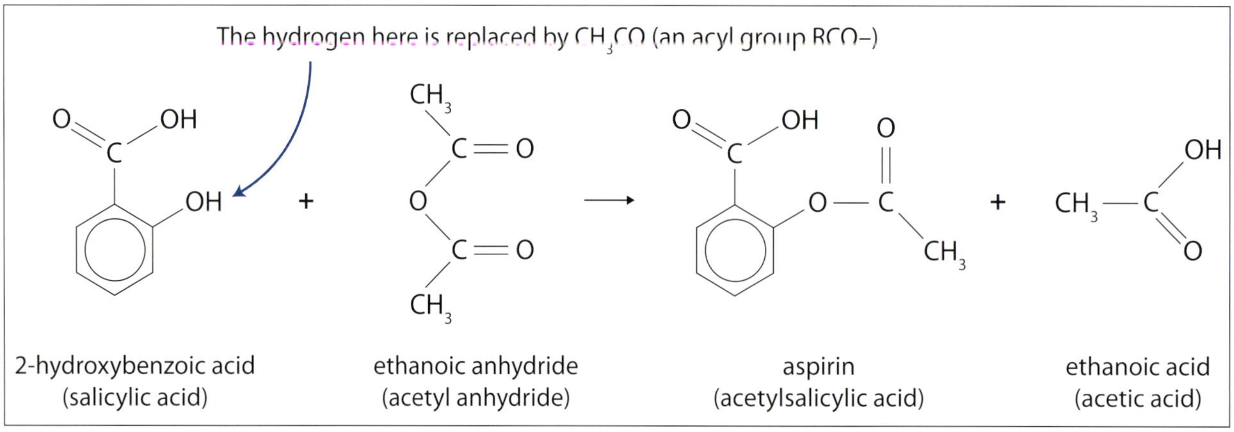

Tip: This equation, written using molecular formulae, is:

$C_7H_6O_3 + C_4H_6O_3 \rightarrow C_9H_8O_4 + C_2H_4O_2$

Preparation of aspirin in the laboratory

The following method can be used to prepare aspirin in the laboratory:

1. Place 1.0 g of 2-hydroxybenzoic acid (salicylic acid) in a pear shaped flask and add 2 cm^3 of ethanoic anhydride (acetyl anhydride). Note that ethanoic anhydride reacts readily with water so all the apparatus must be dry.

Tip: You do not need to learn exact masses and volumes, just the general method.

2. Slowly add 8 drops of concentrated phosphoric(V) acid (a catalyst).

Tip: Conc phosphoric(V) acid is corrosive so wear gloves and goggles when using it, and add it slowly to allow any heat produced to dissipate.

3. Warm by placing a vertical condenser on the flask and putting it in a hot water bath, or heat gently under reflux for 20 minutes.
4. Add water (to hydrolyse any unreacted ethanoic anhydride to ethanoic acid).
5. Pour the mixture onto crushed ice in a beaker.
6. Use suction filtration to remove the crude aspirin (white crystals).

The purification steps then are:

1. Recrystallise to purify by dissolving in the minimum volume of water or ethanol, filter hot by gravity, cool and crystallise and filter by suction filtration.
2. Dry in a low temperature oven or in a desiccator.
3. The melting point is then determined and compared with that of pure aspirin. If the aspirin is pure then the melting point should be sharp with a very small range.

In the industrial manufacture of aspirin cost is important. The manufacturer must choose chemicals which are cheap. They must also determine whether a catalyst is necessary, i.e. is the reduction of reaction time significant enough to justify the price of the catalyst per unit of aspirin produced? Additionally, a catalyst may pose toxicity problems which will incur additional costs.

Checking the purity of aspirin using a chemical test

The purity of aspirin can be tested by the following method:

1. Add a few drops of **ferric chloride** (iron(III) chloride) to a solution of aspirin.
2. If it remains yellow there are no impurities.
3. If it changes to a purple colour, then there may be salicylic acid impurities.

Tip: Ferric chloride is an old name for iron(III) chloride – the (III) is not included.

Percentage yield

Using mole calculations and ratios, it is possible to work out the mass of a chemical which should be produced in a reaction, if the mass of the starting material is given. The **mass of chemical expected**, by calculation, is called the **theoretical yield**. However, less mass is often obtained than what is expected due to experimental error. The mass of chemical **actually** obtained is called the **actual yield**.

The percentage yield of any preparation can be calculated using the equation:

$$\textbf{\% yield} = \frac{\textbf{actual yield}}{\textbf{theoretical yield}} \times \textbf{100}$$

The method to calculate percentage yield is as follows:

1. Work out the moles of the reactant using

   $$\text{number of moles} = \frac{\text{mass}}{M_r}$$

2. Use the ratio in the balanced symbol equation to work out the number of moles of product.
3. Use the equation mass = moles × M_r to work out the mass of product which should form. This is the theoretical yield.
4. Use the equation:

   $$\text{\% yield} = \frac{\text{actual yield}}{\text{theoretical yield}} \times 100$$

Tip: Remember that M_r is the relative formula mass which is calculated by adding the mass of each atom present in the formula.

Worked example

In an experiment 20.0 g of salicylic acid were reacted with an excess of ethanoic anhydride. Calculate the percentage yield given that 17.3 g of aspirin were obtained. Give your answer to 3 significant figures.

$$C_6H_4(OH)COOH + (CH_3CO)_2O \rightarrow HOOCC_6H_4OCOCH_3 + CH_3COOH$$

Answer

Step 1: Calculate the relative formula mass of salicylic acid.

To do this it is best to write the given formula as a molecular formula:

$C_6H_4(OH)COOH$

$= C_7H_6O_3$

$M_r = (7 \times 12) + (6 \times 1) + (16 \times 3) = 138$

Step 2: Calculate the number of moles of salicylic acid.

$$\text{Moles} = \frac{\text{mass}}{M_r} = \frac{20.0}{138} = 0.14493$$

Tip: At this stage make sure you round correctly, and keep more significant figures than you need in the final answer.

Step 3: Calculate the number of moles of aspirin.

The ratio from the symbol equation is 1 mole salicylic acid : 1 mole of aspirin

So the moles of aspirin = 0.14493

Step 4: Then calculate the relative formula mass of aspirin.

aspirin = $HOOCC_6H_4OCOCH_3$

$= C_9H_8O_4$

$M_r = (9 \times 12) + (8 \times 1) + (8 \times 4) = 180$

mass = moles × M_r

$= 0.14493 \times 180$

$= 26.1\text{g}$

This is the theoretical yield.

Step 5: Calculate the % yield.

$$\%\ \text{yield} = \frac{\text{actual yield}}{\text{theoretical yield}} \times 100$$

$$= \frac{17.3}{26.1} \times 100$$

$= 66.28\%$

$= 66.3\%$ (to 3 significant figures)

Tip: The rules for rounding are (a) if the next number is 5 or more, round up (b) if the next number is 4 or less, do not round up. So to round 66.28 to 3 significant figures, look at the fourth number, which is This is greater than 5 so round up to 66.3.

Worked example

A student reacted excess salicylic acid with 6.00 cm^3 of ethanoic anhydride. The reaction produced 6.08 g of aspirin. The density of ethanoic anhydride is 1.08 g/cm^3.

(a) Calculate the mass of ethanoic anhydride used.

(b) Calculate the number of moles of ethanoic anhydride used.

(c) Calculate the maximum mass of aspirin which could be formed.

(d) Calculate the percentage yield of aspirin. Give your answer to 2 significant figures.

Answer

(a) *The question gives a volume of ethanoic anhydride, so first convert the volume to mass, using the density.*

$$\text{density} = \frac{\text{mass}}{\text{volume}}$$

$$1.08 = \frac{\text{mass}}{6.0}$$

$1.08 \times 6.00 = 6.48\text{g}$

(b) *ethanoic anhydride has the formula* $(CH_3CO)_2O$ which is $C_4H_6O_3$

$M_r = (4 \times 12) + (6 \times 1) + (3 \times 16) = 102$

$$\text{Moles} = \frac{\text{mass}}{M_r} = \frac{6.48}{102} = 0.0635$$

(c) *From the balanced symbol equation the ratio is:*
1 mole ethanoic anhydride : 1 mole aspirin.
So 0.0635 moles ethanoic anhydride : 0.0635 mole aspirin
aspirin = $HOOCC_6H_4OCOCH_3 = C_9H_8O_4$
So $M_r = 180$
mass = mol × M_r
= 0.0635 × 180 = 11.43g

(d) *Calculate the percentage yield of aspirin obtained by the student.*

$$\% \text{ yield} = \frac{\text{actual yield}}{\text{theoretical yield}} \times 100$$

$$= \frac{6.08}{11.43} \times 100 = 53.2$$

= 53% (to 2 significant figures)

Tip: Rather than using masses, you can also calculate percentage yield by finding the actual yield in moles and dividing by the theoretical yield in moles.

Why is the percentage yield less than 100% in a preparation?

The **theoretical** reasons why the percentage yield is less than 100% in a preparation are as follows:

- Side reactions occur, so by-products may be produced instead of the expected product.
- The reaction is incomplete.

The **practical** reasons why some solid is lost and the percentage yield is less than 100% in a preparation are as follows:

- Some product is lost in purification steps. For example, in recrystallisation some solid may still be dissolved in the solvent.
- Some product is lost in transferring between vessels. To minimise this loss sometimes rinsing out the vessel is useful.

Improving quality and yield

Recrystallising several times may improve purity. However this may cause decreased yield. Purity can also be increased by washing with iced water. However, this too may cause decreased yield, particularly if the water is not sufficiently cooled in which case some of the aspirin may dissolve.

To increase the yield, ensure that the reactants are pure, and that a minimum volume of hot solvent is used in recrystallisation.

Questions

1. Aspirin is a solid at room temperature. It can be prepared in the laboratory from salicylic acid and ethanoic anhydride.

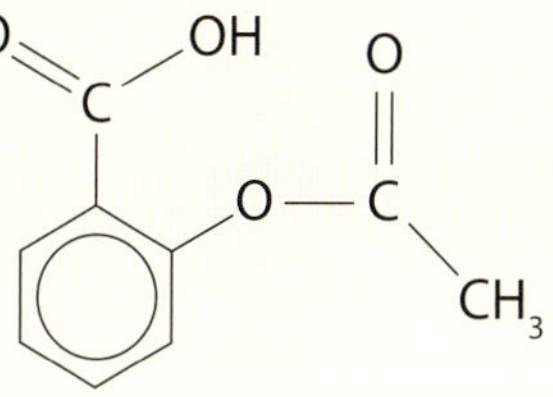

aspirin

(a) Draw the structure of salicylic acid. [1]
(b) Describe the laboratory preparation of a crude impure sample of aspirin from salicylic acid and ethanoic anhydride. **The quality of your written communication will be assessed in this part.** [6]
(c) Describe how you would purify the sample of aspirin by recrystallisation. [4]
(d) Describe how you would determine the melting point of the purified aspirin and decide if it was pure. [4]
(e) Describe how you experimentally show, using a chemical test, if the aspirin prepared contained any salicylic acid impurities. [3]
(f) 10.0 g of salicylic acid were reacted with an excess of ethanoic anhydride. Calculate the percentage yield given that 9.1 g of aspirin were obtained. [3]

2. Aspirin can be prepared by reacting 2-hydroxybenzoic acid with ethanoic anhydride in the presence of concentrated phosphoric acid. The method used was:
Place 20.0 g of 2-hydroxybenzoic acid in a pear shaped flask and add 40 cm³ of ethanoic anhydride. Safely add 5 cm³ concentrated phosphoric acid to the mixture and heat under reflux. Add water to hydrolyse any unreacted reactants. Pour the mixture onto 400 g of crushed ice in a beaker. The product is separated by suction filtration, recrystallised from water and dried in a dessicator. The melting point is then determined.

(a) Suggest the role of the concentrated phosphoric acid. [1]
(b) Explain how you would safely add the concentrated phosphoric acid. [2]
(c) What is meant by the term reflux? [1]
(d) Name the reactant which is hydrolysed by adding water and state the product of this hydrolysis. [2]
(e) Why is the mixture poured onto ice? [1]
(f) Why is suction filtration used rather than gravity filtration to separate the product? [1]
(g) What is meant by the term hydrolyse? [1]

3. 5.0 g of butan-1-ol (M_r 74) was reacted with an excess of hydrogen bromide and 6.4 g of 1-bromobutane (M_r 137) was obtained. For every one mole of butanol used, one mole of brombutane is obtained. Calculate the percentage yield of bromobutane. Give your answer to 2 significant figures. [3]

4. In an experiment 23 g of ethanol, C_2H_5OH, was reacted with excess ethanoic acid and 33 g of ethyl ethanoate, $CH_3COOC_2H_5$, is obtained.

$$C_2H_5OH + CH_3COOH \rightarrow CH_3COOC_2H_5 + H_2O$$

Calculate the percentage yield of ethyl ethanoate. [5]

5. Phenol is converted to trichlorophenol (TCP) according to the equation below.

$$\underset{\text{Phenol}}{C_6H_5OH} + 3Cl_2 \rightarrow \underset{\text{TCP}}{C_6H_2Cl_3OH} + 3HCl$$

In the reaction 50.0 g of phenol produced 97.6 g of TCP. Calculate the percentage yield of TCP to 2 significant figures.

6. 8.0 cm^3 of butan-1-ol (M_r 74) of density 0.80 g cm^{-3} was reacted with an excess of sodium bromide and concentrated sulphuric acid. After purification, 3.7 cm^3 of 1-bromobutane (M_r 137) of density 1.3 g cm^{-3} were obtained. One mole of butan-1-ol produces one mole of 1-bromobutane. Calculate the percentage yield of 1-bromobutane. Give your answer to 2 significant figures. [4]

Unit A2 3:
Medical Physics

8: PHYSIOLOGICAL MEASUREMENTS TO MONITOR HEALTH

Students should be able to:

9.1.1 demonstrate an understanding of core body temperature measurements and compare commonly used thermometers including:

- clinical mercury; ear (tympanic); forehead strip; infrared (IR) and digital; and
- how the thermometer is used to measure body temperature;

9.1.2 demonstrate an understanding of the range of temperatures over which the body can survive including hyperthermia and hypothermia;

9.1.3 demonstrate an understanding of the measurement of blood pressure;

9.1.4 demonstrate an understanding of the sphygmomanometer and investigate its use to collect and evaluate data;

9.1.5 scrutinise a range of blood pressure values and analyse them with reference to values of blood pressure for a normal adult;

9.1.6 develop an experiment to monitor heart activity effectively and compare this critically to how data is collected and analysed using an electrocardiogram (ECG);

9.1.7 recall that brain activity can be monitored using Functional Magnetic Resonance Imaging (fMRI) and Magnetoencephalography (MEG) and explore how it can be monitored using the electroencephalogram (ECG); and

9.1.8 recognise typical EEG traces as alpha (α); beta (β); theta (θ); delta (Δ) and gamma (γ) waves based on frequency ranges and give examples of when you might see each of those during an EEG.

9.2.1 describe the physical principles and application of, and the equipment used in, the following diagnostic imaging techniques:

- magnetic resonance imaging (MRI) scans;
- *Note: the remaining elements of 9.2.1 are covered in chapter 9.*

Tip: Get to know your specification. It tells you exactly what you need to know as you prepare for your exam. It can be found on the CCEA website: www.ccea.org.uk

Temperature

In medicine, core body temperature is one of many clinical indicators that tell us what is going on deep inside the human body. In some sports the body is pushed to extremes. Knowing the core body temperature is essential in such sports if permanent damage to organ systems is to be avoided.

Measuring temperature

Body temperature can be measured in different ways. In this section we will consider six methods: oral, rectal, ear, underarm, infrared and forehead strip.

1. Oral method

In this method, temperature is measured by placing a thermometer in the mouth. Traditionally, mercury-in-glass thermometers were used. However, mercury is very poisonous and, while the risk of cracking the glass and ingesting mercury is small, it is not insignificant. In addition, mercury-in-glass thermometers take several minutes to reach core body temperature and are often difficult to read accurately. For these reasons, mercury-in-glass thermometers are rarely used in western medicine today and are **never** used with infants, small children or patients with impaired mental capacity. Instead a digital thermometer is recommended.

For accurate measurement with an oral thermometer, the patient:

- should be mature enough to cooperate and follow instructions;
- should not have taken any hot or cold food or liquid for some time;
- should be able to breathe in and out normally through the nose.

The procedure is as follows:

1. The thermometer is placed under the tongue and the lips tightly closed around it.

2. The thermometer is left in place until it beeps to indicate completion of reading – this can range from 12 seconds to 60 seconds, depending on the manufacturer, but is generally faster than a mercury-in-glass thermometer.
3. The thermometer is removed from the mouth and the reading recorded.
4. The thermometer is cleaned with a clinical wipe soaked in alcohol and put away for further use.

2. Rectal method

This method is used for infants, small children and people who are unable to hold a thermometer safely in their mouths. Rectal methods give a more accurate measurement of body temperature compared to oral methods, but because they are quite invasive, oral methods are generally preferred.

The procedure for a digital thermometer is as follows:

1. A lubricant such as petroleum jelly is first applied to the bulb of the thermometer to make the insertion of the thermometer easier.
2. The patient is asked to lie on one side and spread their buttocks.
3. The bulb end of the thermometer is inserted about 1 or 2 cm into the anal canal.
4. The patient is asked to close their buttocks to keep the thermometer in place.
5. When the device beeps, the thermometer is gently removed and the reading recorded when the device beeps.
6. The thermometer is cleaned with cool, soapy water, rinsed and then rubbed with a clinical wipe soaked in alcohol and put away for further use.

For obvious hygiene reasons no rectal thermometer is ever used in the mouth, even after cleansing with alcohol.

3. Ear thermometer

This method uses a thermometer specifically designed to be inserted into the ear, and uses infrared radiation to measure temperature.

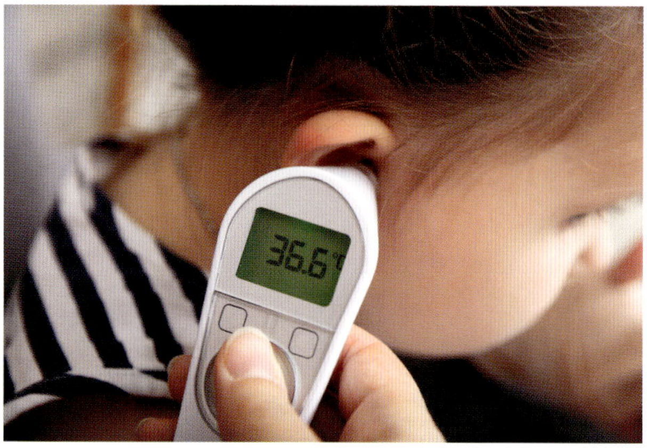

The procedure is as follows:

1. The upper earlobe is gently pulled back to open up the ear canal.
2. The digital ear thermometer is switched on to activate the infrared sensor.
3. The thermometer probe is gently inserted into the ear canal.
4. After a few seconds the thermometer will beep.
5. The probe is removed from the ear canal and the temperature recorded.
6. The thermometer is cleaned with cool, soapy water, rinsed and then rubbed with a clinical wipe soaked in alcohol and put away for further use.

4. Underarm thermometer

Like the ear thermometer, this method uses a thermometer that measures infrared radiation, but from under the patient's arm. It is non-invasive and frequently used with children.

The procedure is as follows:

1. The digital underarm thermometer is switched on to activate the infrared sensor.
2. With the tip of the thermometer pointing at the child, their arm is raised and the thermometer probe is slipped under their arm, with the tip gently pressed against the centre of the armpit.
3. The patient's arm is lowered close against the body so the thermometer stays in place.
4. After a few seconds the thermometer will beep.
5. The thermometer is removed from the armpit and the temperature recorded.
6. The thermometer is cleaned with cool, soapy water, rinsed and then rubbed with a clinical

wipe soaked in alcohol and put away for further use.

5. Infrared thermometer

Although the ear thermometer and underarm thermometer both detect infrared radiation, the term **infrared thermometer** is generally reserved for those which detect radiation from the arm or forehead.

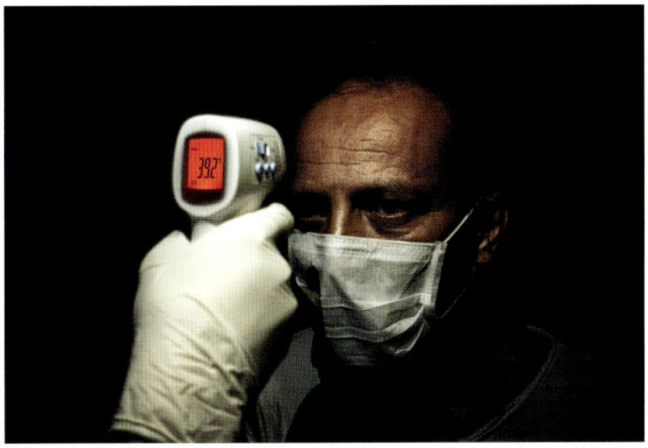

The procedure is as follows:

1. The thermometer is switched on and directed at the patient's arm or forehead.
2. The activation trigger is squeezed and a spot of red light appears on the patient's skin.
3. A few seconds later the instrument beeps and the patient's temperature appears on the thermometer's screen.

6. Forehead strip

Forehead strips are single-use devices used mainly with babies. The strip adheres to the child's forehead and a colour change indicates the surface temperature.

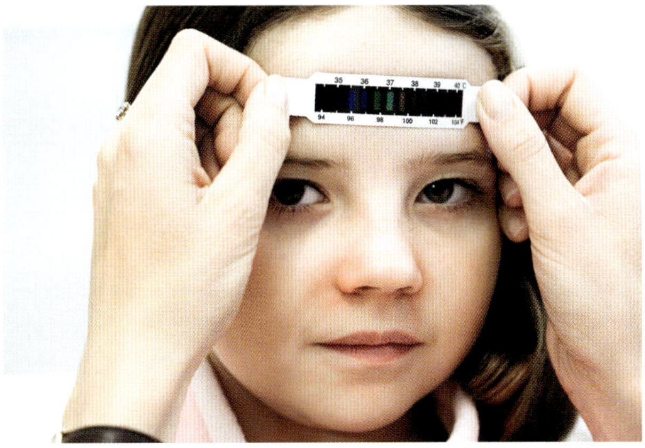

Tip: It is a good idea to make summaries of what you have learned. Start by summarising the material on thermometers by drawing up a suitably-labelled table. Tables make revision much easier.

Human body temperature

Normal human core body temperature is usually between **36.5°C and 37.5°C**. However, this can vary slightly due to age, time of day, physical activity and so on. The measurement may also vary depending on where the reading is taken, i.e. orally, in the rectum, under the arm, in the ear canal or on the forehead. For example, a rectal temperature is typically 0.3°C to 0.6°C higher than that in the mouth.

When core body temperatures stray from the normal range problems occur:

- **Hyperthermia** occurs when the body cannot dissipate enough heat through the normal biological processes, such as sweating and vasodilation. As a result, the core temperature rises. Core temperatures of **41°C** or more are considered life-threatening; temperatures of **44°C** or more are almost invariably fatal.

Tip: Know the difference between vasodilation and vasoconstriction. If the body's core temperature is too high, the blood vessels supplying blood to the skin can swell or dilate – vasodilation. This causes more heat to be carried by the blood to the skin, where it can be lost to the air. If the core temperature is too low, the blood vessels near the skin can shrink – vasoconstriction. This reduces heat loss through the skin and helps the body's core temperature to rise to normal values.

- **Hypothermia** occurs when the body cannot produce enough heat and the core temperature falls. The body responds by shivering, goose bumps, an urge to hug oneself and by vasoconstriction. Core temperatures of **32°C** or less are considered life-threatening; temperatures of **26°C** or less are almost invariably fatal.

Tip: Don't leave revision to the last minute. Revision is a constant process of confirming by reading, writing and solving problems – your exam will test what you need to know, understand and be able to do.

Blood pressure

Blood pressure (often abbreviated to **BP**) is generally measured with a simple, non-invasive device called a **sphygmomanometer**. BP is expressed as two numbers separated by a solidus, for example 120/80, which is read as "one twenty over eighty". The first number gives the **systolic BP** – this is the maximum pressure which occurs in the chambers of the heart over a single heartbeat. The second number is the **diastolic BP** – this is the pressure in the arteries when the heart is relaxed, that is, between the beats.

The sphygmomanometer itself usually consists of a mercury manometer (which measure pressure), plastic tubing, an inflatable cuff and an air pump. Measuring BP with this type of sphygmomanometer also requires the use of a stethoscope to allow the health professional to listen to the blood as it flows in an artery.

The procedure is as follows:

1. The patient sits (or lies) down.
2. The cuff is placed on the upper arm at heart level and the valve is closed.
3. The stethoscope is placed over the brachial artery just below the elbow and the sound of the blood flow is detected.
4. The cuff is inflated rapidly to a pressure around 180 mm Hg using a hand pump. At this pressure blood no longer flows in the brachial artery, that is, no sound is now heard in the stethoscope.
5. The cuff pressure is slowly decreased by opening the valve.
6. When a knocking ('Korotkoff') sound is first heard, the manometer reading is recorded. This is the systolic pressure.
7. The cuff pressure is further reduced at a moderate rate (about 3 mm Hg per second) until the Korotkoff sound is no longer heard.
8. A second reading of the manometer is then taken. This is the diastolic pressure.

This type of BP measurement is extremely accurate and is regarded as the 'gold standard'. However, there is increasing reluctance to use mercury anywhere in medicine because of its toxicity. As a consequence, aneroid devices (which do not contain mercury) are gaining popularity. At the same time, using a stethoscope properly is a clinical skill which requires training and practice. For that reason, sphygmomanometers intended for domestic use employ a different principle which does not require a stethoscope and can be used without extensive training. They are however, slightly less accurate than the method described above.

Tip: Procedures such as the one used to measure BP are often examined in Quality of Written Communication (QWC) questions. Get practice writing continuous prose and checking that your spelling, punctuation, grammar and use of technical terms are all accurate.

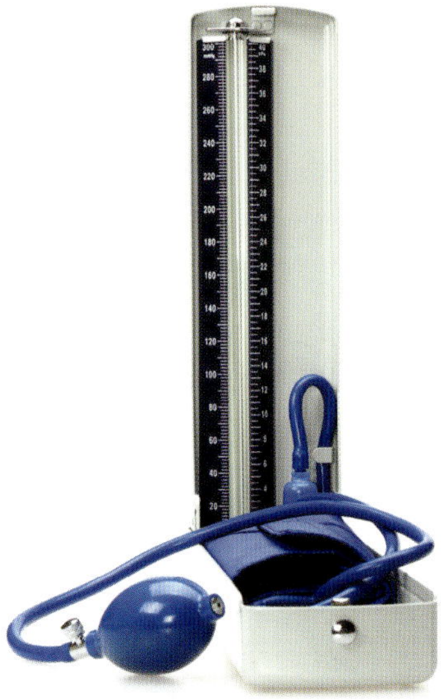

A traditional sphygmomanometer (stethoscope not illustrated)

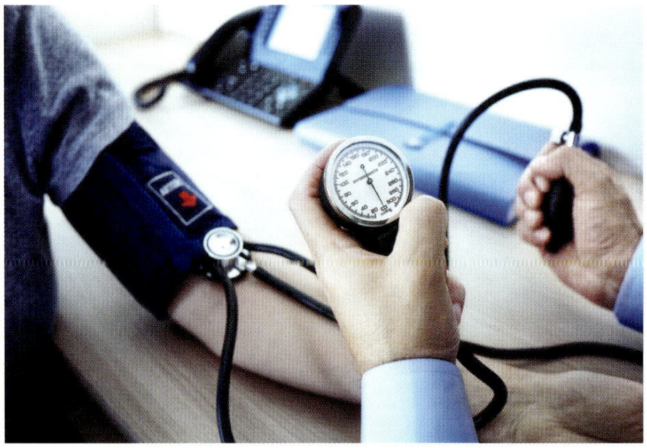

Sphygmomanometer with aneroid meter (stethoscope not illustrated)

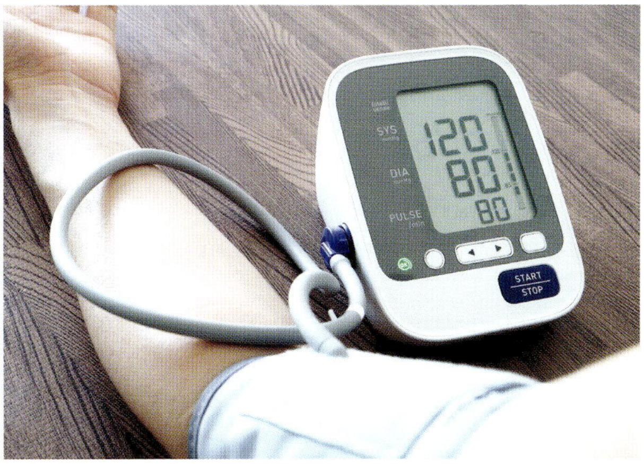

Sphygmomanometer for domestic use (stethoscope not required)

The NHS suggests that:

- **ideal BP** is considered to be between **90/60 mm Hg and 120/80 mm Hg**;
- high BP (**hypertension**) is considered to be **140/90 mm Hg** or higher;
- low BP (**hypotension**) is considered to be **90/60 mm Hg** or lower.

Note that a BP measurement, taken at a single point in time, is just one of many indicators which must be interpreted by a doctor in reaching a clinical diagnosis. Physiological status (age, gender, exercise, medication etc) can give rise to considerable variation in BP values.

Electrocardiograms

An **electrocardiogram (ECG)** is a graph of voltage versus time showing the electrical activity of the heart. It is obtained using electrodes (sensors) placed on the skin. These electrodes detect the small electrical changes that are a consequence of electrochemical changes in the heart as it beats. The output graph is printed on a chart recorder or displayed on a monitor.

ECGs can help detect **arrhythmias** – where the heart beats too slowly (bradycardia), too fast (tachycardia) or in an irregular way. They can also be used to detect coronary heart disease and heart attacks (myocardial infarction). They are non-invasive, can be administered by any appropriately-trained healthcare professional and take only a few minutes.

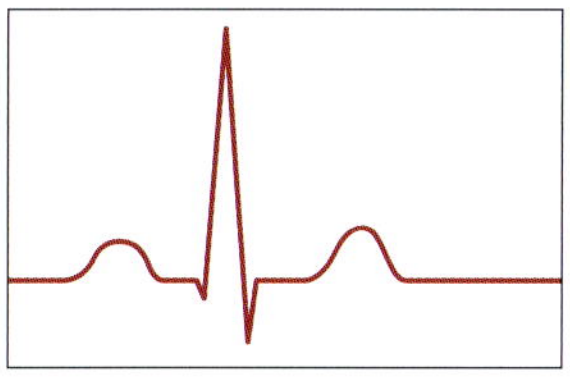

Trace representing a single heartbeat

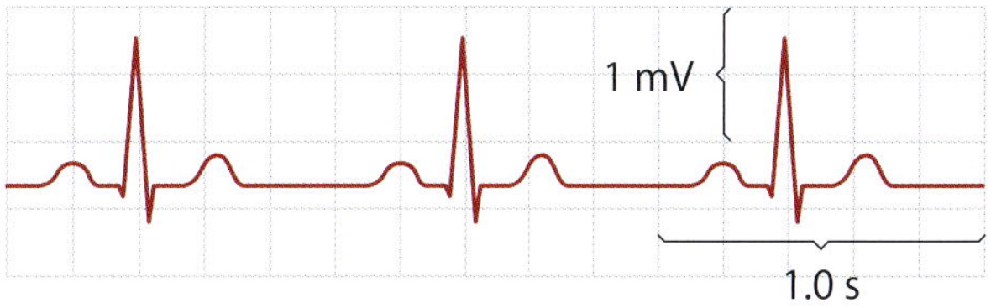

Electrocardiogram (ECG) showing normal behaviour of the human heart

Electrocardiograms have limitations. The trace produced represents the output from the patient's heart at a single point in time. In addition, abnormalities detected are not necessarily due to heart problems. For example, the patient may be on prescribed drugs which can affect the heart's rhythm. It is also possible that the patient suffers from 'white coat syndrome' – a condition in which the patient is psychologically affected by the appearance of a doctor in a white coat and this changes the heart's rhythm.

Practical work

This unit offers rich opportunities for practical investigation. Below are three suggestions for practical investigations – but there are many other possible areas which you might like to study.

Important: For health and safety reasons, all practical investigations should be directed by a teacher and only be carried out under the direct supervision of a teacher or healthcare professional.

1. How does the pulse / BP of students change as a result of physical exercise?
2. How long does it take the pulse / BP of students to return to normal following physical exercise?
3. In what way, if at all, do these physiological changes vary with the body mass, height, BMI or fitness of the students taking the exercise?

Measuring blood pressure, pulse rate and taking an ECG gives a snapshot of different parts of our circulatory system at a point in time. But values outside the normal range are not in themselves conclusive indicators of a heart or circulatory abnormality. For example, all three can be affected if the patient is on prescription drugs or alcohol, is under stress or has undertaken recent physical exercise. The diagnosis of a medical condition is much more complex and should only be done by a doctor.

Tip: Never neglect practical work or think that it is less important than theory. Remember the average student only remembers a small part of what they **read**, but they remember over 90% of what they **do**. Always strive for useful activity in learning.

MRI (Magnetic Resonance Imaging)

What is MRI?

About 60% of the human body is made up of water molecules (H_2O), which consist of hydrogen and oxygen atoms. The nucleus of each hydrogen atom is a **spinning proton**. Protons behave like tiny magnets and are very sensitive to magnetic fields. In the presence of **a very strong magnetic field**, most of the protons in the human body line up in the same direction, in the same way that a magnet can pull the needle of a compass.

If the body is then exposed to a short burst of **radio waves**, a large number of the protons are knocked out of alignment. When the radio waves are turned off, the protons realign. This **realignment causes each proton to emit a characteristic radio wave**. These radio waves are then picked up by **receivers** and provide information about the exact location of the protons in the body. They also help to distinguish between the various types of tissue in the body, because the protons in different types of tissue realign at slightly different speeds, producing slightly different signals.

The signals from the billions of protons in the body are combined, by computer, to create **a very detailed image** of the inside of the body.

Tip: This unit contains a number of important abbreviations – ECG, EEG, MRI and so on. Make sure you know what they all mean. You could make a list of them with their meanings alongside.

Suitability of MRI scans

Almost everyone can have an MRI scan – some exceptions are listed below. MRI scans are non-invasive and the medical consensus is that they pose no risk to human health. However, the magnetic field used is **very, very strong** – around **sixty thousand** times stronger than that of the Earth's magnetic field. This means that MRI scans are not suitable for patients with ferromagnetic implants or ferromagnetic metal fragments inside their bodies. This is due to the enormous force that the scanner's magnet would exert on them. Radiographers take the precautionary approach – accidents have occurred where pieces of equipment, chairs and even medical beds have crashed into MRI scanners due to the force exerted on their ferromagnetic components by the magnets!

Tip: It is important that you use technical words accurately. For example, you should know that ferromagnetic materials contain at least one of the following elements: iron, cobalt and nickel.

An MRI scan will generally not be given to patients if they have:

- **a pacemaker** – a small electrical device used to control an irregular heartbeat;
- **metal plates, wires, screws or rods** – used during surgery for bone fractures;
- **a nerve stimulator** – an electrical implant used to treat long-term nerve pain;
- **a cochlear implant** – a device similar to a hearing aid that is surgically implanted inside the ear;
- **a drug pump implant** – used to treat long-term pain by delivering painkilling medication directly to an area of the body, such as the lower back;
- **brain aneurysm clips** – small metal clips used to seal blood vessels in the brain that would otherwise be at risk of rupturing (bursting);
- **metallic fragments** in or near the eyes or blood vessels (common in people who do welding or metalwork for a living);
- **prosthetic (artificial) metal heart valves**;
- **eye implants** – such as small metal clips used to hold the retina in place;

- **artificial joints** – such as those used for a hip replacement or knee replacement;
- **surgical clips or staples** – used to close wounds after an operation.

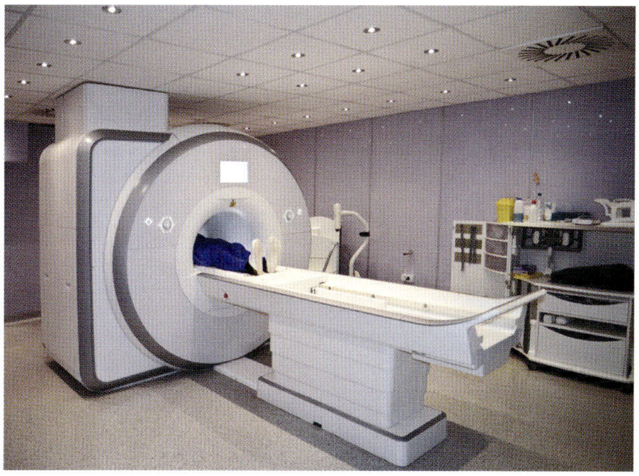

A typical MRI scanner

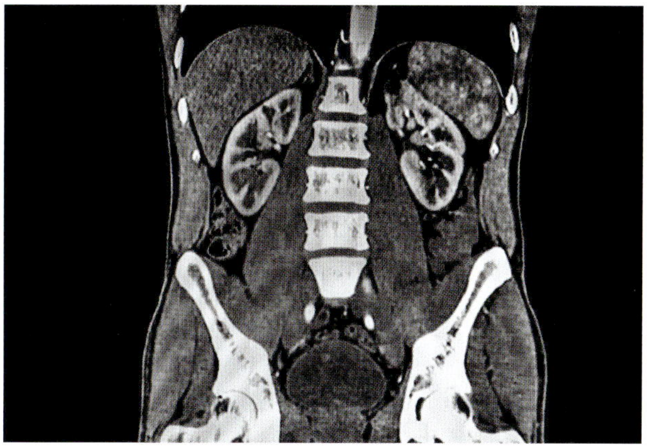

MRI scan of a human abdomen

Procedure

Before entering the scanner room, the patient is asked to remove all items of metal from their person. This includes watches, rings, keys and so on. Generally, the patient lies on a motorised bed that is moved inside the scanner.

The MRI scanner is operated using a computer which is located in a different room to keep it away from the very powerful magnetic field. A radiographer operates the scanner from the adjacent room and can see and hear the patient on a television monitor. The patient is able to talk to the radiographer through an intercom system.

To avoid the images being blurred, it is very important that the patient keeps absolutely still throughout the whole of the scan. For that reason, babies and infants are seldom scanned as they are unable to keep still. In exceptional cases, such patients might be given an anaesthetic to keep them still, but such procedures carry a clinical risk.

Depending on the size of the area being scanned and how many images are taken, the whole procedure will take from a few minutes to one-and-a-half hours. Where the procedure is long, the radiographer would allow the patient to relax and move around between one set of pictures and the next.

Since the scanner may make loud tapping noises from time to time as the current in the scanner coils are turned on and off the patient is often offered earplugs, or headphones through which the patient can listen to music.

Interpretation of the images obtained in an MRI scan is done by a specialist doctor known as a radiologist.

Tip: Many of the medical devices discussed in this book were invented by British scientists, for example Peter Mansfield (MRI) and Godfrey Hounsfield (CT scanner). The portable defibrillator was invented by Professor Frank Pantridge in Northern Ireland. Today AEDs (automatic external defibrillators) can be seen all over the world. If you get the chance, read the fascinating biographies of these people.

Advantages and disadvantages of MRI scans

The main advantages of MRI scans are as follows:

- they require minimal patient preparation;
- they do not use ionising radiation, in contrast to X-rays and CT scans;
- they are non-invasive;
- they can be programmed to produce moving images – so they are useful in cardiac and brain investigations, where study of blood flow is critically important;
- they can be used with all parts of the body.

The main disadvantages of MRI scans are as follows:

- MRI scanners are considerably more expensive to purchase, maintain and operate than other imaging techniques – typically over one hundred thousand pounds for a high-end model;
- some patients experience claustrophobia while lying in the 'tunnel' and cannot remain still;

- greater technological expertise is required to operate an MRI scanner than other scanning techniques;
- patient throughput in an MRI department is slow because scanning can take a considerable length of time.

Functional MRI (fMRI)

Functional MRI allows neurologists to study brain activity by detecting changes associated with blood flow. For a long time it has been known that when the neurons in any part of the brain are excited, the blood flow to that area increases – that is, there is an increase in the flow of oxygen-rich blood to that area of the brain. The oxygen-rich blood gives a different MRI signature to oxygen-poor blood. In this way the active part of the brain can be imaged with an MRI scan. This form of MRI is known as blood oxygenation level dependent (BOLD) imaging or **functional MRI (fMRI)**.

This kind of scanning enables neurologists to discover which parts of the brain are responsible for different physical activities. fMRI has also revolutionised brain imaging and the diagnosis and treatment of strokes, brain tumours and brain haemorrhages.

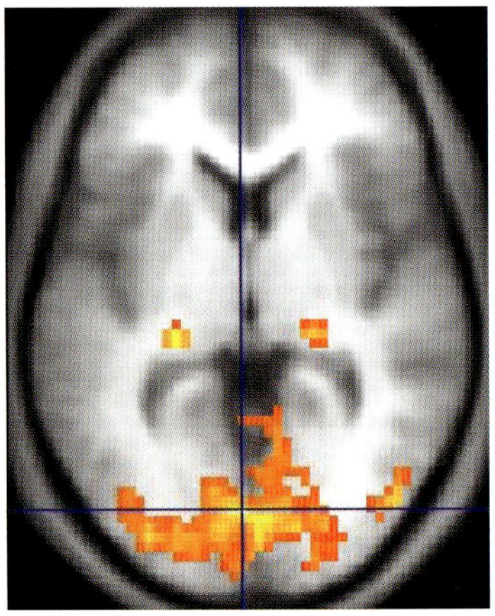

fMRI scan of the brain showing those parts which are neurologically active

Magnetoencephalography (MEG)

Magnetometers are sensors which measure the strength and direction of a magnetic field. In recent years they have been made more accurate and more sensitive, so that today they can detect fields as low as 10 femtotesla, that is 0.000 000 000 000 010 tesla. This is about the strength of the magnetic field produced by the electrical activity in a neuron in the human brain. By comparison, the strength of a typical bar magnet of the type used in schools is about 10 millitesla or 0.010 tesla. So, the field around a bar magnet is about a million million times stronger than that of a neuron.

Nevertheless, the incredibly small field in the human brain can now be measured and doctors and medical physicists can use this technology to obtain a picture of what is happening inside the human brain.

Magnetoencephalography (MEG) is a **functional neuroimaging technique** for mapping brain activity. This is done using very sensitive smart sensors called **SQUID**s (superconducting quantum interference devices) which measure magnetic fields produced by electrical currents occurring naturally in the brain. More than 300 of these SQUID sensors are arranged inside a helmet worn by a patient. The sensors are all connected to a computer.

By analysing the signals recorded by all of these sensors, doctors can identify normally functioning neurons, and can pinpoint malfunctioning neuron systems with great accuracy. MEG is therefore used to identify which parts of the brain are affected in epilepsy, brain injuries, coma, stroke and other conditions where brain function is impaired. This can help them develop more effective treatments for individual patients.

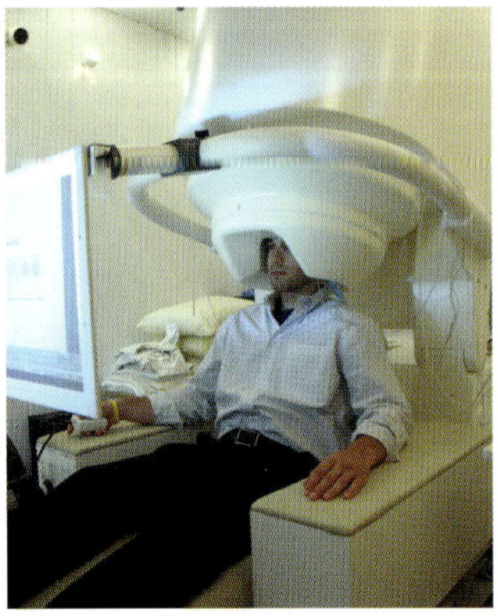

A typical MEG scanner

Electroencephalography (EEG)

Like MEG, **electroencephalography** (EEG) is a technique which is used to measure brain activity. It does this by detecting signals coming from the brain using sensors attached to the scalp. However, in an EEG these signals are electrical, while in a MEG they are magnetic.

An electroencephalogram is a trace, or graph, of voltage against time. This graph enables doctors to diagnose epilepsy, head injuries, brain tumours, sleep disorders and comas.

Unlike ECG traces, brain wave traces do not have a regular pattern with a fixed frequency and amplitude. Some typical traces obtained by EEG are shown in the table below.

Brain Waves	Frequency	Indicator
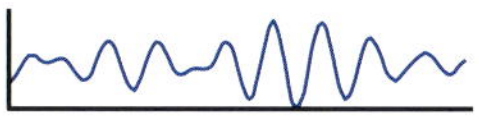	8 – 12 Hz	Alpha (α) waves are dominant when relaxed.
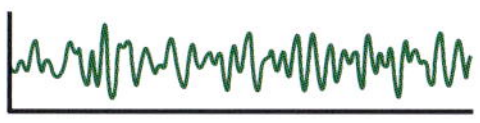	12 – 38 Hz	Beta (β) waves are dominant when alert.
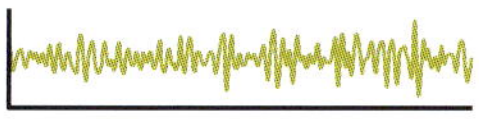	38 – 42 Hz	Gamma (γ) waves are dominant when the brain is in a state of altruism.
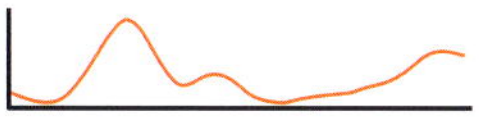	0.5 – 3 Hz	Delta (Δ) waves are characteristic of dreamless sleep.
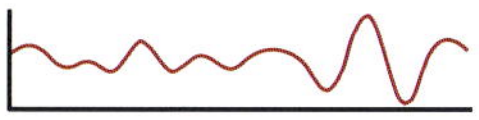	3 – 8 Hz	Theta (θ) waves are characteristic of sleep while dreaming.

Note that magnetic fields are less distorted than electric fields by the skull and scalp. This means that the MEG scan is able to 'see' fine structures inside the brain, that cannot be seen by an EEG. Therefore, MEG results in a better spatial resolution than EEG, which is an important advantage of the technique.

Questions

1. Hypothermia and hyperthermia are serious medical conditions.
   (a) (i) What is hypothermia? [1]
   (ii) What is hyperthermia? [1]
   (iii) What are the temperatures above and below which the human body can no longer stay alive? [2]
   (b) The mercury-in-glass clinical thermometer is now seldom used in medicine in the UK. Explain fully why this is so. [2]
   (c) Suggest a clinical situation in which a healthcare professional might prefer an anal thermometer rather than any other type of thermometer. [1]

2. (a) (i) Identify the apparatus shown below and state its purpose. [2]

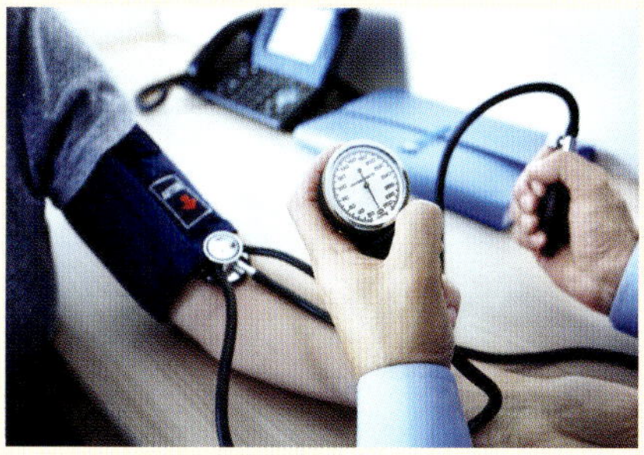

   (ii) What additional piece of medical equipment would be required by a healthcare professional in order to use apparatus shown above? [1]
   (b) A nurse measures the blood pressure of four different male patient at rest and records the data in a table like the one shown below.

	Patient A	Patient B	Patient C	Patient D
Age (years)	15	45	60	80
Systolic BP	115	85	130	145
Diastolic BP	75	55	80	95

   (i) In what units are systolic and diastolic BP measured? [1]
   (ii) What is hypotension? [1]

(iii) Which patient would appear to suffer from this condition? [1]

(iv) Why might the nurse refer Patient D to his doctor? [1]

(c) Describe how you would measure the blood pressure of a patient. **Your quality of written communication will be assessed in this answer.** [6]

3. fMRI is a tool which is being used increasingly in medicine.

(a) What do the letters fMRI stand for? [1]

(b) Not all patients can be given an fMRI.

(i) State three types of patient for whom fMRI would not be suitable. [3]

(ii) What type of electromagnetic wave is involved in fMRI scanning? [1]

(iii) Name three clinical conditions which might be diagnosed / assessed using an fMRI scan. [3]

(c) State a reason why MRI scanners are not more commonly used in medicine. [1]

4. EEG and MEG are used for both diagnosis and therapy in medicine.

(a) What do the letters MEG and EEG stand for? [2]

(b) (i) MEG and EEG are both used to assess the activity in the same organ. Name this organ. [1]

(ii) What is the fundamental difference between MEG and EEG? [2]

(c) The graph below shows the output from an EEG scanner.

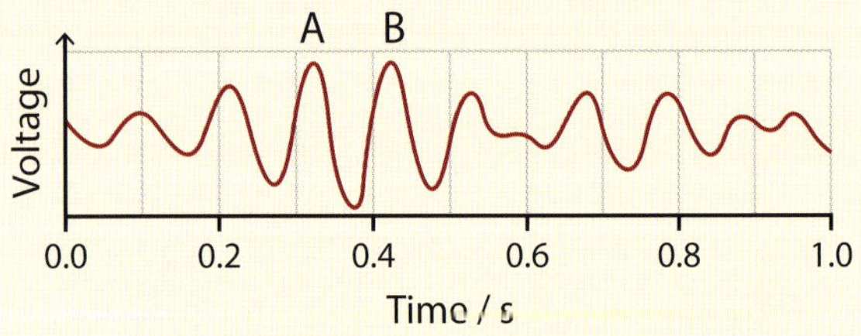

(i) By first finding the time interval between peaks A and B, calculate a typical frequency of these waves. [3]

(ii) Clinically, what type of wave is being illustrated and in what state was the patient when the EEG was taken? [2]

9: DIAGNOSTIC IMAGING TECHNIQUES

Students should be able to:

9.2.1 describe the physical principles and application of, and the equipment used in, the following diagnostic imaging techniques:
- conventional X-rays;
- computerised tomography (CT) scans;
- the flexible endoscope, including the use of lasers and optical fibres;
- ultrasonic A-scans and B-scans;
- conventional gamma ray imaging;
- *Note: magnetic resonance imaging (MRI) was covered in chapter 8.*

9.2.2 recall that the properties of X-rays are ionising radiation of high energy and high frequency and that they are part of the electromagnetic spectrum;

9.2.3 demonstrate an understanding of the functions of the main components in an X-ray tube;

9.2.4 recall that X-rays are absorbed more by tissues of high density than by tissues of low density;

9.2.5 demonstrate an understating of the operation of an optical fibre in the context of endoscopy;

9.2.6 demonstrate an understanding of the terms coherent and incoherent bundles in endoscopes;

9.2.7 recall that a practical endoscope requires several channels, including a channel for target illumination, image collection, irrigation and surgical tools;

9.2.8 define specific acoustic impedance, Z, as the product of the density of the tissue, ρ, and the speed of sound in that tissue, v, using the equation $Z = \rho v$ and use this in numerical calculations;

9.2.9 define the intensity reflection coefficient, R, between tissues of different specific acoustic impedance Z_1 and Z_2 as $R = \left(\frac{Z_2 - Z_1}{Z_2 + Z_1}\right)^2$ and use the equation to calculate R;

9.2.10 recall that, while ultrasound has a frequency greater than 20 kHz, the frequency of the ultrasound used in medical imaging typically lies between 1 MHz and 18 MHz;

9.2.11 recall that deep structures such as liver and kidney are imaged at lower frequencies (1–6 MHz), which give greater penetration than high frequencies but cannot resolve fine structures;

9.2.12 recall that structures nearer the surface such as the breast and thyroid glands are imaged at higher frequencies (7–18 MHz) because they do not have to penetrate deeply into the body, and these can resolve fine structures;

9.2.13 demonstrate an understanding that the intensity reflection coefficient, R, is a measure of the fraction of the incident sound energy which is reflected; and

9.2.14 demonstrate an understanding of the need for a gel between the ultrasound probe and the skin to allow ultrasound waves to be transmitted into and out of the body without large energy loss.

Conventional X-rays

What are X-rays?

X-rays are electromagnetic waves of very high energy, high frequency (around 3×10^{16} Hz to 3×10^{19} Hz) and low wavelength (around 10 nm to 10 pm). X-rays are ionising radiation, that is, they cause atoms in the materials through which they pass to lose one or more electrons and become ions. Because they can readily penetrate human flesh, but are largely absorbed by bone, they have been used for over a century to examine bones and other structures inside the body.

X-ray machines

The diagram below shows a conventional X-ray machine as might be used in the casualty department of a hospital to obtain an image of a broken bone.

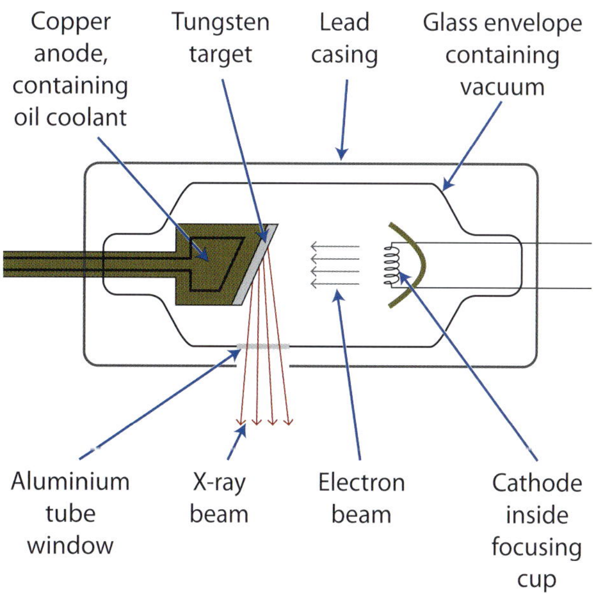

X-rays are produced when high speed electrons strike metal targets with a high atomic number, such as tungsten. In an X-ray machine the electrons are emitted by a cathode which is heated to a very high temperature (until it is white hot) by an electric current passing through the cathode.

These electrons are then accelerated to very high speeds toward a metal anode (the target) by using a very high voltage (typically 100 kV). Upon striking the anode, around 0.5% of the electrons produce X-rays, which form the X-ray beam. The other 99.5% simply heat the anode, which needs to be constantly cooled. In the case of a fixed anode, as shown in the diagram, this cooling is achieved by oil circulating through the anode removing heat by conduction, convection and radiation.

Smaller X-ray tubes, such as those found in a dentist's surgery, use a rotating anode to ensure that the electron beam is not always focused on the same point on the anode, which ensures that the temperature rise is quite small. A lead window not only protects users from stray X-rays, but also removes soft (lower energy, lower frequency) X-rays which are not required.

X-ray photographs

X-rays are absorbed more by materials of high density (like bone) than materials of low density (like flesh). If a human arm is placed between an X-ray source and a detector, more X-rays are absorbed by the bone than the flesh, so a **shadow** is produced on the detector. Hence, in a modern X-ray photograph bones appears white and flesh is dark.

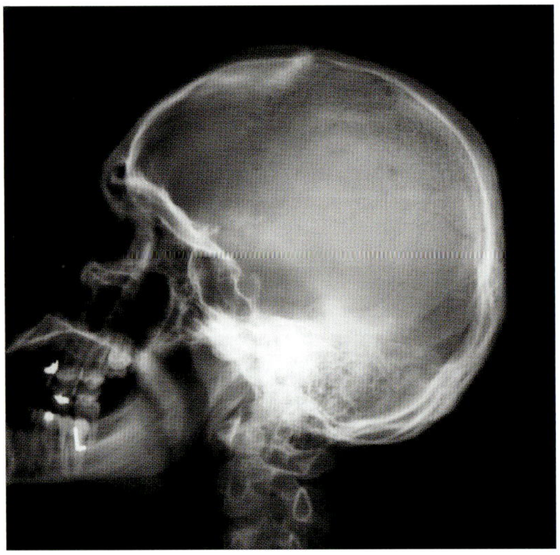

Traditionally, X-ray images were produced on photographic film which had to be developed chemically. This process was expensive and used highly-polluting metals such as silver. Today the detector is an array of charge coupled devices (CCDs). These produce a digital image which can be sent electronically from an X-ray department to the clinician who requested it within minutes.

Precautions with X-rays

Radiographers apply three principles when considering how to maximise their own safety and that of the patient: maintain maximise distance, shield where possible and minimise the X-ray dose. Therefore radiographers:

- maximise their distance from the X-ray source by controlling the equipment from outside the room;
- observe from behind a lead-lined shield/ window and ensure that patients cover those parts of their body not being X-rayed with a lead apron;
- set the exposure in such a way as to minimise the dose experienced by the patient.

The dose experienced by the patient depends on three main factors – the tube voltage (which determines penetration), the tube current (which determines the number or 'quantity' of X-rays), and the exposure time.

Computerised tomography (CT)

A conventional X-ray produces a two-dimensional image. **Computerised tomography (CT)** scanning is a diagnostic imaging procedure that uses X-rays to build cross-sectional images ('slices') of the body.

A CT scanner is shaped like a ring, inside which the patient is placed. Within the ring are X-ray tubes that emit narrow, fan-shaped, monochromatic (single wavelength) beams of X-rays. The X-rays pass through the patient's body towards an array of detectors on the opposite side of the ring. The tubes and the detectors rotate around the stationary patient in the same direction, creating individual pictures that are cross-sections, or slices, of the body.

Tip: The word 'tomography' comes from the Greek word 'tomos' (τόμος) meaning 'slice'.

The images from a CT scan are constructed from the data of X-ray intensity from the sensors – this is now usually done by computer software. At this stage the images are black, white and grey, as with ordinary X-rays, but they can be digitally colour-coded to highlight different tissue densities.

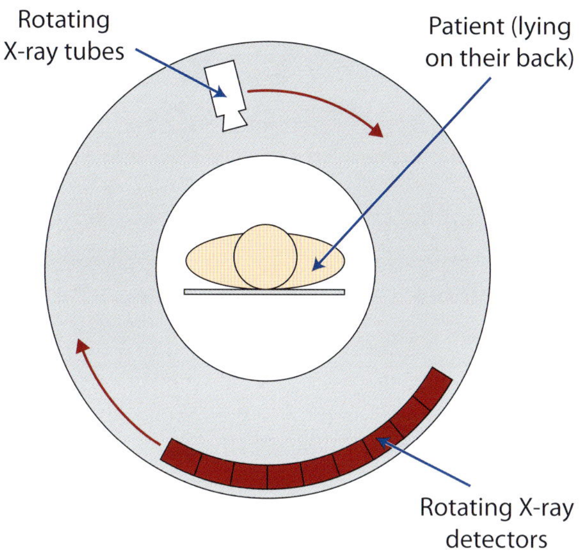

Cross-section of a CT scanner

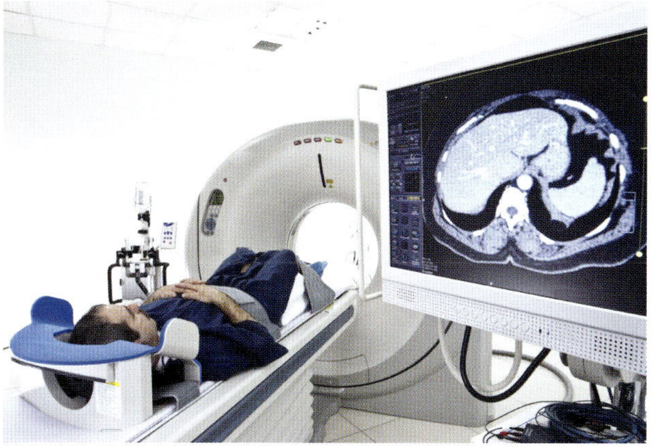

A typical CT scanner

Computer software is then used to join the 'slices' together to generate three-dimensional views of the inside of the body, allowing doctors to see the length, breadth and depth of tissues. Such views are much more detailed than might be produced by conventional X-rays.

The amount of time the patient spends in the CT scanner and the preparations made beforehand vary depending on which part of the body is being scanned. However, use of multiple X-ray tubes within the same scanner means that detailed scans can often be done in a matter of seconds.

Disadvantages of CT scans

Even though the X-ray fan allows several 'slices' to be done at one time – reducing the time of the scan – CT scanning always results in the patient's body being subjected to a dose of radiation that may be a hundred times higher than that for a conventional X-ray. This is because the scan may take hundreds of 'shots' to construct the final image. Doctors always have to weigh up the advantage of carrying out a CT scan (remarkable images which could lead to a better diagnosis) with the disadvantage (potential damage done to the body by harmful radiation).

Conventional gamma ray imaging

What are gamma rays?

Gamma (γ) rays are electromagnetic waves of high energy and high frequency. In fact, their frequency range overlaps with those of X-rays. However, while X-rays are emitted as a result of transitions between electron shells, gamma rays are emitted by **unstable nuclei**. They are another example of an ionising radiation.

The gamma ray camera

A gamma ray camera is a device that can construct an image by detecting gamma rays coming from a source, often a radioactive compound, injected into a patient. The camera is typically used to observe the internal structure of a particular part of the body, such as a muscle or lung.

At the heart of every gamma ray camera is an array of **scintillation counters** and **photomultipliers**, as shown in the diagram on the following page. A scintillant, such as sodium iodide, is a material which gives out a flash of visible light when struck by high energy radiation, in this case a gamma ray coming from the source. This light is directed on to a photocathode which causes it to emit an electron for each photon that hits it.

These electrons are accelerated in a **photomultiplier** tube and made to collide with electrodes called dynodes. The dynodes are made of materials which emit several electrons for every incident electron. In this way a significant current can be produced from a single gamma ray photon striking the scintillator. The electrical signals from multiple photomultiplier tubes are then analysed by a computer to produce an image.

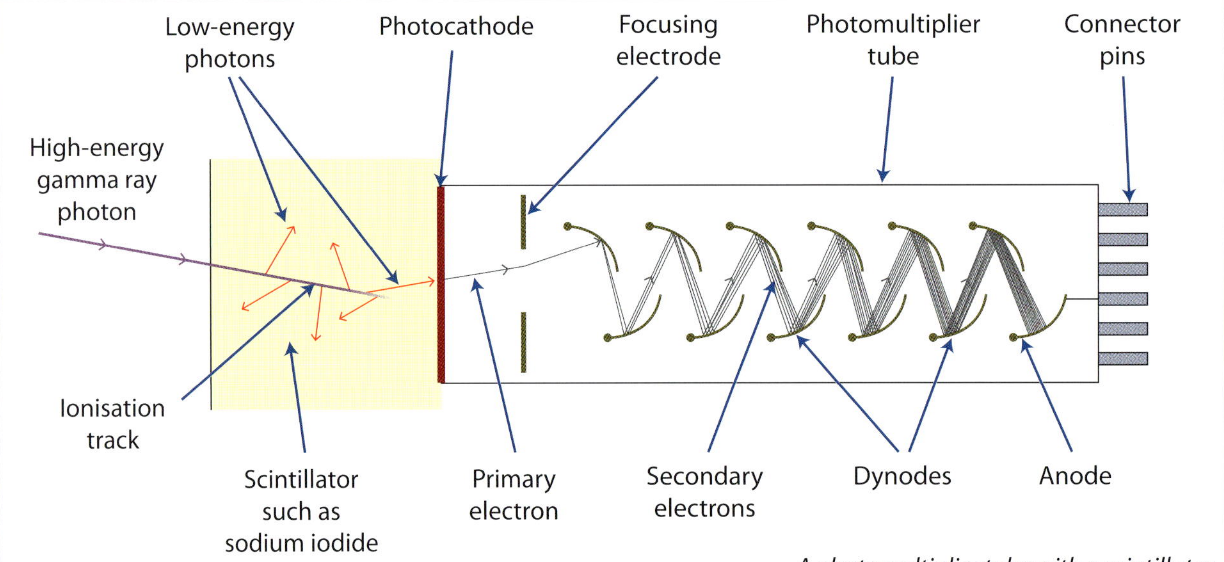

A photomultiplier tube with a scintillator

Procedure

In order to construct the image, the computer needs some way to correlate the detected gamma ray photons with their point of origin in the source. To achieve this, a device called a **collimator** is normally placed between the patient and an array of photomultipliers. The collimator consists of a thick lead sheet– up to 75 mm thick – with thousands of small holes through it.

> **Tip:** The CCEA specification does not require students to know details of the collimator's construction.

The collimator and camera are positioned adjacent to the patient, as shown below.

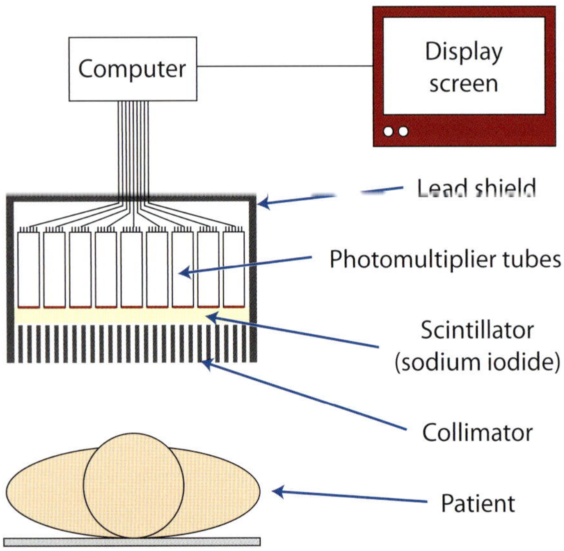

The gamma rays from the patient are detected by the camera, interpreted by a computer and displayed on a screen.

The source of the gamma rays

The source of the gamma rays can be:

- a radioisotope injected into the patient's body;
- an external radioactive material;
- a positron emitting nuclide (used in PET scanning, discussed below).

A gamma ray camera can cope with all three.

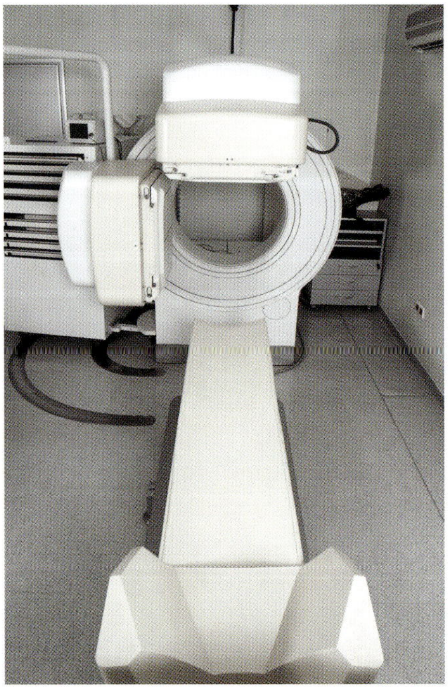

A portable gamma ray camera

Positron emission tomography (PET)

Certain elements emit particles of antimatter called **positrons** (positive electrons). When positrons collide with electrons they annihilate each other. All of the mass of the positron and the electron is converted into gamma ray photons. To conserve momentum, the process must produce exactly two gamma ray photons which travel in opposite directions. Detection of these gamma rays and computer analysis can be used to obtain a 3D image of parts of the human body. The technique is called **positron emission tomography** or **PET** scanning.

The source of the positrons is a radiopharmaceutical which is administered to the patient intravenously. A radiopharmaceutical is a drug which contains a radioactive element. One of the radiopharmaceuticals used in PET scanning today is rubidium chloride in which the normal rubidium has been replaced with the **positron-emitting isotope ^{82}Rb.** This radioisotope is extensively used in cardiac perfusion testing where the clinician is interested in how well the blood flows into and out of the muscles in the heart.

> **Tip:** A radioisotope is a radioactive isotope (form of an element). Isotopes are discussed in more detail in chapter 10.

When undergoing a PET scan, the patient lies very still on a bed which is moved into the scanner. The scanner, shown in the diagram below, is ring-shaped

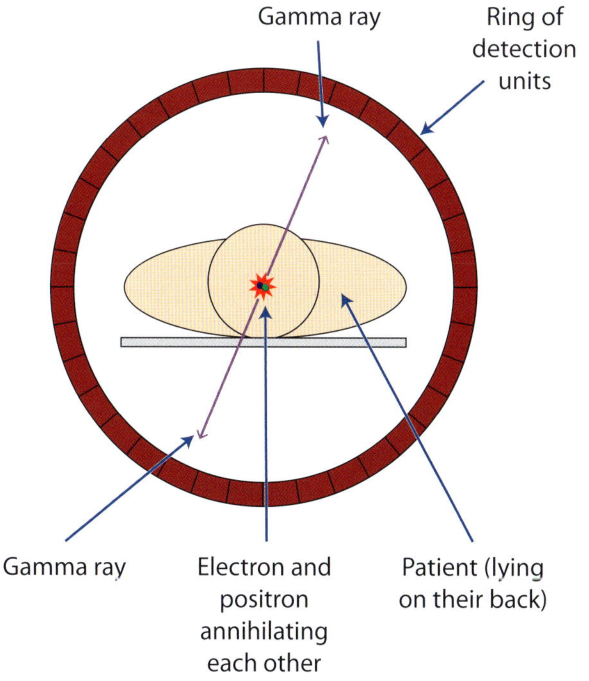

Cross-section of a PET scanner

and looks very like a CT scanner. The gamma rays pass through the patient's body towards an array of detectors on the opposite sides of the ring. The gamma rays from a single event are detected simultaneously. Computer calculations identify the points from which the gamma rays originated and these are used to build an image. The whole procedure lasts about thirty minutes.

Endoscopes and endoscopy

What is an endoscope?

An **endoscope** is a flexible tube that allows a clinician to look into the body. The development of the optical fibre in the 1960s allowed the construction of practical endoscopes that were both flexible and of a small diameter. In some cases, for example when it is to be inserted into the abdomen to study the liver, spleen or other organs, a small incision is required. This is known as keyhole surgery or laparoscopy. In many cases no surgery is required, for example when it is used to view the gastrointestinal tract (oesophagus, stomach and duodenum).

Principle of the endoscope

The endoscope uses the principle of **total internal reflection**. When light travels from glass into air it is

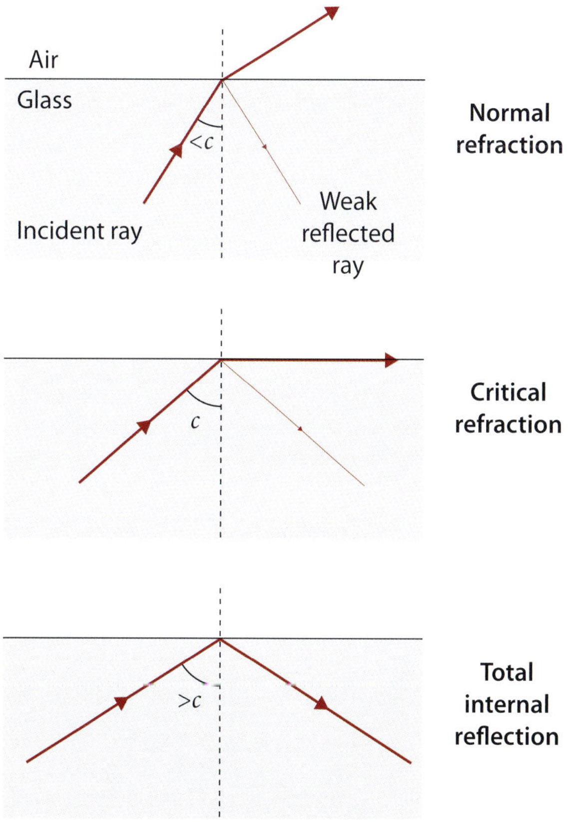

refracted away from the normal. However, if the angle of incidence in the glass exceeds the critical angle *c*, then total internal reflection takes place.

By using total internal reflection repeatedly, it is possible to make light travel along the length of a glass rod, as shown below. If the glass rod is flexible – as in an optical fibre – and the angles through which it is bent are not too great, the light will pass out of the end of the fibre.

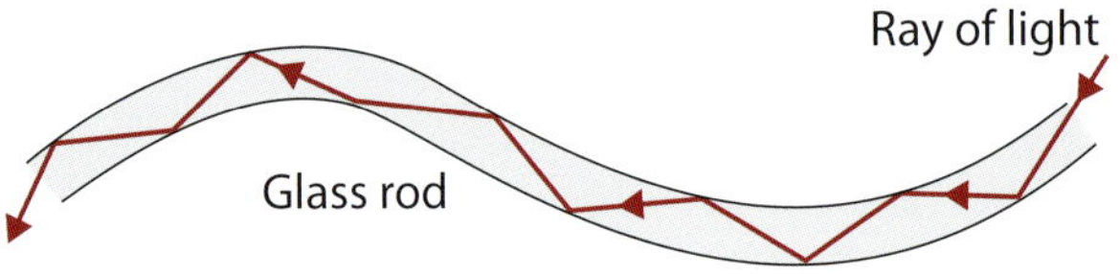

The endoscope has two bundles of optical fibres:

- the **illumination bundle**, which carries light to the object being viewed;
- the **image bundle,** which carries back the reflected light to produce an image. The optical fibres inside the image bundle are carefully arranged **parallel to each other** to create what is termed a **coherent bundle**.

Using an endoscope

The image is viewed or photographed through a magnifying eyepiece, as shown below. Often a TV camera is attached and the image displayed on a monitor and recorded on a hard disk drive. The information obtained by an endoscope examination provides direct, and often very clear, evidence of conditions such as bleeding ulcers, constrictions, benign and malignant tumours and cirrhosis of the liver.

Most endoscopes have **at least four channels** (tubes which pass along the length of the endoscope), two of which carry the optical fibres:

- the **illumination channel**, which carries the inexpensive illumination bundle of optical fibres to the target;
- the **image channel**, which carries the coherent image bundle of optical fibres from the target;
- the **irrigation channel** through which water is carried to wash the distal end of the optical fibres;
- the **surgical tools channel** which can carry a range of equipment such as:
  - forceps, controlled from the viewing end, to allow a surgeon to remove a sample of
  - tissue (a biopsy) for detailed analysis;
  - electrodes that can be used to apply heat to stop bleeding;
  - different types of extractor that can be used to remove foreign objects from the gastro-intestinal tract, for example drugs hidden in the lower bowel of smugglers.

Tip: Distal means most **distant** from the eyepiece.

In more recent years, keyhole surgery has involved **the use of lasers with endoscopes**. Lasers are suitable for such surgery because:

- very high intensity light can be passed down an endoscope and used to cut or destroy tissue;

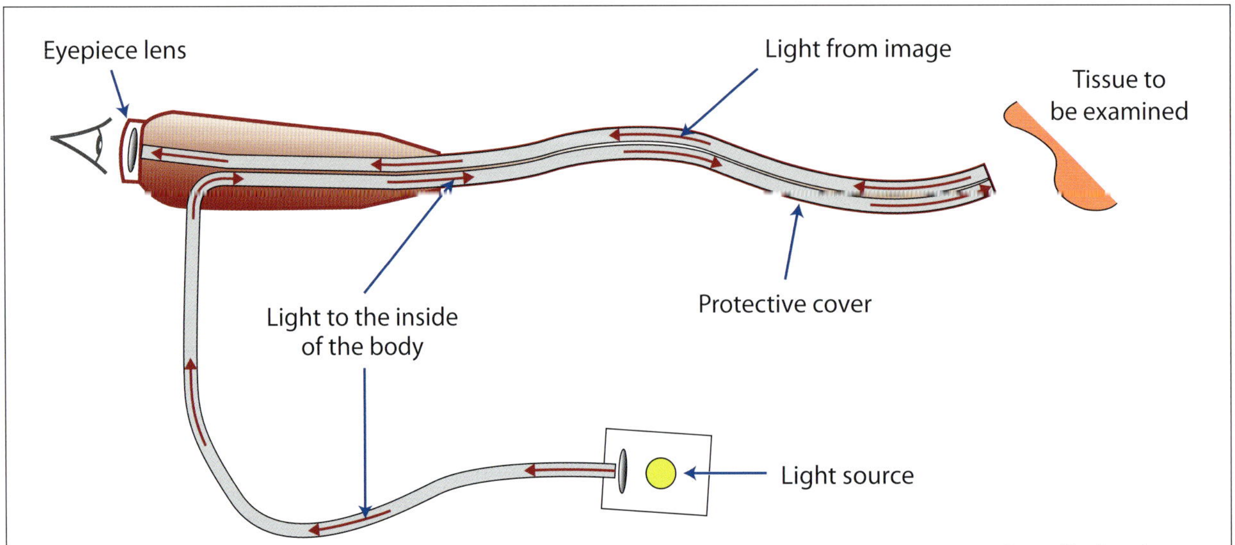

A medical endoscope

- lasers produce heat that causes the tissue around the cut to seal and prevents bleeding;
- the beam is narrow and can therefore make very precise cuts;
- different frequencies of laser beam can be used, depending on the area being targeted.

Ultrasonic imaging

What is ultrasound?

The range of human hearing is approximately **20 Hz to 20 kHz**. Sound waves with a frequency greater than 20 kHz are called **ultrasound**. Ultrasound waves are longitudinal pressure waves. Typical diagnostic ultrasound frequencies used in medicine are in the range **1 MHz to 18 MHz**.

Low intensity ultrasonic waves pass through tissue without causing harm, unlike X-rays which cause ionisation and can damage cells. Ultrasonic waves are reflected, however, at the boundaries between biological structures. These reflections allow images of internal organs to be created by an ultrasound scanner.

Unlike X-rays and gamma rays, ultrasound is not an ionising radiation. Therefore it is very safe to use and presents no safety issues when imaging, for example, unborn babies in the womb.

Ultrasound scans

All ultrasound scans involve a medical professional moving a transceiver over the surface of the patient's skin, as shown in the picture below.

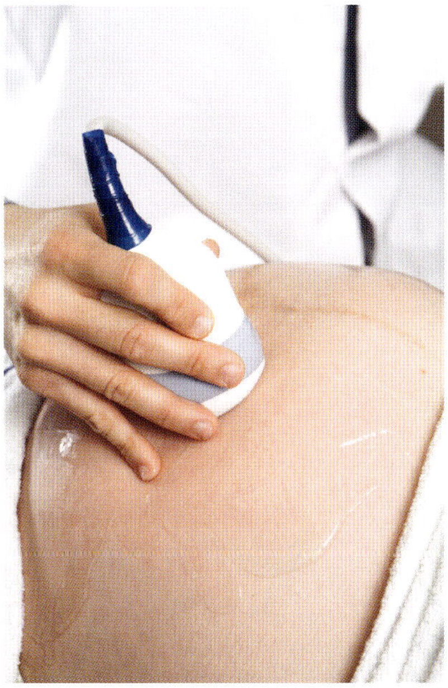

This device produces the ultrasound which passes into the patient's body. Some of this ultrasound is reflected from the structures within the body and out again to the transceiver. These pulses of reflected ultrasound are detected and are used to generate an image.

One complication is that ultrasound waves are strongly reflected at the air-skin boundary (we say the **air-skin boundary has a high intensity reflection coefficient**). To overcome this problem, a water based cellulose **jelly is smeared on the skin**. This jelly acts as a coupling agent to ensure that most of the ultrasound enters the body.

The problem with air reflection is not limited to the air outside the body. Considerable amounts of air are found in the **lungs** and other gases are found in abundance in the **bowel**. This means that **ultrasonic imaging cannot be used with such organs**.

There are two main types of ultrasound scan – the A-scan, and the B-scan.

The A-scan

The 'A' in **A-scan** means **amplitude**. When used in this way, a pulse of ultrasound is sent into the body and its reflection is displayed as a graph on a screen. The horizontal axis on the display represents time and the vertical axis represents the amplitude of the reflected wave.

In the diagram below, an ultrasound scanner is being used to scan a foetus. The ultrasound waves are reflected from various structures within the womb. The display shows a typical A-scan of a foetal head. A measure of the diameter of the baby's head is an indicator of the age and the development of the

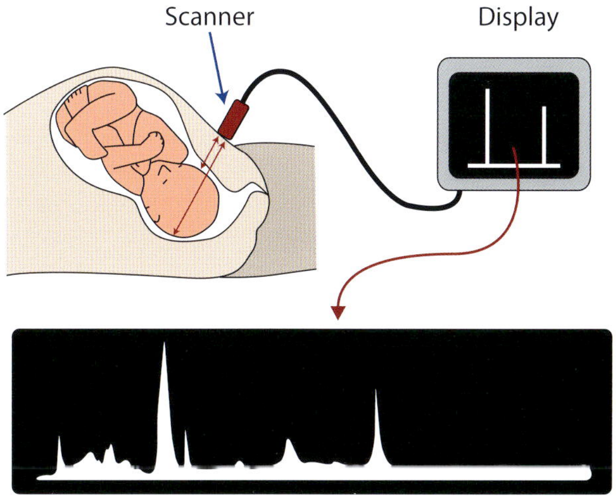

Typical display for an A-scan

foetus. The measure is based on the time interval between the peaks. The worked example that follows shows how such a scan can be used to measure the diameter of the foetal head.

Worked example

The diagram shows a simplified version of an actual ultrasound display. The vertical lines represent the echoes from two structures within the body. A scan is made of the head of a foetus, as shown. Estimate the diameter of the head. The speed of ultrasound in the body is around 1500 m s^{-1}.

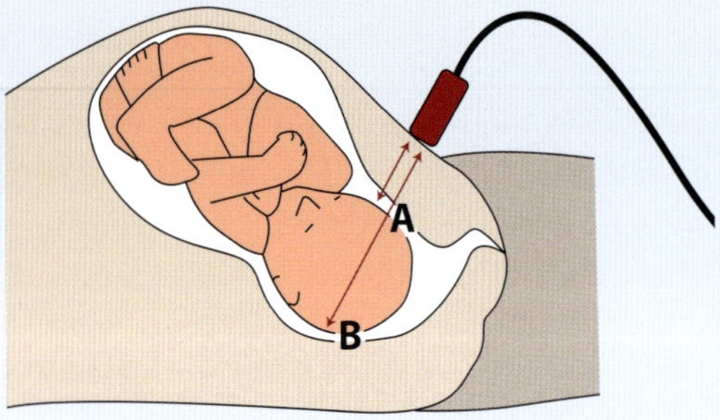

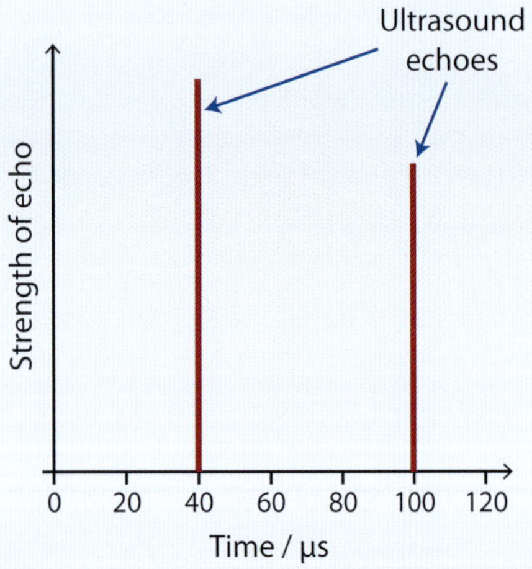

Answer

From the graph, the time between the pulses is the time taken for ultrasound to travel from A through the baby's head to B and then back to A again. Time = 100 – 40 = 60 μs = 6×10^{-5} s.

This trace indicates that the separation of the two structures is:

$\frac{1}{2} \times 1500 \times 6\times10^{-5} = 0.045$ m (45 mm)

> **Tip:** When carrying out echo calculations look out for the factor of 2. Remember that distance = ½ × speed of wave × total time of wave in the organ.

> **Tip:** Any exam with Physics in its name is sure to have mathematics problems. Unit A2 3 is no exception. The best way to prepare for these questions is to practise, practise, practise.

The B-scan

The 'B' in **B-scan** means **brightness**. A B-scan produces an image that is easier for a human to interpret. The ultrasound probe is scanned across the body in a series of lines. The strength and position of the reflected ultrasound are stored electronically. The data stored are then used to produce an image on a TV screen. The strength of the signal is employed to determine the brightness of the spots on the screen. The picture below shows a B-scan of a foetus.

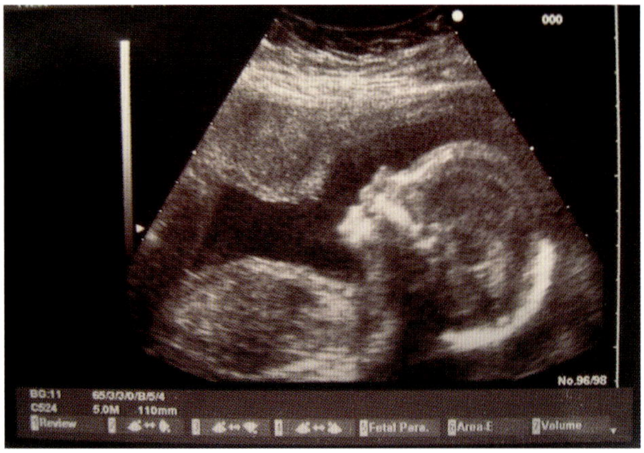

B-scans are commonly used by obstetricians and gynecologists to monitor foetal development. They can also be used to identify tumours in the liver and other organs, and enable cardiologists to see the functioning of the valves of the heart in real time.

Specific acoustic impedance, *Z* and intensity reflection coefficient, *R*

As we have seen, a coupling gel is required between the transceiver and the skin when using ultrasound for medical imaging. This is due to the tissue's **specific acoustic impedance**, a measure of how much resistance an ultrasound beam encounters as it passes through.

Specific acoustic impedance, Z, is defined as the product of the density of the tissue, ρ, and the speed of ultrasound in the tissue, v, by the equation:

$$Z = \rho \times v$$

Since the unit for density is kg m^{-3} and the unit for speed is m s^{-1}, the unit for Z is:

kg m^{-3} × m s^{-1} = kg m^{-2} s^{-1}

Tip: You need to remember the equation for Z. It is good if you can also remember the unit in which Z is measured, but it is better still if you can work it out yourself.

Now consider a pulse of ultrasound passing from one material into another. If the specific acoustic impedance in both materials is the same, then none of the sound is reflected – it is all transmitted from one material into the other. However, the larger the difference between the Z-values for each material, the more reflection occurs at the boundary between them. This allows us to define the **intensity reflection coefficient**, R, between tissues of different specific acoustic impedance Z_1 and Z_2 by the equation:

$$R = \left(\frac{Z_2 - Z_1}{Z_2 + Z_1}\right)^2$$

Note that R is dimensionless; that is, it has no unit. R represents the fraction of the incident intensity at the boundary that is **reflected**. Often R is expressed as a percentage. Thus, the percentage of the incident intensity that is **transmitted** is given by:

100% – R (%)

Tip: Questions on specific acoustic impedance will demand knowledge of standard index form and the use of a calculator. If you are not sure of the mathematics, ask your teacher.

Worked example

An ultrasound beam travels at a speed of 1.5 km s^{-1} through soft tissue.

(a) If the specific acoustic impedance of soft tissue is 1.65×10^6 kg m^{-2} s^{-1}, calculate the density of the soft tissue.

(b) A parallel beam of ultrasound passes normally through a layer of muscle and fat as shown in the diagram below.

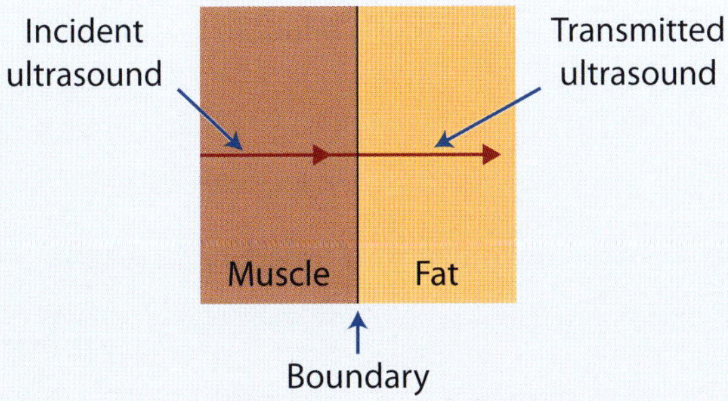

The table shows the specific acoustic impedance for muscle and fat.

	Specific acoustic impedance, Z / kg m^{-2} s^{-1}
muscle	1.7×10^6
fat	1.3×10^6

Calculate the percentage of the intensity of the ultrasound that is **transmitted across the boundary** from the muscle into the fat.

Answer

(a) $\rho = \frac{Z}{v} = \frac{1.65\times10^6}{1.5\times10^3} = 1100 \text{ kg m}^{-3}$

(b) $R = \left(\frac{Z_2 - Z_1}{Z_2 + Z_1}\right)^2$

$= \frac{(1.3 - 1.7)^2}{(1.3 + 1.7)^2}$

$= 0.0178 = 1.78\%$

This means 1.78% of the incident intensity is reflected, so:
100% – 1.78% = 98.22% of the incident intensity is transmitted.

Tip: Always show your full working in calculations. By doing so you may pick up marks for a correct method even if your final answer is incorrect.

Ultrasound frequency in scanning

As we have noted, the frequency of ultrasound waves used in medicine lies between 1 MHz and 18 MHz. As ultrasound passes through the body it spreads out and is scattered and absorbed by the molecules it strikes.

Lower frequency, higher wavelength ultrasound is more penetrating than high frequency, low wavelength ultrasound. On the other hand, high frequency ultrasound has a much greater resolution (that is, the structures which can be imaged are much smaller) than low frequency ultrasound. In practice, therefore, there has to be a compromise between resolution and penetration when choosing a frequency for a particular application:

Ultrasound frequency	Penetration	Resolution
High	Low	High
Low	High	Low

In most cases, the optimum frequency is one for which the organ is at a depth of 200 wavelengths. Suppose, for example, a surgeon wanted to image part of the ear 2.0 cm below the surface. Then the optimum wavelength is 2.0×10^{-2} m ÷ 200 = 1×10^{-4} m. In such tissue ultrasound travels at 1500 m s^{-1}, therefore the optimum frequency, *f*, is 1500 ÷ 1×10^{-4} = 15 MHz.

Tip: You have about two years to learn your way around a scientific calculator. Get to know it well. Do not buy a calculator with which you are not familiar a few weeks before your exam!

Deep structures, such as the liver and kidney, are therefore imaged at lower frequencies (1–6 MHz) which give greater penetration but are unable to resolve fine structures. On the other hand, structures nearer the surface such as the breast and thyroid glands are imaged at higher frequencies (7–18 MHz) because they do not have to penetrate deeply into the body, and these frequencies can resolve fine structures.

Ultrasound 'listening time'

The diagram below shows two pulses of ultrasound such as might be emitted by an ultrasonic transceiver in a hospital. The four waves on the left side and the four waves on the right side of the diagram are ultrasonic. For waves with a frequency of 10 MHz, the pulse duration would be 0.4 microseconds. It is critically important that the pulse is short enough to ensure that the leading edge of the pulse returns well after the trailing edge departs.

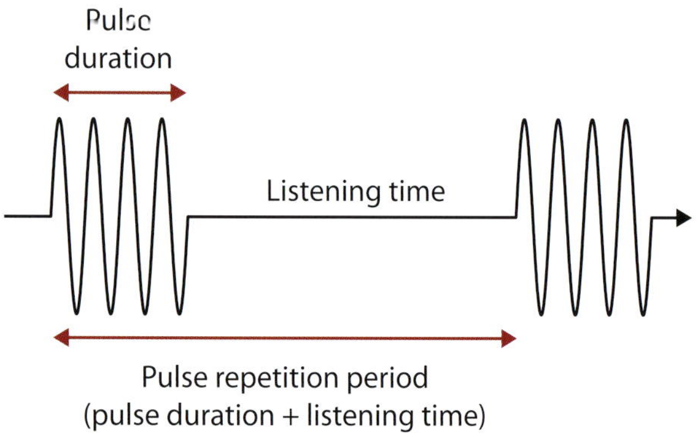

By contrast, the time between the pulses typically lasts between 100 microseconds and 1000 microseconds. This is called the 'dead time' or '**listening time**' and is set by the radiographer. **It is during this time that the echoes from the target are received**. The listening time is necessary because the echoes from the target organ must not interfere with the waves being emitted by the transceiver. Clearly, the deeper the target organ the longer the listening time has to be.

Tip: Some things you have just got to remember – but don't rely on memory alone. The students who do best learn principles and techniques rather than rely on memory.

Questions

1. The diagram shows an X-ray tube, of the type found in a modern hospital.

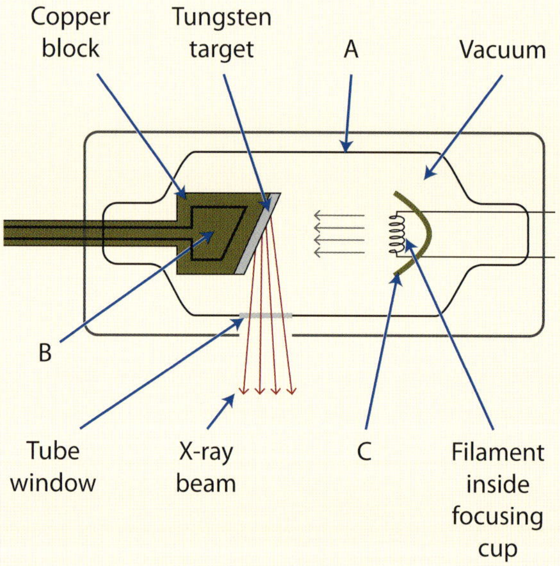

(a) (i) Identify the particles which move between the hot filament and the tungsten target. [1]

These particles are accelerated to very high speeds.

(ii) What brings about their acceleration? [1]

(iii) What happens to the kinetic energy of these particles when they hit the target? [1]

(iv) Why is the tungsten target embedded in a large copper block? [2]

(v) Why is oil made to circulate within the copper block? [1]
(vi) Why is it essential for there to be a vacuum in the X-ray tube? [1]
(vii) Identify the structures labelled A, B and C in the diagram. [3]
(viii) What prevents most of the X-rays from leaving the tube? [1]
(ix) The tube window is made of aluminium. Suggest why this is so. [1]

(b) X-rays are an important tool used by doctors in the diagnosis of disease.
(i) What are X-rays? [1]
The diagram shows an X-ray image of a human foot and ankle.

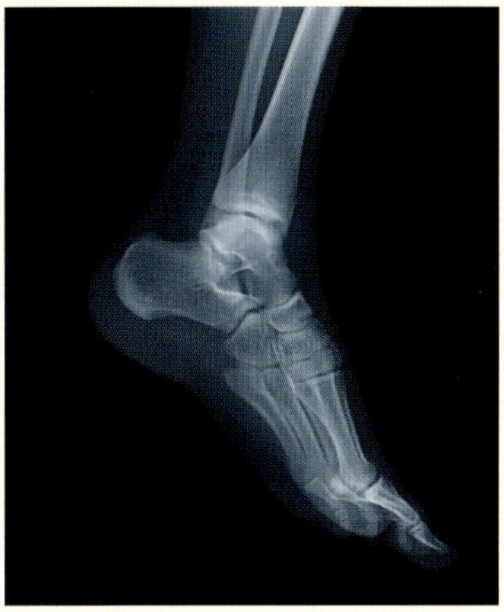

(ii) Explain why the bones appear to be almost white, but the surrounding tissue is quite dark. [3]
X-rays are described as ionising radiation.
(iii) What is meant by ionising radiation? [2]
(iv) What is the main danger associated with the use of ionising radiation? [1]

2. As part of the process of medical diagnosis a patient may have a CT scan.
(a) What do the letters CT stand for in the phrase 'a CT scan'? [1]
(b) In what ways are the procedure used and dose to the patient in a CT scan different from that used to produce a conventional X-ray image? [4]
(c) State one similarity and one difference between the images produced in conventional X-ray images and in CT scans. [3]

A 25-year-old woman is undergoing tests to identify the cause of pain in her lower abdomen. A CT scan is considered as part of the diagnosis process, but after a conversation with the patient, this course of action is abandoned.
(a) Suggest
(i) a possible reason why the CT scan may not be suitable for this patient;
(ii) an alternative diagnostic procedure which might now be considered. [2]

3. Ultrasound is finding increasing use in medicine.
(a) (i) What is ultrasound? [1]
(ii) What is the frequency range of ultrasound used in medicine? [1]
(iii) State the difference between an ultrasound A-scan and a B-scan. [2]
(b) (i) Explain why the pulses of ultrasound used in medical imaging must be of short duration. [2]
(ii) State two processes which reduce the strength of the reflected signal received by the probe. [2]
(c) An ultrasonic investigation is made on an organ in a patient's abdomen. The diagram below shows the path of the ultrasound into and out of the patient's body.

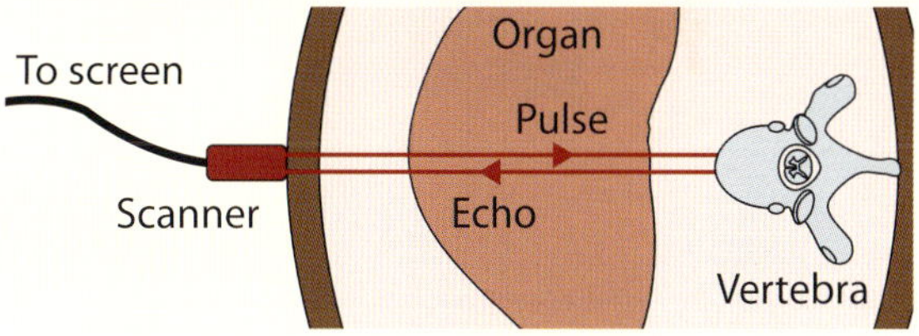

The graph below shows the display on an oscilloscope screen of the ultrasound signal. The speed of sound in the organ is 1200 m s^{-1}.

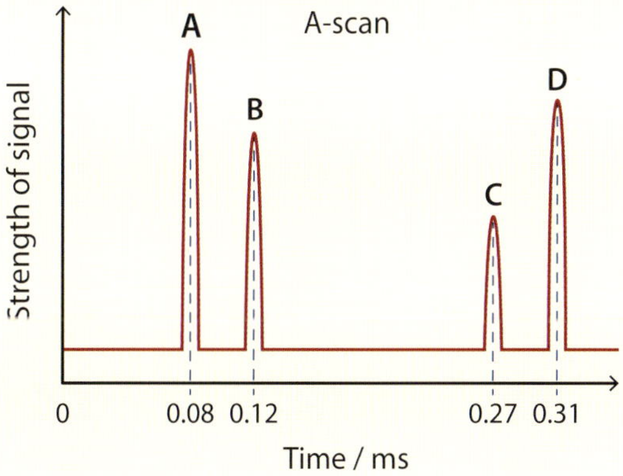

(i) Use your knowledge of ultrasound to interpret the peaks labelled A, B, C and D. [4]
(ii) Suggest why pulse D has a higher amplitude than pulse C. [1]
(iii) Calculate the width of the organ. [4]

4. A patient is to have a PET scan. A small amount of radioisotope is injected into the patient's bloodstream. The patient then lies on a horizontal table and is moved into the scanner. The scanner has many detectors positioned in a vertical circle around the patient.
(a) (i) State what is meant by a radioisotope. [1]
(ii) What do the letters PET stand for? [1]
(b) The diagram shows the head of the patient, 18 cm across, placed centrally between two of the detectors in a PET scanner.

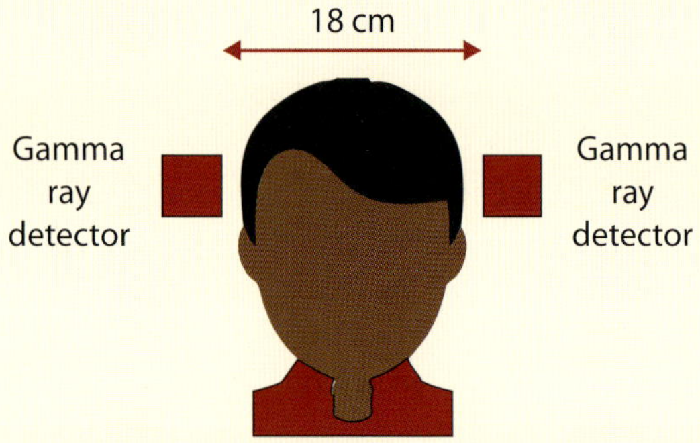

To find where the gamma photons are produced between the detectors, the scanner measures the time interval between the triggering of the first detector and the triggering of the second detector. Take the speed of gamma rays in the head to be 3×10^8 m s^{-1} and ignore the distance between the outside edge of the patient's head and the detector. Calculate the **maximum** value of this time interval. [4]

5. When ultrasound travels across a boundary from blood to the wall of a blood vessel there is a decrease in acoustic impedance across the boundary. This results in 0.0625% of the intensity of the incident ultrasound being reflected at the boundary. Calculate the acoustic impedance of the tissue comprising of the wall of the blood vessel, given that the acoustic impedance of blood $= 1.64\times10^6$ kg m^{-2} s^{-1}.

10: MEDICAL USES OF RADIATION

Students should be able to:

9.3.1 investigate the use and detection of the types of radiation used in medicine for diagnosis and therapy;

9.3.2 demonstrate an understanding of properties of alpha (α), beta (β) and gamma (γ) radiation;

9.3.3 identify the dangers of each type of radiation;

9.3.4 investigate experimentally, or develop a mathematical model of, the process of radioactive decay;

9.3.5 recall that the activity, *A*, of a radioactive material is measured in Becquerel (Bq) and that 1 Bq represents one disintegration in a second;

9.3.6 define the physical half-life of a radioactive material as the time taken for the activity of that material to decrease to half of its original activity;

9.3.7 recall that the physical half-life of a radionuclide, $T_{½}$, is related to the decay constant, λ, by the equation $T_{½} = 0.693 / \lambda$ and use this in numerical calculations;

9.3.8 observe and describe an experiment to determine the half-life of protactinium;

9.3.9 define biological half-life of a radioisotope as the time it takes for half of that radioisotope to be removed from the body by natural metabolic processes;

9.3.10 categorise the uses of radiation in medical diagnosis and treatment;

9.3.11 critically evaluate the precautions taken by medical physicists when using radiation;

9.3.12 compare the use of different radiopharmaceuticals and evaluate their specific properties which enable their use in diagnostic nuclear medicine, including:

- technetium-99 – a gamma emitting radioactive tracer used in medical imaging;
- rubidium-82 – a pharmaceutical rapidly taken up by the heart muscle and used in positron emission tomography (PET) perfusion imaging;
- thallium-201 in the form of thallium chloride for cardiac imaging and the detection of cancers;
- iridium-192 – implant used after initial cancer treatment to deliver an additional dose of radiation; and
- iodine-131 – absorbed by the thyroid and used in the destruction of cells in the thyroid that are overactive;

9.3.13 demonstrate an understanding of how the medical use of radiation contributes to the background count;

9.3.14 demonstrate an understanding of how background radiation is taken into account in experimental investigation; and

9.3.15 recall and use the equations for radioactive decay

$A = A_o e^{-\lambda t}$ and $\ln A = \ln A_o - \lambda t$

and use these equations to calculate *A* (activity at time *t*), A_o (original activity), λ (decay constant) and *t* (elapsed time).

Radioactivity

Radioactive decay occurs when an unstable nucleus loses energy by emitting **ionising radiation**. Radioactive decay is a spontaneous, random process and it is impossible to predict when a particular nucleus will decay.

Three different types of ionising radiation are emitted from the nuclei of radioactive materials – **alpha** (α), **beta** (β) and **gamma** (γ) radiation. Their properties are listed in the table on the next page.

Dangers of alpha, beta and gamma radiation

Alpha particles have negligible penetration in any human tissue, though an ingested source will cause catastrophic damage to cells because of the density of the internal ionisation. Beta particles have a wide range of penetrations and because of their unpredictable paths their depth of penetration in tissue cannot be defined accurately. Gamma rays do not have a definite penetration in tissue. However, their intensity falls off in a predictable way (exponentially) like X-rays.

The degree of danger from radiation depends on whether or not the source is outside or inside the body.

Inside the body

If the radioactive source is inside the body, **alpha radiation is the most dangerous** because it has much greater ionising power than the others and causes more cells to mutate (and potentially cause cancer). Because alpha radiation is very short range the damage is not widespread, but it can be catastrophic where it does occur. Beta and gamma radiation are

	alpha (α)	beta (β)	gamma (γ)
Nature	helium nucleus (particle)	fast electron β^- (or positron β^+) (particle)	high frequency electromagnetic wave / photon
Relative charge*	+2	–1 (or +1)	none
Relative mass*	4	1/2000	none
Ionisation mechanism	collision with orbiting electrons	ejection of electrons	at low energy mainly by photoelectric emission †
Number of ion-pairs produced per mm of air	1000	10	1
Radiation absorbed by:	0.1 mm aluminium, or thin paper, or a few cm of air	a few mm of aluminium	a few cm of lead

* compared to the proton

† different mechanisms occur at high energy

Types of ionising radiation

not as dangerous because they have a smaller ionising power, they are much more penetrating and are just as likely to pass right through a given cell as they are to cause it to mutate.

Outside the body

If the radioactive source is outside the body, alpha radiation is not as dangerous, because it is has such a short range that it is unlikely to reach living cells inside the body. However, **beta and gamma radiation are the most dangerous sources** because they can penetrate the skin, disrupt DNA and cause cells to become cancerous.

Background radiation

Radiation is all around us – it can still be detected even when all known radiation sources have been removed. There are many sources for this **background radiation**, including radon in the air, radioactive rocks in the ground (particularly uranium ores and granite), cosmic rays from space, discharges from nuclear power stations, nuclear weapons tests etc. Background radiation can interfere with experiments so, before any experiment is carried out, it is essential to obtain a measure of the background radiation. This background count is then subtracted from any readings of radiation coming from a specific source. In this way, we can ensure that we are recording the count due solely to the specific source.

GM counter

Radiation can be measured with a GM counter. The photograph opposte shows a portable, battery-operated counter with its GM tube. Each time an alpha or beta particle enters the GM tube the number displayed on the screen, called the count, increases by 1. Together the two pieces of apparatus are called a Geiger counter, or GM counter. GM is short for Geiger-Müller, in honour of the two scientists, Hans Geiger and Walther Müller, who first invented it.

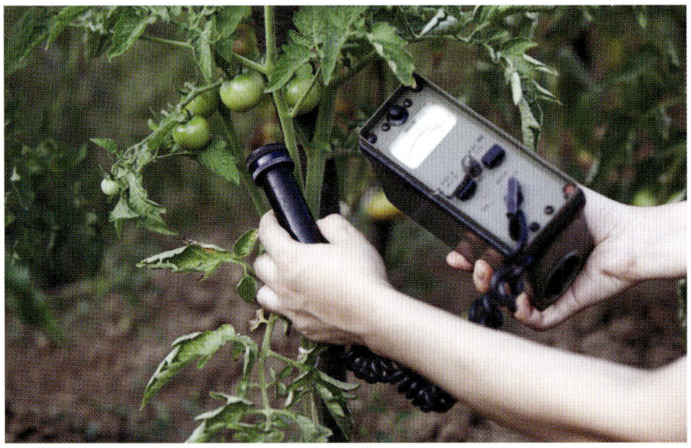

The method for measuring background radiation is as follows:

- First remove known sources of radiation from the laboratory, then set the GM counter to zero.
- Switch on the counter and start a stopwatch.
- After 30 minutes read the count on the counter.
- Divide the count by 30 to obtain the background count rate in counts per minute. A typical figure in Northern Ireland is around 15 counts per minute.

Tip: This is a good experiment that everyone can do in a lab because it does not require radioactive material.

Law of radioactive decay

The rate at which a source of radiation decays, A, is directly proportional to the number of radioactive nuclei in the source, N. This is known as the **law of radioactive decay** and can be written as the equation:

$A = -\lambda N$ where λ = the decay constant for the source, measured in s^{-1}

The rate A is measured in disintegrations per second, commonly denoted by the unit Becquerel, Bq. The minus sign is necessary because the quantities A and N both decrease as time passes.

Tip: You must remember this formula and be able to use it in numerical calculations.

Tip: Never use solidus notation when expressing units. For example, the unit for activity is always written as Bq or counts s^{-1}, **never** as counts/second.

Physical half-life, $T_{½}$

The **physical half-life** of a radioactive sample is the time taken for the activity of that radioactive sample to decrease to half of its original value. We refer to **physical** half-life to distinguish it from biological half-life which will be discussed later. Most textbooks ignore biological half-life, but in medical physics it is essential to make the distinction.

Using differential calculus, the law of radioactive decay and the definition of physical half-life, it can be shown that:

$$T_{½} = \frac{0.693}{\lambda}$$

$A = A_0 e^{-\lambda t}$ where A_0 = the activity at time $t = 0$

Tip: You must remember these formulae and be able to use them in numerical calculations.

Worked example

(a) A small volume of a solution containing a radioactive isotope has an activity of 1.2×10^4 disintegrations per minute. This solution is injected into the bloodstream of a patient. After 24 hours a 1 cm^3 sample of the blood is found to have an activity of 0.65 disintegrations per minute. Estimate the volume of blood in the patient. The half-life of the isotope is 15 hours.

(b) Another radioisotope of the same activity and emitting the same type of radiation of the same energy but having a much longer half-life is available. Discuss briefly the reason why the radioisotope with a half-life of 15 hours is preferred.

Answer

(a) Total initial activity = 1.2×10^4 disintegrations per minute

Since $T_{½}$ = 15 hours, then the decay constant

$$\lambda = \frac{0.693}{T_{½}} = \frac{0.693}{15} = 0.0462 \text{ hour}^{-1}$$

Total activity after 24 hours

$= A_0 e^{-\lambda t}$

$= 1.2 \times 10^4 \times e^{(-0.0462 \times 24)}$

= 3959 disintegrations per minute

Activity in 1 cm^3 of blood

= 0.65 disintegrations per minute

So total volume of blood is:

$3965 \div 0.65 = 6091$ cm^3 (just over 6 litres)

(b) A very long half-life means that the radioactivity is likely to remain in the patient for a long time causing radiation damage to the internal organs. However, the radioisotope half-life must be long enough for the radioactive agent to emit sufficient radiation be measured accurately shortly after full dilution in the blood, a process which may take around 24 hours.

Worked example

A certain isotope used in medical physics has a half-life of 3.0 minutes. When taken from a locked cupboard it has an activity of 794 Bq. When prepared for injecting into a patient's vein the isotope has an activity of 500 Bq. Calculate the time which elapsed between removing the isotope from the cupboard and its preparation for injecting into the patient.

Answer

Decay constant

$$\lambda = \frac{0.693}{T_{½}}$$

$$= \frac{0.693}{3}$$

$$= 0.231 \text{ minutes}^{-1}$$

To find t when activity is 500 Bq:

$$\ln A = \ln A_0 - \lambda t$$

$$\ln 500 = \ln 794 - 0.231t$$

$$t = (\ln 794 - \ln 500) \div 0.231$$

$$t = (6.677 - 6.215) \div 0.231$$

$$t = 2 \text{ minutes}$$

Tip: You need to be familiar with the use of logs, natural logs and their inverse functions. Practise using them on your calculator and remember that the complete list of mathematical skills needed for LHS can be found in Appendix 1 of the specification – which can be downloaded from the CCEA website.

Experiment to verify the law of radioactive decay and find the half-life of radioactive protactinium

Tip: This is a prescribed experiment that means you must either observe it being done in your school or on an online platform like *YouTube*. Observe and remember.

This experiment uses protactinium-234 as a radioactive source. By measuring its radioactivity over a period of time, the law of radioactive decay and be verified. The experiment also allows the half-life of protactinium to be determined.

Setting up the protactinium source

Protactinium-234 is one of the decay products of uranium-238 and any compound of uranium-238 will have within it traces of protactinium. These traces may be conveniently extracted from it by chemical means.

To set up the source, a thin-walled polythene bottle is filled with equal volumes of an acid solution of uranyl nitrate and pentyl ethanoate. When the liquids are shaken up together, most of the protactinium is dissolved in the organic pentyl ethanoate. As the solutions are not miscible, the protactinium remains in the upper layer once the liquids have separated.

The protactinium decays by β^- emission into another long-lived isotope of uranium (uranium-234) which is itself α–emitting. The very long half-life indicates low radioactivity, and in any case, it is not enough to interfere with this experiment. Moreover, the α–particles which are emitted will not penetrate the polythene bottle containing the protactinium.

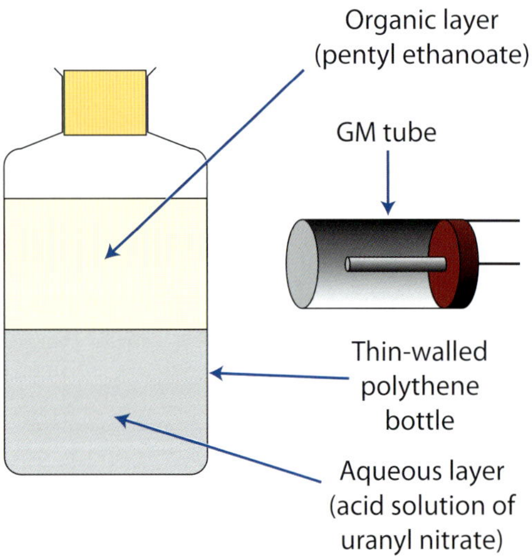

Procedure

The experiment is carried out as follows:

- The practical arrangement is as shown in the diagram above.
- The Geiger-Muller (GM) tube is attached to a ratemeter, clamped about a centimetre from the bottle opposite the upper organic layer and switched on.
- The count-rate of the β–activity of the protactinium is observed on the ratemeter, and is recorded at 10 second intervals.

- Allowance is then made for the background count – if, say, the measured rate with the GM tube and ratemeter is 32 counts minute^{-1} and the background rate is 15 counts minute^{-1}, then the corrected count rate is 32 – 15 = 17 counts minute^{-1}.

Treatment of the results to find the half-life of protactinium

The corrected count rate of the protactinium is taken as a measure of its activity, A.

By the law of radioactive decay:

$A = A_0 e^{-\lambda t}$

Taking natural logs of both sides gives:

$\ln A = \ln A_0 - \lambda t$

Comparing this equation with that for a straight line, $y = mx + c$, we see that a graph of ln A (y-axis) against time, t (x-axis) will be a straight line of gradient $-\lambda$ and y-axis intercept $\ln A_0$.

Therefore we can plot a graph of ln A (y-axis) against time, t (x-axis) and draw the straight line of best fit. We then determine its gradient, which is $-\lambda$, and hence find λ. An example of such a graph is shown below.

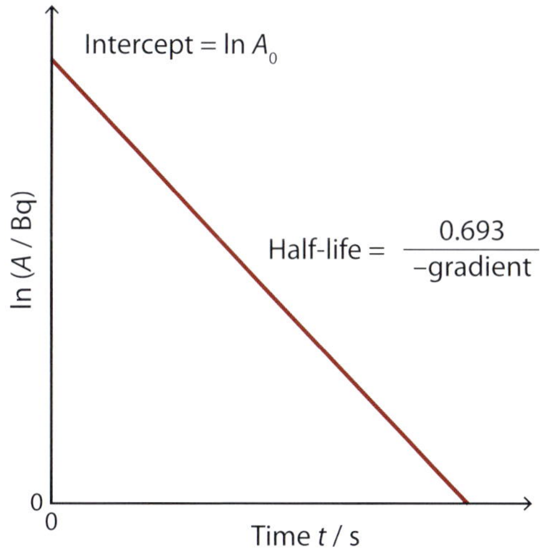

We can then find the half-life by calculating the value of 0.693 ÷ λ. The generally accepted value for the half-life of protactinium-234 is 68 seconds.

Obtaining this straight line is also (indirect) proof of the law of radioactive decay.

Tip: Note that A has units of Bq, but ln A has no units – that is why the brackets in ln (A / Bq) are essential – ln A / Bq is wrong because it suggests ln A has units of Bq.

Demonstrating the exponential form of the law of radioactive decay

It is also possible to demonstrate the exponential form of the law of radioactive decay ($A = A_0 e^{-\lambda t}$) by plotting the graph of activity, A against time, t. An example of such a graph is shown below.

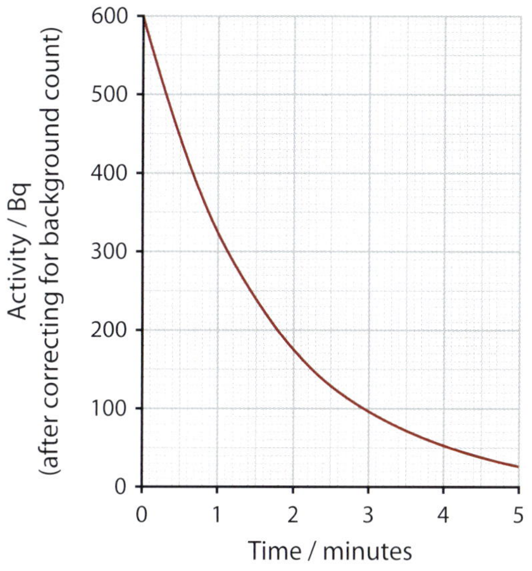

From this curve the student can see that the activity halves every minute, that is, the half-life is 68 seconds.

In the equation $A = A_0 e^{-\lambda t}$, the units for λ and t must be complementary. For example, if λ is in s^{-1}, then t must be in seconds; if λ is in hours^{-1}, t must be in hours. Similarly, A and A_0 must be in the same units as each other, although not necessarily linked to the units for λ and t. For example, A and A_0 could both have units of disintegrations per minute, while λ and t have units of seconds^{-1} and seconds.

Biological half-life

When a radioactive substance is injected into the human body, various biological processes will remove it. This includes respiration, urination and defecation. The **biological half-life** of a radioisotope, T_B, is defined as the time it takes for half of that radioisotope to be removed from the body by natural metabolic processes.

This means that the **effective half-life**, T_E, of a radioisotope in the body is less than the physical half-life, $T_{½}$, from radioactive decay alone.

The effective half-life is then given by:

$$\frac{1}{T_E} = \frac{1}{T_B} + \frac{1}{T_{½}}$$

where T_E = effective half-life
T_B = biological half-life
$T_{½}$ = physical half-life

Worked example

Suppose a radiopharmaceutical is injected into the bloodstream of a patient as part of a blood test. The radiopharmaceutical has a physical half-life of 13 hours and a biological half-life of 21 hours. Calculate its effective half-life.

Answer

$$\frac{1}{T_E} = \frac{1}{T_B} + \frac{1}{T_{½}}$$

$$\frac{1}{T_E} = \frac{1}{21} + \frac{1}{13} = 0.1245$$

$$T_E = \frac{1}{0.1245} = 8 \text{ hours}$$

Tip: There are two common mistakes when using the equation for effective half-life. The first is forgetting to ensure that the physical and biological half-lives are measured in the same unit. The second is omitting the final step. Don't forget to use the reciprocal button (x^{-1}) on your calculator at the end!

Nuclear medicine

Radiopharmaceuticals

Radiopharmaceuticals are radioactive substances which are administered to patients in the course of their diagnosis or treatment. CCEA Life and Health Science students are required to know about the application of **five** particular radiopharmaceuticals in a diagnostic or therapy setting. These are listed in the table at the bottom of the page.

When considering which radiopharmaceutical to use, the radiologist must consider several factors. The preparation must:

- be **chemically available**, with **high purity** and in a suitable pharmaceutical form;
- have **suitable biological behaviour**, distributing itself in the organ or metabolic pathway in an efficient way;
- contain a radionuclide with suitable **radiation characteristics** as regards radiation emitted and half-life.

Technetium-99 ($^{99}Tc^m$) is the metastable product of the β^- decay of the radioactive element molybdenum-99. The 'm' in the symbol means 'metastable'. Metastable technetium-99 is also radioactive, decaying by the emission of gamma rays, and having a half-life of 6 hours. Technetium-99 is a tracer. This means it is used to produce an image of an organ. In this case the image is predominantly in bone and brain scans. For bone scans, it is used directly to diagnose the nature of skeletal injury. In brain scanning, it is useful for the detection of strokes and dementia. It is also used to identify the predominant lymph nodes draining a cancer, such as breast cancer or melanoma.

Rubidium-82 is injected into a patient's vein in the form of rubidium chloride. The Rubidium-82, a β^+ emitter, is rapidly taken up by the heart muscle where the positrons combine with electrons to produce gamma wave pairs which are then detected using a Positron Emission Tomography (PET) scan. It can be

Radiopharmaceutical	Radiation	Application
technetium-99	gamma	radioactive tracer used in medical imaging
rubidium-82	positrons, which give rise to gamma radiation	a pharmaceutical rapidly taken up by the heart muscle and used in positron emission tomography (PET) perfusion imaging
thallium-201	gamma (by electron capture)	in the form of thallium chloride for cardiac imaging and the detection of cancers
iridium-192	beta and gamma	implant used after initial cancer treatment to deliver an additional dose of radiation by brachytherapy
iodine-131	mainly beta	absorbed by the thyroid gland and used in the destruction of cells in the thyroid that are overactive

employed in myocardiac perfusion testing, that is, testing the blood flow to the muscles of the heart as part of an ischemic study. The half-life of the rubidium-82 is only 1.27 minutes, so it is very rapidly lost from the body.

Thallium-201, an emitter of gamma rays, has a half-life of just over 3 days. It is mainly used with a conventional gamma ray camera in imaging the heart and the coronary arteries. Very little of the drug is taken up by the brain or spinal cord, but it is absorbed by brain and spinal cord tumours – this makes it very effective for detecting and imaging brain and spinal cord cancers.

Iridium-192 has a half-life of 106 days and decays by β^- and gamma emissions. Its long half-life makes it particularly suitable for brachytherapy – a treatment in which 'seeds' (ribbons or capsules that contain the iridium-192) are placed inside the body in or near the tumour. It is used primarily to treat cancers of the head, neck, breast, cervix, prostate and eye. Brachytherapy allows doctors to deliver higher doses of radiation to specific areas of the body, compared with the conventional form of radiation therapy (external beam radiation) which projects radiation from a machine outside the patient's body. Brachytherapy often causes fewer side effects and the overall treatment time is usually shorter than is the case with external beam radiation.

Tip: The word 'brachytherapy' comes from the Greek word 'brachys' (βραχύς) meaning 'short distance'.

Iodine-131 has a half-life of 8 days, decays by β^- (and gamma) emissions and is usually administered orally. Iodine accumulates in the thyroid gland and therapy with this isotope is often used to kill cancerous cells there (or destroy cells in an overactive gland). More recently, however, iodine-123 has been used instead of iodine-131 – mainly because its lower half-life of 13 hours leads to a much lower dose of radiation being given to the patient.

Medical use of radiation and the background count

The pie chart opposite shows the sources of the UK background radiation count. Note especially that about 14% of it comes from the use of ionising radiations in medicine, most of which comes from X-rays and the use of radioisotopes in nuclear medicine. For most people the average annual dose due to background radiation is about 2.6 millisieverts per year.

Tip: A millisievert is a measure of radiation dose. CCEA Life and Health Sciences students need not be concerned about the detail of what a millisievert is.

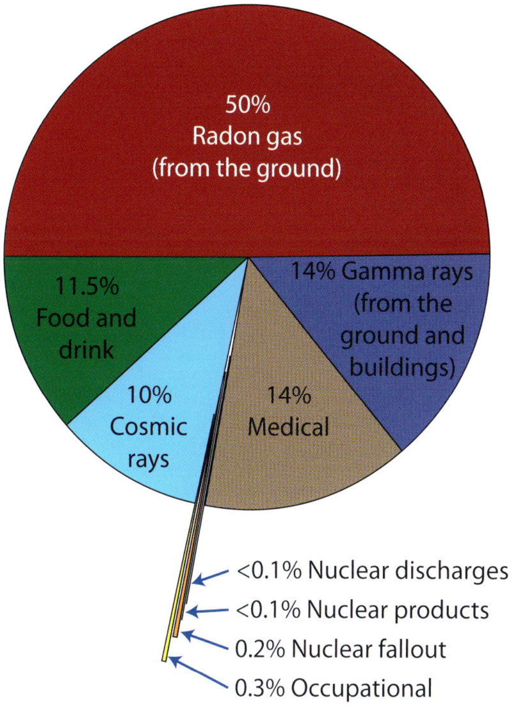

When we have a procedure involving ionising radiation, we receive an additional dose over and above the background count. The tables on the next page detail the additional dose for different types of procedure. There are two important points to note:

- Conventional X-rays (such as might be given in a fracture clinic to detect broken bones or in a dentist's surgery to detect a tooth abscess) make little appreciable change to the total radiation dose received over a year.
- Procedures which involve multiple imaging (to create a 3D picture or a dynamic, moving image) give a significant increase in the total amount of radiation received by the patient. These include CT scans and gamma ray scans.

Diagnostic procedure	Typical effective doses (millisieverts)	Equivalent period of natural background radiation	Lifetime additional risk of fatal cancer per exam
X-ray – teeth	< 0.01	< 1.5 days	1 in a few million
X-ray – chest	0.02	3 days	1 in a million
X-ray – pelvis	0.7	4 months	1 in 30 000
X-ray – abdomen	0.7	4 months	1 in 30 000
CT – head	2	1 year	1 in 10 000
CT – chest	8	3.6 years	1 in 2500
CT – abdomen/pelvis	10	4.5 years	1 in 2000

Radiation doses from X-ray and CT procedures

Diagnostic procedure	Typical effective doses (millisieverts)	Equivalent period of natural background radiation	Lifetime additional risk of fatal cancer per exam
Thyroid scan (Technectium-99m)	1	6 months	1 in 20 000
Bone scan (Technectium-99m)	4	2 years	1 in 5000
Dynamic cardiac (Technectium-99m)	6	2.7 years	1 in 3300
Myocardial perfusion (Thallium-201)	18	8 years	1 in 1100

Radiation doses from nuclear medicine procedures

Data amended from https://www.gov.uk/government/publications/medical-radiation-patient-doses/patient-dose-information-guidance

For this reason, radiologists and other healthcare professionals take the decision to give a patient a CT scan or involve them in a procedure involving nuclear medicine very seriously, and only consider doing so when the risks of doing so are less than the potential benefits.

Tip: If you want to know where students do well in LHS exams (and where they don't!) read the Chief Examiner's Reports. You can find them on the CCEA website.

Precautions taken by medical physicists when using radiation

There is little concern about alpha radiation because it has a very short range and is so easily absorbed. Beta radiation is also readily absorbed, although it has a significant range in air. **The major concerns are X-rays and gamma rays.**

Three principles guide the precautions taken by all healthcare professionals when using **X-rays and gamma rays**:

- **Minimise time** of exposure to the radiation. As the time spent in a radiation area increases, so does the radiation dose received. Therefore, it is best to minimise the time spent in any radiation area. If a healthcare professional's assigned duties involve working in and around radiation areas, then the activity should be organised and planned in advance to limit the time spent in the radiation area.
- **Maximise distance** from the source. As the distance from a radiation source increases, the radiation exposure decreases rapidly. Doubling the distance between a person and the radiation source reduces the radiation exposure to one quarter of the original exposure. It is good practice to keep as much distance between the healthcare professional and the radiation source as is reasonably possible. Operating theatre or A&E nurses are not always able to leave a patient unattended during a procedure using ionising radiation, but they can move away from the source as much as possible.

- **Maximise shielding** between the source and personnel. A material which absorbs the radiation is called a **shield**. The thicker the shielding, the less radiation reaches the person. Lead and concrete are the most commonly used materials for shielding X-rays and gamma rays as they are very effective in stopping or blocking the radiation beam. The walls of X-ray rooms are lead-lined to reduce the radiation exposure to those on the other side of the wall. Lead aprons are commonly used to shield body parts from X-rays and gamma rays, as shown in the picture below, which shows a patient receiving an ankle X-ray, with the rest of their body shielded by a lead apron.

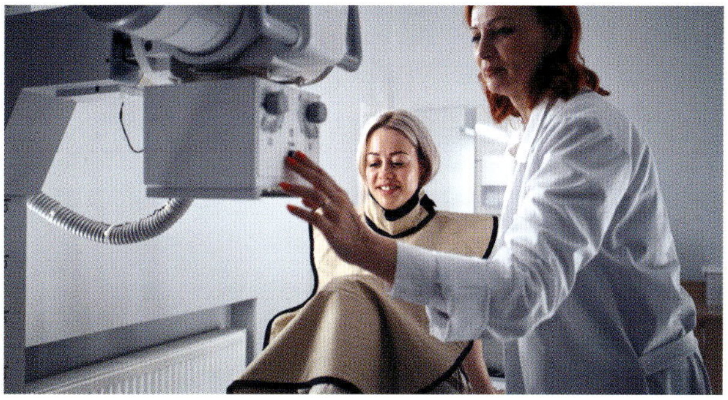

Questions

1. (a) Compare and contrast the nature, charge, mass and range of α, β and γ radiation. [12]

(b) Explain why alpha particle sources are so damaging to human health if ingested, but are relatively harmless outside the human body. [2]

(c) Define what is meant by (i) the physical half-life and (ii) the biological half-life of a radioactive substance. [2]

(d) Phosphorus-32 decays by the emission of b-radiation and is used in the treatment of bone cancer. The physical decay constant of ^{32}P is 0.0475 days^{-1} and its biological half-life is 1455 days.

(i) Show that the physical half-life of P is approximately 14.6 days. [1]

(ii) Suggest one metabolic process by which P might be excreted from the body. [1]

(iii) Use the equation $(T_{effective})^{-1} = (T_{physical})^{-1} + (T_{biological})^{-1}$ to calculate the effective half-life of P. [1]

(e) A radiopharmaceutical with an effective half-life of 2.5 hours and an activity of 1000 Bq is injected into the body of a patient at exactly 8.00 am. The patient is required to remain in isolation in the hospital until the activity of the radiopharmaceutical is 100 Bq or less. Calculate the earliest time at which the patient might leave the hospital. [4]

2. (a) Describe, in detail, how data may be collected from which the half-life of protactinium may be determined. Include in your description how the protactinium is prepared and state the equipment used to collect the data. **Your quality of written communication will be assessed in this answer.** [6]

(b) A student carried out the experiment to determine the half-life of protactinium and plotted a graph of ln (A / Bq) against time t / s, as shown below. A represents the corrected activity.

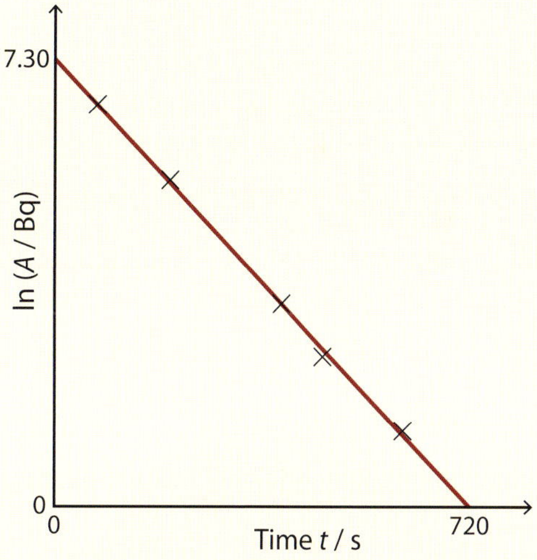

Use the graph to find:

(i) the corrected activity of the protactinium in Bq at times t = 0 s and t = 720 s; [2]

(ii) the half-life of protactinium; and [2]

(iii) the time taken for the corrected activity to fall from its initial value to 500 Bq. [2]

(c) Explain what is meant by *corrected* activity. [1]

3. Rubidium-82 is a pharmaceutical rapidly taken up by the heart muscle and used in positron emission tomography (PET) perfusion imaging.
   (a) Compare and contrast the properties of a positron with those of an electron. [2]
   (b) What happens when a positron collides with an electron? [2]
   (c) What is meant by cardiac perfusion imaging? [1]

   PET uses a gamma ray camera. The main components of a gamma ray camera are a **collimator**, a **scintillant**, an array of **photomultiplier tubes**, a **computer** and a display system.

   (d) State the functions of the four components in bold type in the paragraph above. [8]

4. (a) Discuss the precautions taken by healthcare professionals when using ionising radiation. **Your quality of written communication will be assessed in this answer.** [6]

   Medical physicists are sometimes asked to prepare radiopharmaceuticals for injection into a patient's body.

   (b) (i) What is a radiopharmaceutical? [1]
   (ii) Discuss the use of ^{131}I (Iodine-131) in the treatment of a patient with a cancerous thyroid gland. [2]

5. The pie chart below shows the major contributors to background radiation.

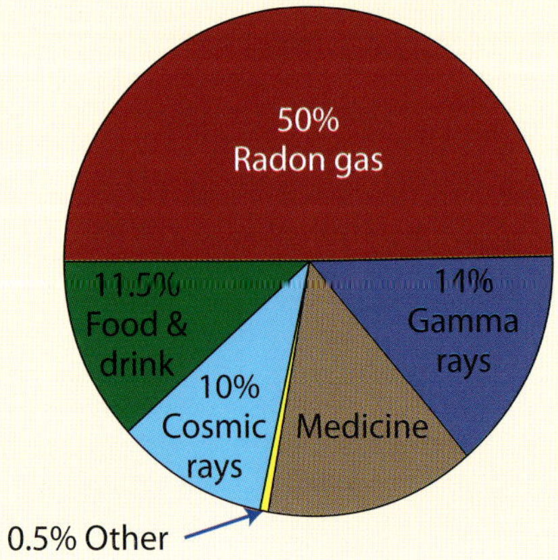

   (a) Calculate the percentage contribution to background radiation made by medicine, giving your answer to the nearest whole number. [1]
   (b) What medical procedures make the biggest contribution to background radiation? [2]

   When a spill of radioactive material has been dealt with, the final check made by medical physicists is to confirm that there is no significant local increase in the background radiation.

   (c) Describe how you might measure the background count in the laboratory. **Your quality of written communication will be assessed in this answer.** [6]

6. Thallium-201 is a radiopharmaceutical with a physical half-life of around 3 days. When used as a chloride salt in solution it has a biological half-life of about 3 minutes. It is used a tracer.
   (a) What is meant by the statement that thallium is a tracer, in the context of nuclear medicine? [1]
   (b) Discuss the properties of thallium-201 which make it suitable for use as a tracer. In your discussion refer to:
   - the nature of the radiation produced by the thallium and how this makes it appropriate to use as a tracer;
   - the significance of its biological half-life and its effective half-life in the body;
   - the risks associated with its use and how they are minimised; and
   - the patients for whom its use would be ill-advised.

   Your quality of written communication will be assessed in this answer. [6]

Unit A2 4:
Sound and Light

11: WAVES

Students should be able to:

- **10.1.1** differentiate between transverse and longitudinal waves, and manipulate computerised simulations of these wave forms, such as in Virtual Physics Laboratory;
- **10.1.2** recognise examples of transverse and longitudinal waves;
- **10.1.3** calculate amplitude and wavelength from displacement-displacement graphs;
- **10.1.4** explain time period from displacement-time graphs and how it relates to the frequency of the wave;
- **10.1.5** calculate wave speed, recalling and using $v = f\lambda$;
- **10.1.6** calculate frequency from time period;
- **10.1.7** demonstrate an understanding of the concept of phase difference;
- **10.1.8** calculate the phase difference between two waves of identical wavelength and speed;
- **10.1.9** appreciate that visible light is a constituent part of the electromagnetic spectrum;
- **10.1.10** recall the regions of the electromagnetic spectrum in order of wavelength and compare the similar features of electromagnetic waves;
- **10.4.1** demonstrate an understanding of how a standing wave can be created when two identical waves travel in opposite directions and describe an experiment to demonstrate the phenomenon;
- **10.4.2** appreciate that when a standing wave is created there is an increase in amplitude and this is called resonance;
- **10.4.3** distinguish between node and antinode positions in a standing wave;
- **10.4.4** draw different standing wave harmonics on a stretched string or closed pipe;
- **10.4.5** calculate wavelength from a standing wave diagram; and
- **10.4.6** perform and evaluate an experiment to measure the speed of sound using a resonance tube.

What are waves?

Waves are everywhere. We encounter sound waves when we listen to a radio, which itself detects radio waves. We see the world around us because our eyes are sensitive to visible light waves. You might even have used a microwave oven to cook your breakfast.

A wave that transports energy through which it moves is called a **progressive** wave. Mechanical waves, such as sound and water waves, do this by causing vibrations in the substance (medium) through which they travel. Electromagnetic waves do not require a medium through which to travel, but are associated with oscillating (vibrating) electric and magnetic fields.

Waves which are not progressive waves are called standing or stationary waves. Standing waves will be discussed later in this chapter.

Transverse and longitudinal waves

Progressive waves can be categorised as either **transverse** or **longitudinal**.

Transverse waves are those in which vibrations of the medium are **perpendicular** to the direction of propagation of the wave.

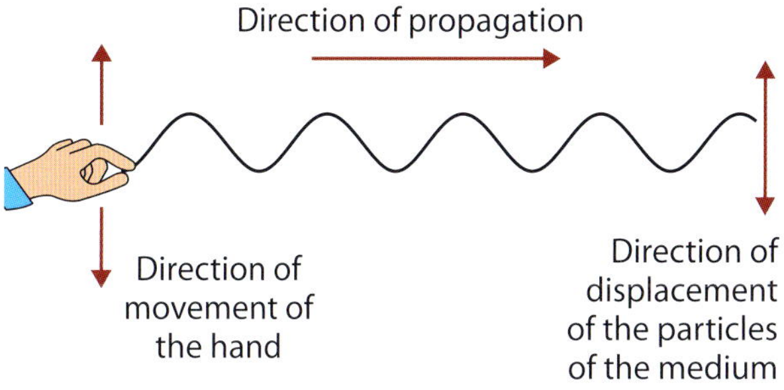

Most waves that you will encounter at A-level are transverse. Examples include water waves, waves on strings, S-type seismic (earthquake) waves and electromagnetic waves (γ-waves, X-rays, ultraviolet light, visible light, infrared light, microwaves and radio waves).

Electromagnetic waves are unique in that they are the only waves that can travel through a vacuum. At first sight this appears to contradict the definition of transverse waves. However, they are classified as transverse because they comprise oscillating electric and magnetic fields, both of which are perpendicular to the direction of propagation.

Longitudinal waves are those in which vibrations of the medium are **parallel** to the direction of propagation of the wave. Examples include sound and ultrasound.

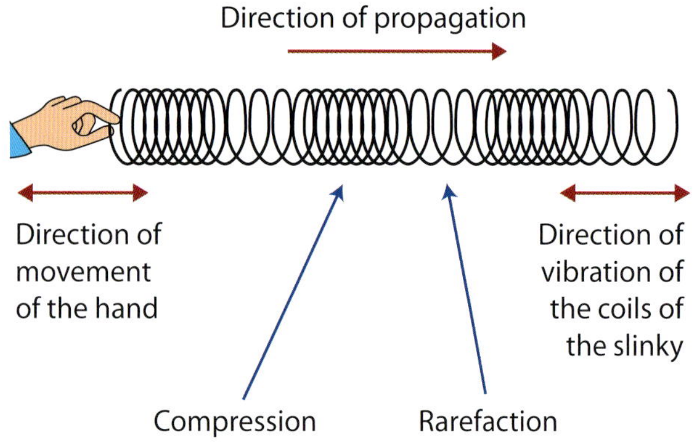

Tip: A slinky spring can be used to demonstrate both transverse and longitudinal waves. For that reason, it is best not to quote it if asked for an example of a transverse (or a longitudinal) wave.

Wavelength (λ) and amplitude (*A*)

In the case of transverse waves, the **wavelength** (λ) of a wave is the distance between successive crests (or troughs). For longitudinal waves, the wavelength is the distance between the centre of one compression and the centre of the next.

The **amplitude** of a wave refers to the maximum displacement of a particle of the medium from its equilibrium (or rest) position. You can think of the amplitude as the distance from the equilibrium position to the crest or from the equilibrium position to the trough.

Both wavelength and amplitude are measured in metres (or multiples or submultiples of metres). The graph below shows both the wavelength and amplitude of a transverse wave.

Periodic time (*T*) and frequency (*f*)

The **periodic time** (*T*) is the time taken for one complete wave/oscillation to pass a stationary point. Periodic time is often simply called the **period**. The following graph shows the periodic time of a wave.

Tip: Remember that you cannot obtain the wavelength from a graph of displacement against time, or the periodic time from a graph of displacement against displacement. But you can obtain the amplitude from either of these graphs.

Frequency (*f*) refers to the number of complete waves passing a point in one second. It is measured in units called Hertz (Hz). For example, a frequency of 100 Hz means 100 waves pass a fixed point per second. Therefore, in this case, the time taken for one wave to pass the same point is $1/100^{th}$ of a second (0.01 s).

It follows that relationship between period, *T*, and frequency, *f*, is:

$$T = \frac{1}{f}$$

where T = period (s)
f = frequency (Hz)

Tip: You must remember and be able to use this equation.

The wave equation

The velocity of the wave can be calculated from its wavelength and frequency using the following equation:

$$v = f \times \lambda$$

where v = velocity
f = frequency (Hz)
λ = wavelength

Tip: You must remember and be able to use this equation.

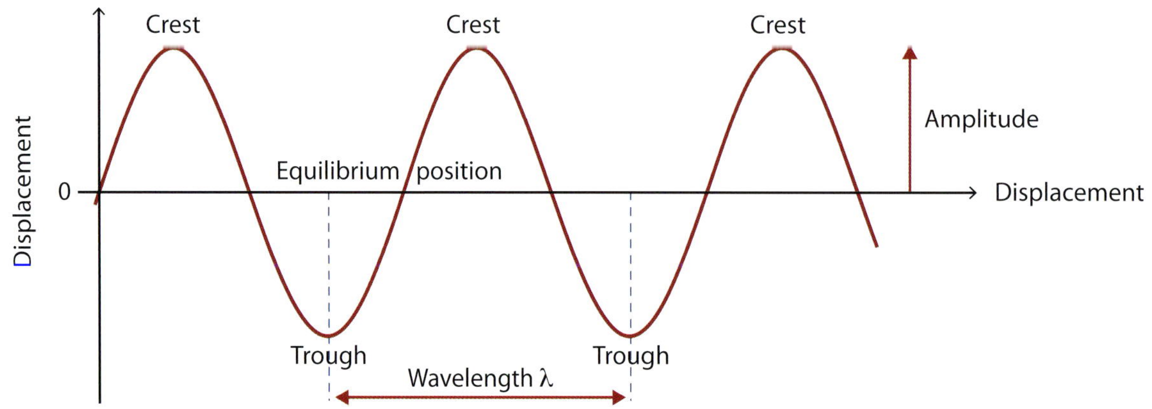

Wavelength and amplitude of a transverse wave

Tip: When using the wave equation, take great care with units. Frequency must always be in Hz. However, the units for wavelength and speed are linked. If wavelength is in metres, speed would be in m s^{-1}, if in centimetres then speed is in cm s^{-1} and so on.

Worked example

The graphs below refer to the same transverse wave.

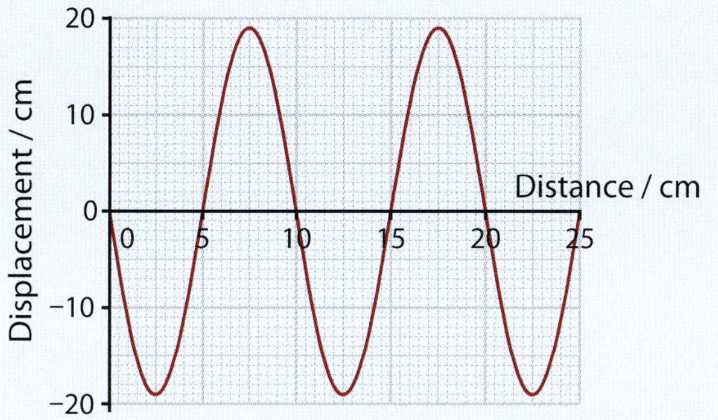

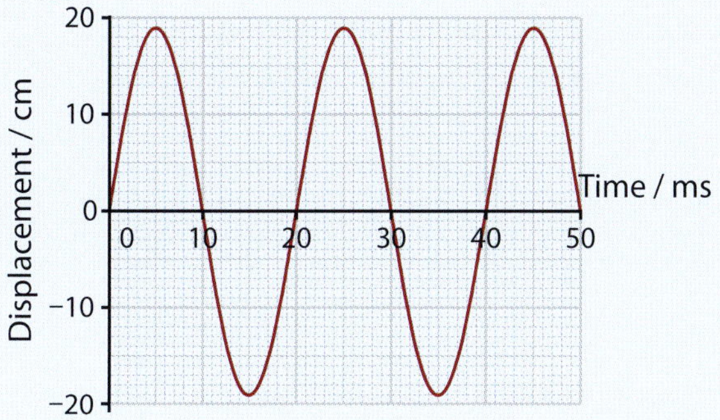

Use the graphs to find (a) the amplitude, (b) the wavelength, (c) the period, (d) the frequency and (e) the speed of these waves.

Answer

(a) *We can find the amplitude from either one of these two graphs.*
Amplitude = maximum displacement from equilibrium
= maximum height of wave
= 19 cm

(b) *To find the wavelength, we use the first graph.*
Over the 25 cm distance there are exactly 2.5 waves.
Wavelength λ = distance between crests
= 25 ÷ 2.5
= 10 cm

(c) *To find the period, we use the second graph.*
In a time of 50 ms, there are exactly 2.5 waves.
Period T = time between peaks
= 50 ÷ 2.5
= 20 ms

(d) To find the frequency, we use the equation

$$T = \frac{1}{f}$$

Rearranging this gives:

$$f = \frac{1}{T}$$

$$= \frac{1}{0.020} \text{ s}$$

$$= 50 \text{ Hz}$$

(e) To find the speed, we use the wave equation:
Speed $v = f \times \lambda$
$= 50 \times 10$
$= 500$ cm s^{-1}

Phase difference

The particles of the medium through which a wave passes vibrate. If two particles are vibrating so that at the same instant they are at the same distance from their equilibrium positions (same displacement), and moving in the same direction, they are said to be **in phase**. In the example below, the points with the same letter are in the same phase.

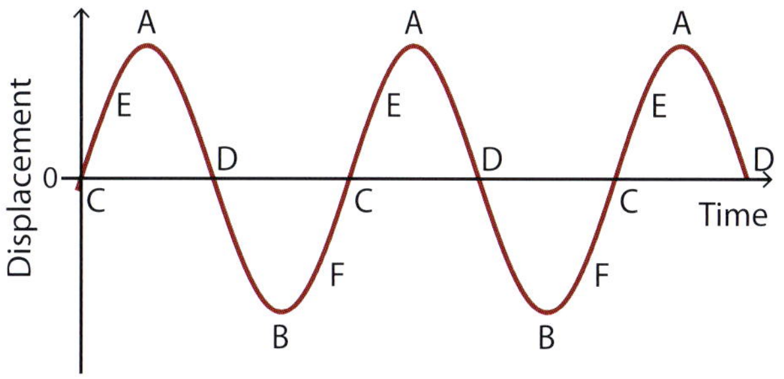

Phase difference is the difference in wavelengths or fractions of a cycle that one point on a wave leads or lags another. Phase difference is expressed as a fraction, or as an angle in degrees. One complete wave is said to represent 360 degrees (like the angle in a circle).

Tip: 'Lags' means 'follows at a later time'.

Consider the following graph.

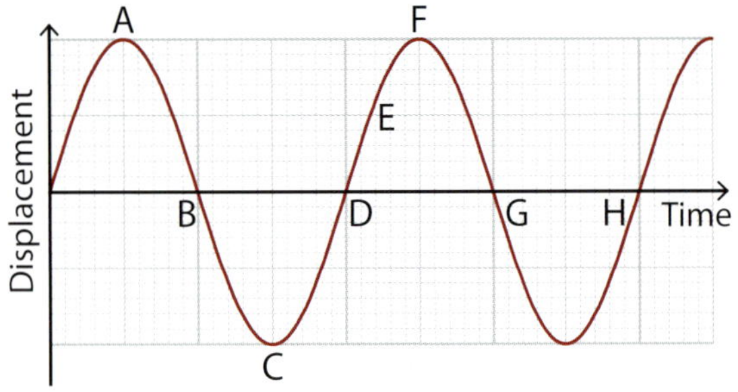

Points A, B, C, D and E are clearly not in the same phase. But by what angle are they out of phase with each other?

Point A is at a peak half a period before C. So we say A leads C by $\frac{T}{2}$ or 180° or C lags A by 180°. A phase difference of 180° has a special meaning – we say that such points are exactly out of phase with each other or, less commonly, that they are in anti-phase. Similarly, point A leads B by $\frac{T}{4}$ or 90°; A leads D by $\frac{3T}{4}$ or 270°; and A leads E by $\frac{7T}{8}$ or 315°.

There are 1¼ waves between point A and point G, so we could say that A leads G by 450°. However, phase differences of more than 360° are always avoided, by subtracting an integral multiple of 360°. So we would say A leads G by 90° (not 450°) and A leads H by 270° (not 630°). We would also say that there is zero phase difference between A and F, rather than 360°.

The table below summarises the phase difference of the points in the graph.

	B	C	D	E	F	G	H
A leads by / °	90	180	270	315	0	90	270

Phase difference – the general case

Phase difference is generally given the symbol ϕ and, so far, we have discussed only the points where ϕ represents a simple fraction of a wavelength. The general case is illustrated below for points within a given wavelength, λ, or period, T.

Within a given wavelength

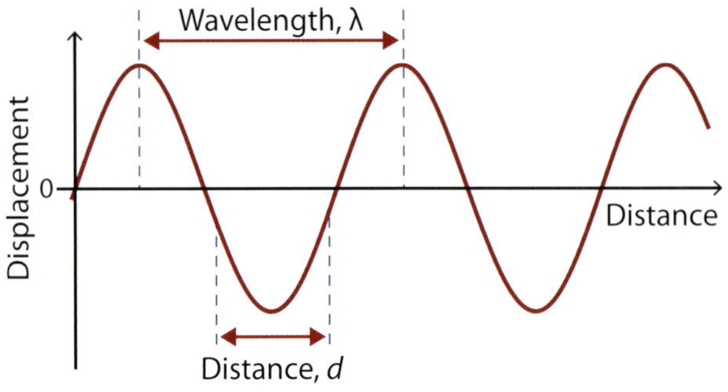

$$\phi = \frac{d}{\lambda} \times 360°$$

Within a given period

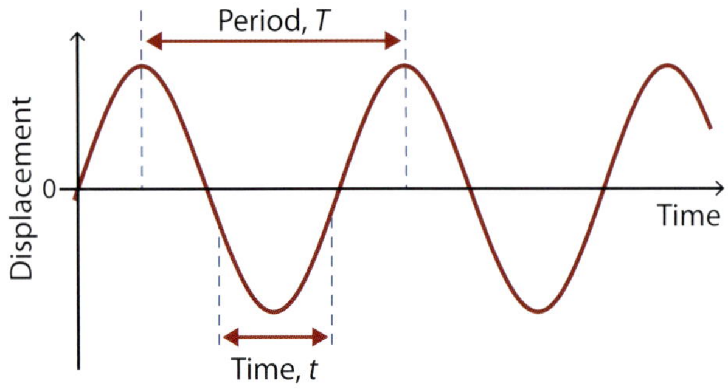

$$\phi = \frac{t}{T} \times 360°$$

Worked example

(a) Find the wavelength of the wave drawn on the grid below.

(b) Calculate the phase difference between points A and B, giving your answer to two significant figures.

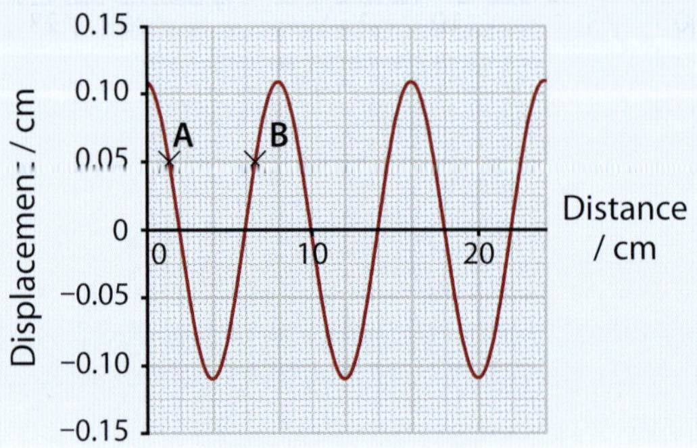

Answer

(a) On the graph there are 5 large squares representing 20 cm, so 1 large square represents 4 cm. The distance between the first and second peaks is 2 large squares. Therefore the wavelength is 8 cm.

(b) Each small square represents 0.4 cm, so the distance AB is just less than 5.6 cm.

$$\phi = \frac{d}{\lambda} \times 360°$$

$$= \frac{5.6}{8} \times 360°$$

$$= 252°$$

$$= 250° \text{ (to 2 s.f.)}$$

Phase difference: A leads B by approximately 250°.

Phase difference between superposing waves

When two waves overlap in time and space they are said to **superpose**. If they have different wavelengths (or different periods) their phase difference will change from moment to moment and from place to place. However, if their wavelengths and periods are the same, their phase difference is constant and they are travelling with the same speed. From their graphs we can find this phase difference using the equation.

The graph below shows two such waves.

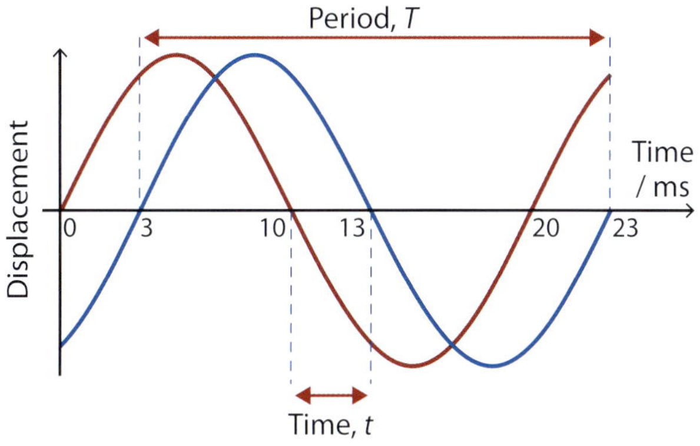

Looking at the times when each crosses the time axis, we see that the red wave is leading the blue wave by 3 ms and that the period, T, of both waves is 20 ms. We can therefore write:

$$\phi = \frac{t}{T} \times 360° = \frac{3}{20} \times 360° = 54°$$

So red leads blue by 54°.

The electromagnetic spectrum

Electromagnetic waves were mentioned earlier in this chapter in the context of transverse waves. We will now examine their properties in greater detail.

Electromagnetic (EM) waves are composed of electric and magnetic fields which oscillate at right angles to the direction of propagation of the wave. They are unique because they are the only waves which can travel through a vacuum. Moreover, in a vacuum, they all travel at the same (enormous) speed of 3×10^8 m s^{-1}. It is easy to read that speed quickly without appreciating its size. This is a speed of 300 000 000 m s^{-1}, which means they can travel around the Earth more than 7 times in one second! In space, they can travel from the Earth to the Moon, and back, in less than 3 seconds!

EM waves are generally classified into seven different regions, according to their wavelength, as given in the table below. Note that the boundaries are not precisely defined – they merge into each other like the colours of the rainbow. Nevertheless, you should remember the broad range of each region, and particularly the wavelengths of the visible spectrum.

Increasing wavelength ↓

Name of wave	Wavelength range (approx.)	Uses
gamma (γ) rays	Less than 10 pm	Gamma ray imaging, PET scans, cancer treatment, sterilising equipment
X-rays	10 pm to around 10 nm	CT imaging, cancer treatment
Ultraviolet	10 nm to around 400 nm	Skin cancer therapy (lymphomas)
Visible light	400 nm to around 700 nm	Endoscopy
Infrared	700 nm to around 1 mm	Thermography (detecting hot spots and cold spots in the body)
Microwaves	1 mm to around 1 m	Thermal ablation (local destruction of cells)
Radio waves	1 m to around 100 km	MRI scanning

Tip: 1 pm = 10^{-12} m; 1 nm = 10^{-9} m; 1μm = 10^{-6} m; 1 mm = 10^{-3} m

Tip: The table does not give the frequency range of the various members of the EM spectrum. However, it is easy to find using the wave equation, $v = f\lambda$, where $v = 3\times10^8$ m s^{-1}.

Standing waves

We have already classified waves as being either transverse or longitudinal. We can also classify them as being either **progressive** or **standing**.

A **progressive wave** is one in which the wavefront moves outwards away from the initial source of vibration, with the wave transferring energy in the direction of propagation as it does so. There are no points in a progressive wave which are permanently at rest.

A **stationary (or standing) wave** is a wave formed by the superposition in time and space of two progressive waves of the same speed, frequency and amplitude, travelling in opposite directions.

Tip: You should memorise this definition of a standing wave.

Standing waves can be demonstrated using **Melde's apparatus** as shown in the diagram below. A wire, about a metre long and connected to a vibration generator, passes over a pulley and is held taut using slotted masses. The vibration generator is connected to an oscillator whose frequency can be varied.

When the oscillator is switched on, a wave generated by the vibration generator passes along the wire towards the pulley where it is reflected back towards the generator. As it does so it superposes on waves travelling in the opposite direction. These waves interfere with each other and produce a standing wave.

What is observed depends on the frequency of the waves being generated. As the frequency rises **resonance** is observed. This occurs when **the amplitude of the vibrations on the wire is a maximum.** The vibration in the wire at the lowest resonance frequency, f_o, is called the **fundamental** mode or **first harmonic.** At a frequency equal to **twice the fundamental frequency**, we see the second mode of vibration or **second harmonic**. At three times the fundamental frequency, we see the third harmonic and so on.

The shape of the waveform in each of these vibration modes is illustrated in the following sketches.

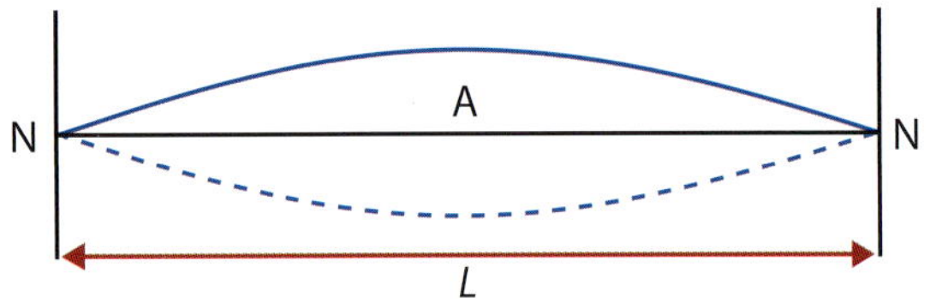

Fundamental resonance
(first harmonic – 1 loop)

$f = f_o$

$L = \frac{\lambda}{2}$ or $\lambda = 2L$

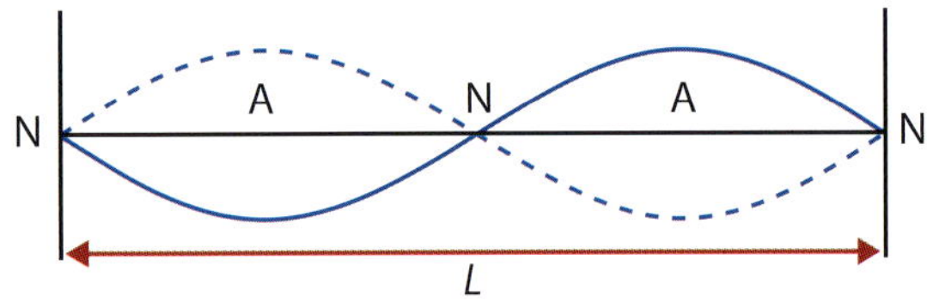

Second mode of vibration
(second harmonic – 2 loops)

$f = 2f_o$
$L = \lambda$ or $\lambda = L$

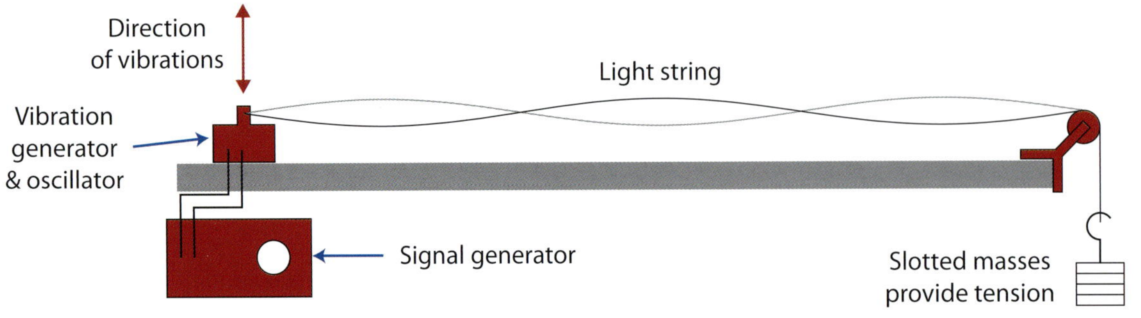

Melde's apparatus

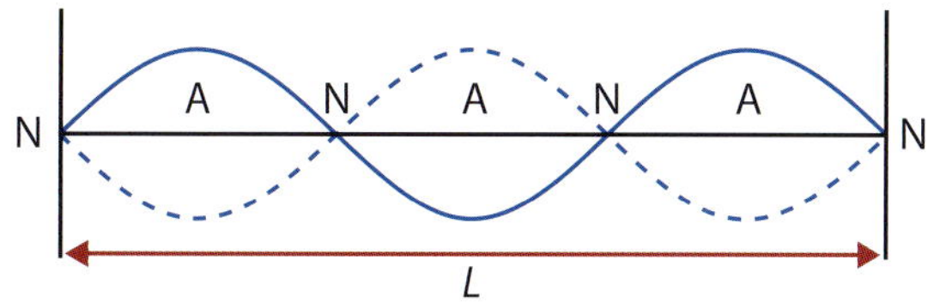

Third mode of vibration
(third harmonic – 3 loops)

$f = 3f_o$

$L = \frac{3\lambda}{2}$ or $\lambda = \frac{2\lambda}{3}$

Notice particularly that:

- the string is at rest at certain fixed points in the wire – these points are called **nodes**, labelled **N**;
- there are **always nodes at the ends** of the wire;
- the harmonic number is equal to the number of complete loops which are seen;
- the points **where the amplitude is a maximum** occur mid-way between consecutive nodes and are called **antinodes**, labelled **A;** and
- the **distance between consecutive nodes** (and between consecutive antinodes) is **half a wavelength**, as shown below – we will use this fact later to measure the speed of sound in air.

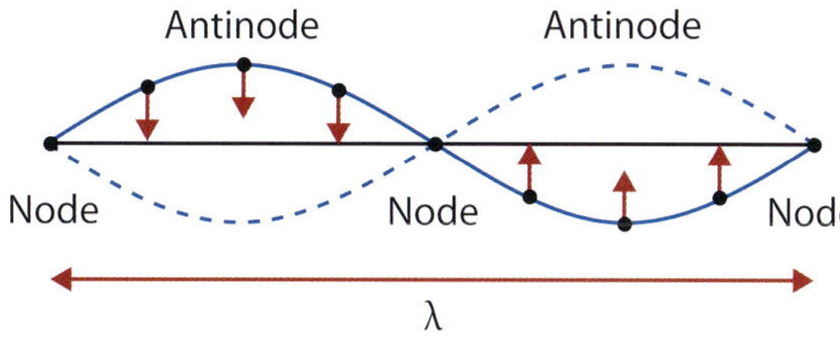

Tip: If you do not see Melde's experiment in school, you might like to look at a video demonstration on the web. A good place to start is to type *Institute of Physics* in your favourite search engine.

Differences between progressive and standing waves

The following table shows the differences between progressive and standing waves.

Tip: The CCEA specification does not specifically mention comparison between progressive and standing waves. However, the table is included for completeness and because understanding the differences will enhance student understanding of standing waves.

Progressive waves	Standing waves
Energy is transferred in the direction in which the wave is propagating.	Energy is not carried away from the source – instead it is stored in the vibrating particles.
There are no points which are permanently at rest. Crests and troughs are at rest only for an instant.	Points called nodes are permanently at rest.
All points in a given wavelength have the same amplitude.	The amplitude varies between a maximum at the antinodes and zero at the nodes.
Adjacent points within a given wavelength have a different phase.	All points between a given pair of consecutive nodes vibrate in phase with each other. However, the points between the next pair of nodes are vibrating ½λ out of phase with these points.

Standing waves in air columns

Standing waves can also be demonstrated with sound using a long glass tube closed at one end. This is commonly known as a **resonance tube**. Sound waves are generated at the top of the air column using a loudspeaker or tuning fork, as shown in the diagram below.

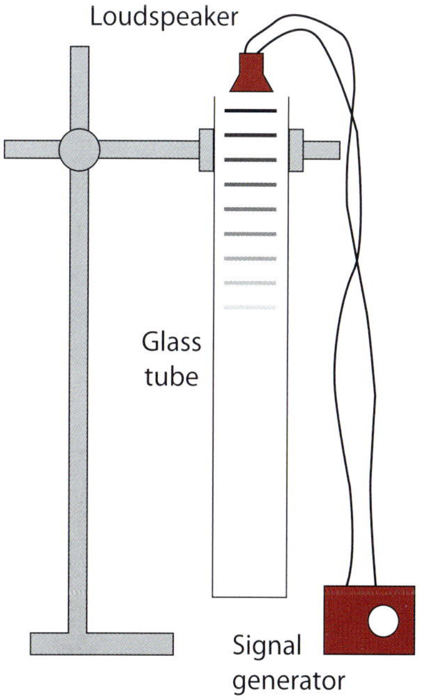

Sound waves from the speaker or tuning fork meet the reflected waves from the bottom of the air column and a standing wave is created. At particular frequencies we have **resonance** and the sound is at its loudest. This is easily checked by removing the glass tube. If a standing wave was present there should be a very noticeable decrease in the loudness of the sound.

As with waves on strings, the different frequencies at which this happens are called **harmonics**. The lowest frequency of sound which creates a standing wave for a particular length of air column is called the **fundamental**.

The diagram below shows three air molecules at three different positions along the air column in the glass tube. Sound is a longitudinal wave, so the vibrations are along the length of the air column, parallel to the direction of propagation of the sound wave.

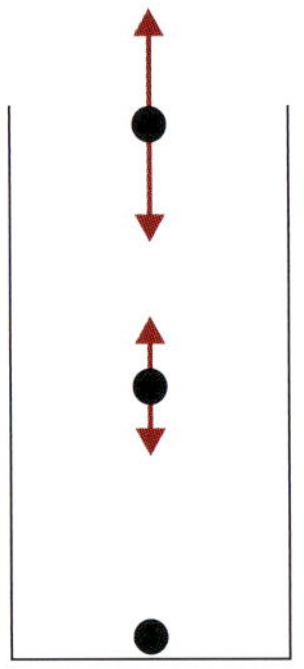

The air molecule at the closed end is not vibrating: this is a **node**. The air molecule at the open end is vibrating with maximum amplitude: this is an **antinode**. The air molecule further down the pipe is vibrating with an amplitude less than that of the molecule at the open end. As we move from the node to the antinode the amplitude of vibration of the air molecules increases.

One way to represent a wave is a graph showing how the displacement of the particles varies with distance along the tube. When this is done for the fundamental mode of vibration of the air in the column we have the graph shown below.

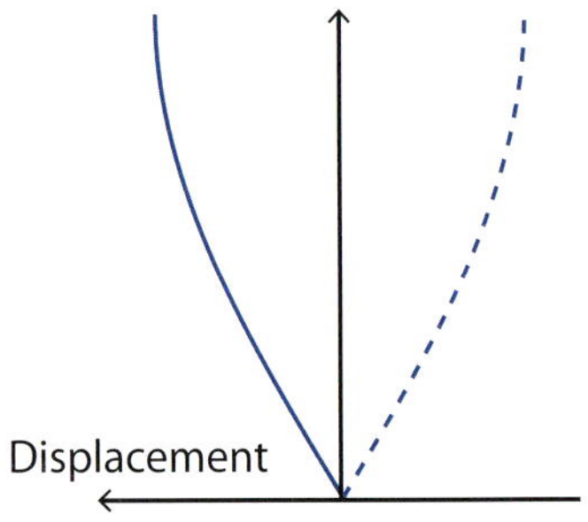

The displacement of the particles gradually increases from the closed end to the open end. The dotted line represents the displacement of the particles half a period later.

Tip: Remember that the distance between a node and an adjacent antinode is a **quarter** of a wavelength.

Note that because the part of the wave at the closed end of the tube must be a node, and the open end of the tube must be an antinode, **only odd numbered harmonics can be observed in a pipe closed at one end.**

Measuring the speed of sound in air

Standing waves provide a means of measuring the speed of sound in air. There are two methods.

Method 1: Using the fundamental mode

In this approach tuning forks of known frequencies are used to create standing waves. The tuning fork is made to vibrate and then held over the open end of a glass tube. The other end of the glass tube is placed in a container of water. The tube can be moved up and down in the water, allowing the length of the air column to be adjusted.

The glass tube is raised or lowered until the fundamental mode of vibration is produced. The fundamental mode is the shortest length of the air column at which the sound becomes noticeably loudest. The length of the air column is then measured.

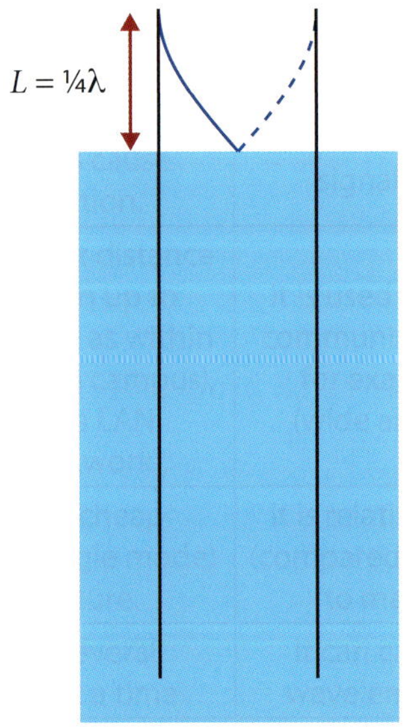

This procedure is repeated for a number of tuning forks of different frequencies.

Recall that in the fundamental mode of vibration the length of the air column, L, is one quarter of the wavelength of the sound, as shown in the diagram.

Using this fact, $\lambda = 4L$, in the wave equation gives:

$v = f\lambda = 4Lf$

Hence:

$$L = \frac{v}{4f}$$

Now compare this to the equation of a straight line passing through the origin, $y = mx$.

This shows us that a graph of L (y-axis) against $\frac{1}{f}$ (x-axis) will yield a straight line through the origin with a gradient $\frac{v}{4}$, from which we can determine a value for v.

Tip: In almost every straight-line graph you will plot in this unit of the specification, you have to go through a mapping exercise, linking the physics equation to $y = mx + c$. This is a skill which you must learn if you are to get the highest possible grades.

Typical measurements and the corresponding graph from such an experiment are shown below.

Frequency / Hz	Length of air column, L / m	$\frac{1}{f}$ / Hz^{-1}
256	0.335	3.91×10^{-3}
304	0.28	3.29×10^{-3}
362	0.235	2.76×10^{-3}
480	0.18	2.08×10^{-3}
512	0.165	1.95×10^{-3}

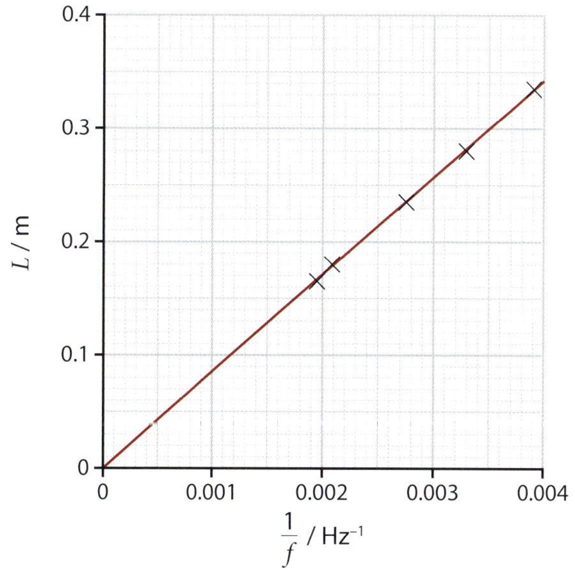

These measurements give a gradient of 86 m s^{-1}. Therefore the speed of sound obtained is 4×86 = 344 m s^{-1}.

Method 2 – Using the first and second positions of resonance

This method uses the same apparatus. First the fundamental mode of vibration is found as before. This is also known as the first position of resonance. The length, L_1, of the air column at the first position of resonance is measured. Using the same frequency, the next shortest length, L_2, at which the loudest sound is heard is recorded. This is the second position of resonance.

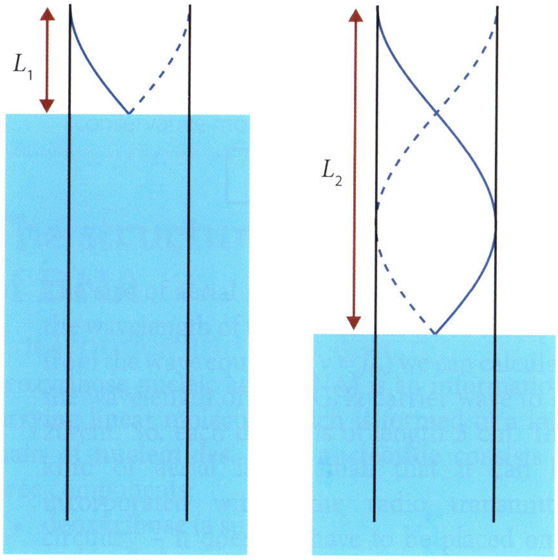

$L_1 = \frac{\lambda}{4}$ and $L_2 = \frac{3\lambda}{2}$

So:

$\Delta L = L_2 - L_1 = \frac{\lambda}{2}$

Rearranging this gives:

$\lambda = 2(L_2 - L_1)$

Using the wave equation, the velocity v can be found since the frequency f and the lengths L_2 and L_1 are known:

$v = f\lambda$

$= 2f(L_2 - L_1)$

This method should be repeated for a number of frequencies and an average value for the velocity of sound calculated.

Alternatively, a graph of ΔL (y-axis) against $\frac{1}{f}$ (x-axis) could be plotted. This will yield a straight line through the origin of gradient $\frac{v}{2}$.

Questions

1. Gamma rays, **X-rays**, **radio waves** and **ultrasound** are all used in medicine in diagnostic imaging. **Visible light** is used in medical endoscopy, **microwaves** are used in the thermal destruction of cells and **infrared** is used in medical thermography.
   (a) Which of the waves in bold type above is/are:
      (i) electromagnetic waves? [5]
      (ii) longitudinal waves? [1]
   (b) The graph below shows a progressive wave of frequency 7.5×10^{9} Hz.

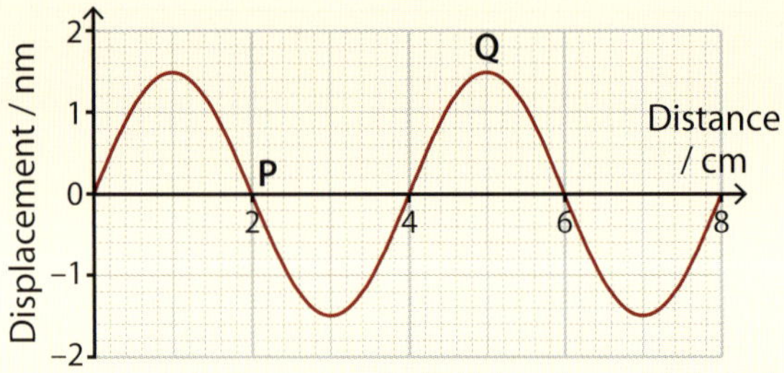

      (i) State the amplitude of this wave. [1]
      (ii) Use the graph to find the wavelength of the wave. [1]
      (iii) State the phase difference between points P and Q. [2]
      (iv) Calculate the period and the speed of this wave. [2]
      (v) To which part of the electromagnetic spectrum does this wave belong? [1]

2. Ultrasound is used in medicine to accelerate the healing of bone fractures. A particular ultrasound wave with a frequency of 1.5 MHz and a wavelength of 1000 micrometres travels through bone. A different pulse of ultrasound has a frequency of 2.0 MHz. Assuming that the two pulses travel at the same speed in bone, calculate the wavelength of the second ultrasound pulse. [4]

3. The following graph is a representation of a sound wave. Copy the diagram and on the same grid, draw a graph of a wave of the same frequency, half the amplitude and leading the wave shown with a phase difference of 60°.

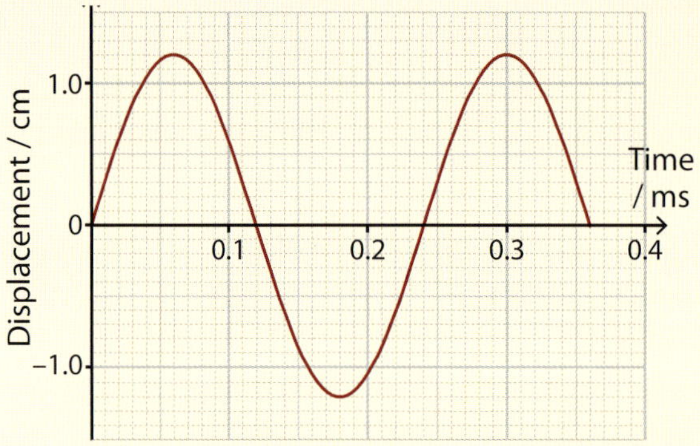

[4]

4. A student started to draw up a table of the members of the electromagnetic spectrum in order of increasing wavelength. After entering the names of three such members, her list looked like Table 1 below.

Table 1

Increasing wavelength ↓	
	X-rays
	Visible light
	Microwaves

The student knew that the typical wavelengths of the remaining members were as shown in Table 2 below.

Table 2

A	1 μm
B	250 nm
C	1 pm
D	100 m

   (a) Copy Table 1 and enter the letters A, B, C and D in the appropriate places. [4]
   (b) What are the names of the members corresponding to A, B, C and D? [4]

5. The diagram shows the apparatus used in a demonstration of standing waves on a stretched wire of length 90 cm.

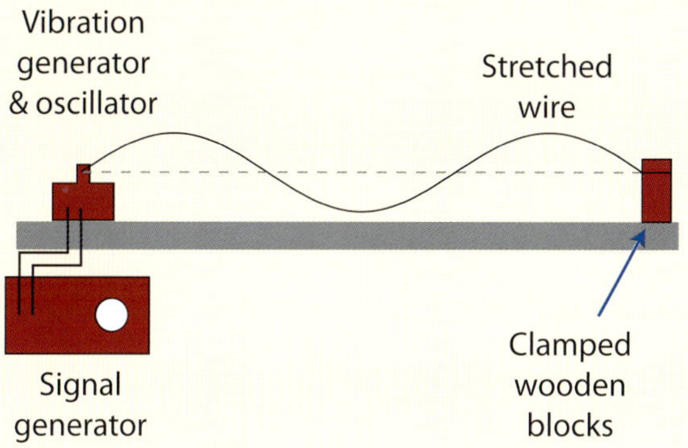

(a) What is a standing wave? [2]
(b) Copy the diagram and on it mark all the nodes with a letter **N** and all the antinodes with a letter **A**. [2]
(c) Which harmonic is illustrated by the diagram? [1]
(d) Calculate the wavelength of the waves on the wire. [2]
(e) If the oscillator shows the vibration generator is operating at 250 Hz, calculate the speed of the waves along the wire. [2]

The student carrying out this experiment increases the tension in the wire and the speed of the waves increases also. Resonance is then no longer observed.

(f) In what way should the student adjust the oscillator to restore the pattern shown in the diagram above? Explain your answer. [3]

6. Standing waves can be observed in a pipe closed at one end. A loudspeaker, attached to a signal generator, is placed at the open end of a tube, as shown in Diagram A (on the right), and the frequency is adjusted to produce resonance.

(a) How does the observer know when resonance has been achieved? [1]
(b) Copy Diagram B (on the right) and on it draw a graphical representation of the standing wave pattern for the first harmonic. [1]
(c) Mark all the nodes and antinodes on your diagram. [2]

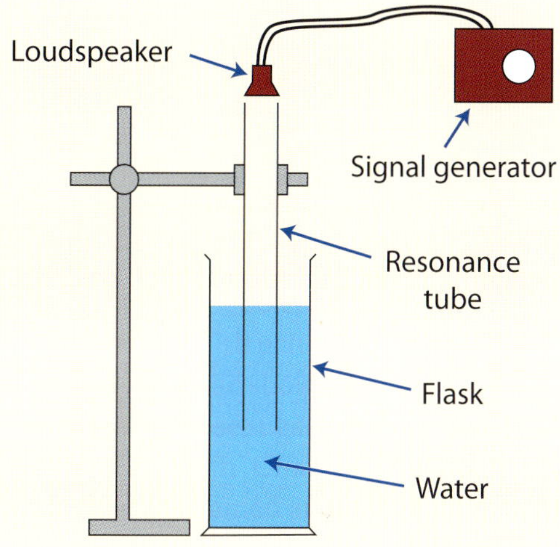

Diagram A

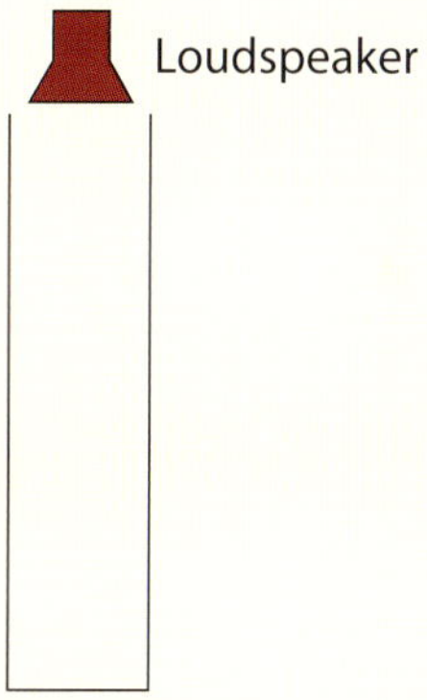

Diagram B

(d) What should the student do with the apparatus in Diagram A to obtain higher harmonics? [3]
(e) The student finds that he can obtain the third, but not the second, harmonic. Explain why this is so. [1]

The length of the tube in the diagram is 420 mm at the first harmonic. On the day the experiment is carried out the speed of sound in air is 336 m s^{-1}.

(f) Calculate the frequency of the sound coming from the speaker when the third harmonic is produced in the 420 mm tube. [3]

7. The human ear is most sensitive at frequencies around 3 kHz – 4 kHz. This is due to resonance in the ear canal. A student estimates the length of her ear canal to be 2.6 cm. If the speed of sound on a particular day is 338 m s^{-1}, calculate the approximate frequency to which this student's ear is likely to be most sensitive. (Hint: find the fundamental frequency in her ear canal.) [2]

8. A student is given a set of tuning forks and a resonance tube arrangement like that illustrated below. All but one of the tuning forks have their frequency marked on them.

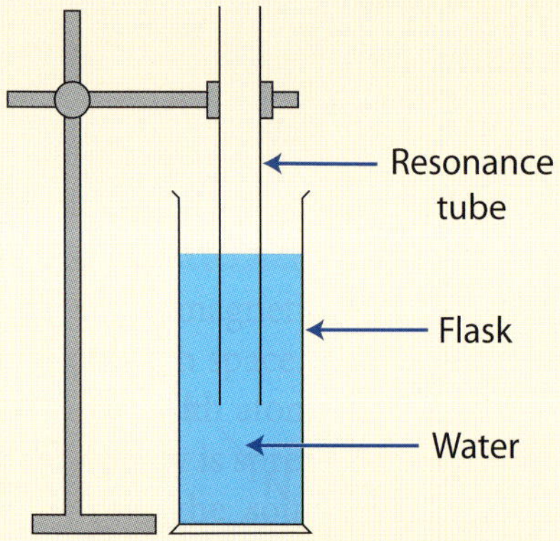

Use your knowledge of fundamental resonance in a tube closed at one end to suggest, in outline, how the student might find the unknown frequency of the unmarked tuning fork.
Your quality of written communication will be assessed in this answer. [6]

12: THE EAR AND HEARING

Students should be able to:

10.2.1 describe the functions of the main parts of the outer ear and label these parts on a diagram, including:
- pinna (auricle);
- auditory canal; and
- tympanic membrane (ear drum);

10.2.2 describe the function of the main parts of the middle ear and label these parts on a diagram, including:
- ossicles – malleus, incus and stapes; and
- Eustachian tube;

10.2.3 describe the function of the main parts of the inner ear and label these parts on a diagram, including:
- oval window;
- cochlea;
- auditory nerve; and
- semi-circular canals;

10.3.1 explain sound intensity and state its units as $W\,m^{-2}$;

10.3.2 perform an experiment to investigate their personal threshold intensity and state the threshold intensity, I_o, for human hearing as $1\times10^{-12}\,W\,m^{-2}$;

10.3.3 recall and use the equation:

$$\text{dB level} = 10\log_{10}\frac{I}{I_o};$$

10.3.4 recall and use the arrangement of 10.3.3 as:

$$I = I_o \times 10^{\frac{\text{dB level}}{10}};$$

10.3.5 demonstrate an understanding of the logarithmic nature of the decibel scale, that each increase of 10 corresponds to a 10-fold increase in intensity;

10.3.6 demonstrate an understanding of the reasons why a logarithmic scale is useful, as human hearing covers a wide range of intensities;

10.3.7 recognise that identical changes in decibel level correspond to identical fractional changes in intensity;

10.5.1 perform an experiment to measure the most sensitive frequency for human hearing;

10.5.2 demonstrate an understanding of how hearing response is frequency dependent and that maximum sensitivity occurs between 3 and 4 kHz and corresponds to resonance in the auditory canal;

10.5.3 appreciate that, due to 10.5.2, loudness is a subjective measure;

10.5.4 interpret graphs of frequency and intensity response for the ear;

10.5.5 demonstrate an understanding of what a phon is and how it can be established experimentally;

10.5.6 interpret and explain equal loudness curves on frequency-intensity response graphs; and

10.5.7 demonstrate an understanding of hearing aids and that they consist of a microphone, amplifier and loudspeaker.

The human ear

Humans hear only when sound waves enter the ear. A labelled diagram of the ear is shown on the next page. It is normally divided into three sections – the outer ear, middle ear and inner ear.

The outer ear

The **outer ear** consists of the pinna (auricle), the auditory canal and the tympanic membrane (ear drum).

Pinna (auricle)

The pinna is the only visible part of the ear. Its function is to act as a funnel to direct the sound further into the ear, rather like the horn of an old gramophone directing sound into the room.

Auditory canal

The auditory canal has two primary functions: helping us to hear by funnelling sound toward the eardrum and protecting the ear drum from injury. The part of the canal closest to the pinna is made of cartilage which has tiny hairs and contains sweat glands. The sweat glands play a defensive role, producing an oily wax which assists in lubricating the canal, keeping it clean and trapping bacteria and fungi which would otherwise cause infection.

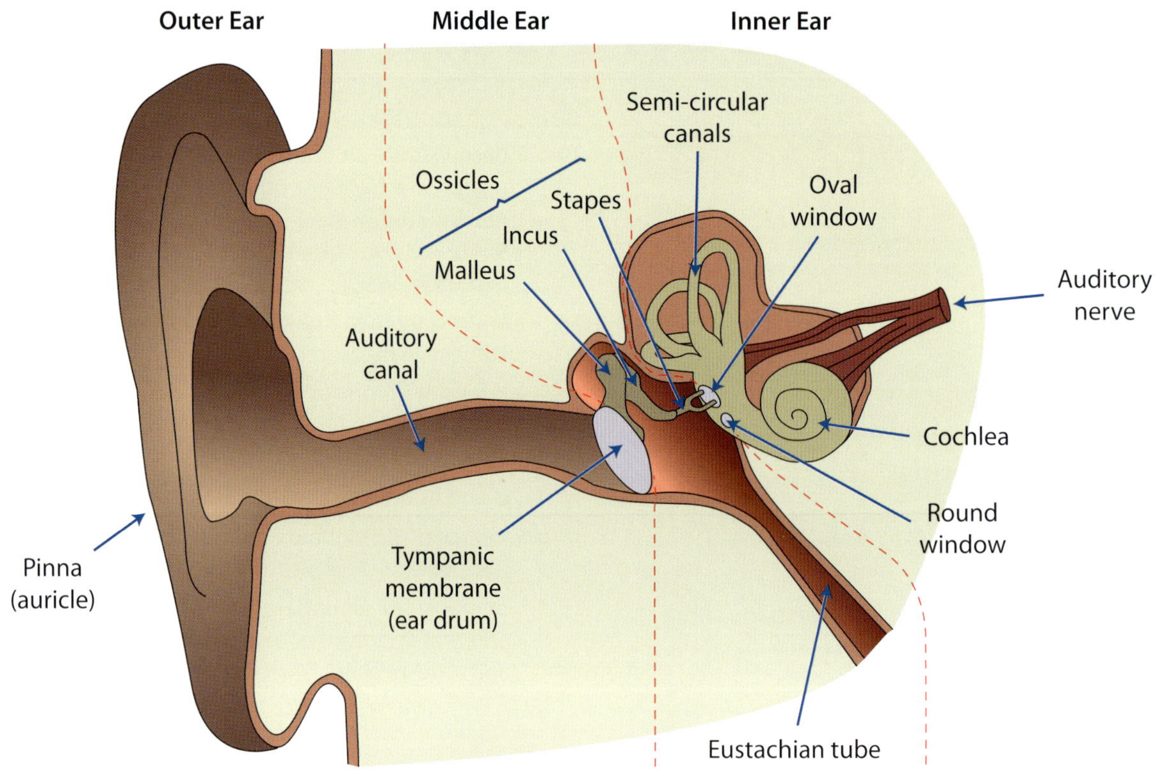

Tympanic membrane (ear drum)

The tympanic membrane is a thin layer of tissue at the bottom of the auditory canal. Sound passing down the canal causes the membrane to vibrate. These vibrations pass from the membrane to the auditory ossicles, which are tiny bones in the middle ear.

Tip: This unit contains a lot of factual information which you must be able to recall. The material is straightforward – but take responsibility for your own learning and remember it.

The middle ear

The **middle ear** consists of the ossicles and the Eustachian tube.

Ossicles

The ossicles are three bones in the middle ear and are the smallest bones in the human body. They have two functions:

- working collectively, they amplify the vibrations from the tympanic membrane by a factor of about ten; and
- they transmit vibrations from the eardrum to the fluid-filled labyrinth called the cochlea.

The shapes of these bones resemble a hammer, an anvil and a stirrup. For that reason, they are commonly known as **malleus**, **incus** and **stapes**, which are the Latin words for hammer, anvil and stirrup respectively.

Eustachian tube

The Eustachian tube is about 3–4 cm long and 3 mm in diameter. It connects the middle ear with the back of the nose. The middle ear is normally filled with air. This air is constantly being absorbed by the body, so fresh supplies of air are needed from time to time. The air cannot get into the middle ear through the ear drum, so it gets in via the Eustachian tube.

The Eustachian tube is normally closed, but it opens whenever we swallow, yawn or chew. This has two results:

- it allows air to get into the middle ear – this is essential to keep the air pressure equal on either side of the eardrum, so that it can vibrate properly and hence the vibrations can be transmitted to the cochlea via the ossicles; and
- it allows any mucus to drain from the middle ear which makes it less susceptible to infection.

Inner ear

The **inner ear** consists of the oval window, the cochlea, the semi-circular canals and the auditory nerve.

Oval window

The oval window is a connective tissue membrane located at the end of the middle ear and the beginning of the inner ear. It connects the stirrup bone (stapes) of the middle ear to the upper part of the cochlea.

Cochlea

The cochlea is the part of the inner ear involved in hearing. It is a spiral-shaped cavity in a bony labyrinth. The cochlea is filled with fluid and is connected to the middle ear by two membrane-covered openings, the oval window and the round window.

> **Tip:** The name 'cochlea' derives from the Ancient Greek word 'kokhlias' (κόχλιας) meaning 'spiral'.

Inside the cochlea is the 'organ of Corti', a structure of highly specialised cells that translate sound vibrations into electrical nerve impulses. The cells of this organ have tiny hair-like strands (cilia) that protrude into the fluid of the cochlea. Different parts of the cochlea respond to different frequencies.

When sound enters the ear, the sound vibrations are relayed from the tympanic membrane (ear drum) by the ossicles in the middle ear to the oval window, where they set up corresponding vibrations in the fluid of the cochlea. These vibrations move the cilia of the organ of Corti, which then sends electrical impulses to the brain.

> **Tip:** The round window provides a means of equalising pressure between the inner ear and the ear canal. However, the CCEA specification does not require you to have knowledge of its function.

Auditory nerve

Electrical impulses relating to hearing are sent to the brain along the auditory nerve.

Semi-circular canals

The semi-circular canals are three tiny, fluid-filled tubes in the inner ear. They **play no role** in hearing but rather help a person keep a sense of balance. When a person moves, the liquid inside the semi-circular canals also moves, like water in a bottle. Tiny hairs that line each canal translate the movement of the liquid into electrical impulses that are sent to the brain via the same auditory nerve that the cochlea uses. The brain can then tell the body how to stay balanced. We need three such canals, so that the brain can be informed of our motion in three-dimensional space.

Sound measurement

Sound intensity and decibel level

Sound **intensity** is a measure of the sound energy passing per second through an area of 1 m^2. Its units are therefore J s^{-1} m^{-2} or W m^{-2}.

Humans hear a very wide range of sound intensities. The smallest detectable sound intensity for humans, **the threshold of hearing**, is given the symbol I_0 and **is generally** taken to be **1×10^{-12} W m^{-2}**. By comparison, the intensity of sound at the front row of a rock concert might be around 1×10^{-1} W m^{-2} – which is 100 000 000 000 times the threshold of hearing!

The ear's perception of loudness depends on the relationship between the intensity and the threshold intensity. That is, the ear responds to **differences** in intensity, rather than **total** intensity. It is useful, therefore, to define a quantity called the **intensity level** which is closely related to what we might call 'loudness'.

Intensity level is defined by the equation:

$$\text{intensity level (in bels)} = \log_{10} \frac{I}{I_0}$$

where I = sound intensity
I_0 = threshold of hearing

The unit for intensity level is the bel and is given the symbol B. However, the bel is a rather large unit, so it is much more common to use the decibel, symbol dB, where 1 B = 10 dB.

The equation that students must remember and be able to use is:

$$\textbf{dB level} = 10 \log_{10} \frac{I}{I_0}$$

> **Tip:** In the latest LHS specification, 'intensity level' is called the 'dB level'. However, when looking at examination papers prior to 2022, students will see reference to the earlier term 'intensity level'. The terms are interchangeable.

There are two reasons why physicists use a logarithmic scale to measure sound intensity level:

- a logarithmic scale means that an **addition** of 10 in the dB level corresponds to a **10 fold** increase in sound intensity; and
- the range of audible sound intensities is so vast that a non-logarithmic scale is impractical.

We can also obtain the intensity from the decibel level by rearranging the equation above. This produces the equation:

$$I = I_o \times 10^{\frac{\text{dB level}}{10}}$$

Tip: This is an equation which students must remember and be able to use.

Tip: Students often find it difficult to do the unusual mathematics introduced in this unit. Get as much practice as you can solving problems involving the use of logarithms on your calculator.

Worked example

(a) Show that the decibel level for sound at the threshold intensity of human hearing is 0 dB.

(b) The decibel level of the sound from an alarm clock at a distance of 1 metre is approximately 80 dB. Calculate the intensity of the sound from the alarm clock.

(c) Contrast the increase in the intensity of the sound with the increase in the intensity level.

(d) Show that when the intensity of sound doubles, the decibel level increases by about 3 dB.

Answer

(a) $\text{dB level} = 10 \log_{10} \frac{I}{I_o}$

$= 10 \log_{10} \frac{1\times10^{-12}}{1\times10^{-12}}$

$= 10 \log_{10} 1$

$= 10 \times 0$

$= 0 \text{ dB}$

(b) $I = I_o \times 10^{\frac{\text{dB level}}{10}}$

$= I = 1\times10^{-12} \times 10^{\frac{80}{10}}$

$= 1\times10^{-4} \text{ W m}^{-2}$

(c) Increase in intensity is by a factor of 100 000 000, or 10^8. However, the increase in decibel level is by an addition of 80 dB.

(d) From (a) the dB level at threshold intensity is 0 dB. Consider doubling the threshold intensity:

New dB level $= 10 \log_{10} \frac{2\times10^{-12}}{1\times10^{-12}}$

$= 10 \log_{10} 2$

$= 10 \times 0.301$

≈ 3

Tip: A consequence of the definition of the decibel as a unit of sound intensity is that identical changes in decibel level correspond to identical fractional changes in intensity. For example, doubling the sound intensity always produces the same increase in the dB level – in this case an increase of 3 dB. Increasing the intensity level from 80 dB to 83 dB has the same effect on the intensity as increasing it from 12 dB to 15 dB – it doubles it.

Sound sources and intensity

The table on the next page lists some typical sources of sound, illustrating how the dB level increases with increasing intensity. The important point to notice is that the increase in intensity is extremely large in comparison with that of the decibel level.

Hearing response

Investigating personal threshold intensity

This investigation might be carried out in school if the appropriate equipment is available. Alternatively, the school might want to develop a relationship with an audiologist who can demonstrate the procedure at the audiologist's premises.

The sound signal is normally delivered via headphones to each ear in turn. At each frequency, ranging from about 20 Hz to about 10 000 Hz (depending on the person listening to the sound), the

Source	Intensity / W m^{-2}	Decibel level / dB	Number of times greater than threshold of hearing
Threshold of hearing	1×10^{-12}	0	10^0
Rustling leaves	1×10^{-11}	10	10^1
Whisper	1×10^{-10}	20	10^2
Normal conversation	1×10^{-6}	60	10^6
Busy street traffic	1×10^{-5}	70	10^7
Vacuum cleaner	1×10^{-4}	80	10^8
Unmuffled road drill	1×10^{-3}	90	10^9
Boombox maximum level	1×10^{-2}	100	10^{10}
Front rows of rock concert	1×10^{-1}	110	10^{11}
Threshold of pain	1×10^{1}	130	10^{13}
Military jet taking off	1×10^{2}	140	10^{14}
Instant perforation of eardrum	1×10^{4}	160	10^{16}

Typical sources of sound

minimum detectable sound intensity is measured and plotted. The graph, known as an **audiogram**, shows the frequency response of the human ear. The graph for a typical young adult is shown below.

Tip: The questions at the end of this chapter show you the depth of the skills and knowledge you will need in this topic. Be sure to do all of them and check your answers.

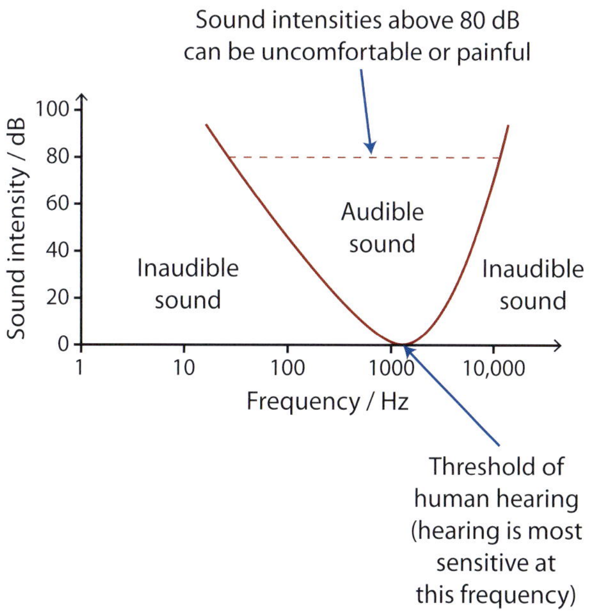

Audiogram for a typical young adult

There are several points to note from the audiogram:

- the graph looks like a 'bucket', within which sound can be heard;
- sound is inaudible outside the 'bucket';
- the frequency scale is logarithmic, because of its huge range;
- as the intensity level increases, the range of audible frequencies increases, but it is most marked at lower frequencies because the graph is asymmetrical;
- the ear is most sensitive at a frequency between 3 kHz and 4 kHz, but the precise figure varies from person to person; and
- the frequency at which the ear is most sensitive broadly corresponds to that at which we get resonance in the auditory canal.

The significance of an asymmetrical audiogram

Consider the effect of increasing the intensity level of a sound from 30 dB to 60 dB. Of course, the sound becomes much louder. But there is another effect. The increase in the lower frequencies which become audible is much greater than the increase in the higher frequencies. This is a consequence of the way in which the ear responds to sound, and is reflected in an asymmetrical response graph.

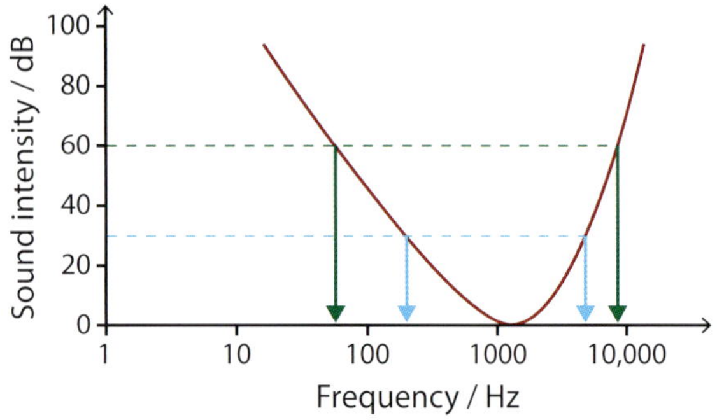

An asymmetrical response graph

During the procedure to obtain an audiogram, the person under test is asked to indicate the loudness of the sound. However, the same sound may be perceived to be louder by one person than another. Therefore we say that **loudness is a 'subjective measure'**, that is, it varies from person to person and is highly frequency dependent.

The phon

Since the loudness of a sound is subjective, physicists were obliged to find a better way of measuring it. The solution is to measure perceived loudness against a **1 kHz reference tone** of adjustable sound intensity level.

The dB level of the 1 kHz reference tone is slowly increased until it is perceived by the listener to be equally as loud as the sound being measured. The loudness level, given in **phons**, of the measured sound is then equal to the dB level of the adjusted reference sound, as measured on a decibel meter.

If this is repeated with sounds across the full range of audible frequencies, we will notice that at some frequencies the sound needs to have a higher sound intensity to be perceived to be as 'loud' as sounds at other frequencies. A line connecting together the sound intensities that a person perceives as equally loud across the range of frequencies is known as an **equal loudness curve**.

Three equal loudness curves are shown on the right, at 0 phons (a very soft sound), 60 phons and 120 phons (a very loud sound).

Note that the response to very loud sounds is much more uniform (flatter) than to very soft sounds. Notice that at all three levels of loudness, there is a greater sensitivity around 3 kHz, consistent with resonance in the ear canal. The 'dips' between 2 kHz and 5 kHz mean that a smaller sound intensity is required to perceive the same loudness as the 1 kHz reference tones.

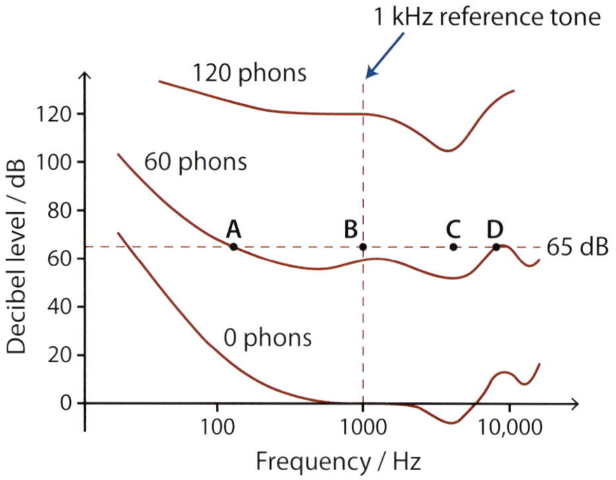

An equal loudness curve

Now consider the 0 phons curve, the very soft sound. The rise to the left of 1000 Hz shows the inability of the ear to discriminate loudness at very low frequencies. There is a significant rise in the sound intensity (in dB) required for a person to perceive the sound at 100 Hz to be just as loud as that at 50 Hz. This is also seen in the 60 phons curve to the left of point A.

Points A to D are all marked at a sound intensity of 65 dB. Points A and D have the same loudness (60 phons). Although B and C have the same intensity (65 dB) they do not have the same loudness as A and D. They are above the 60 phons curve so would, therefore, be perceived as louder than A and D. Point C is the loudest of the four because it is the furthest vertically from the equal loudness curve.

Tip: It is important that you can interpret equal loudness curves. This is a skill that can be learned, but it needs as much practice as you can get in your busy schedule!

Tip: Remember that at 1000 Hz the dB level and the number of phons are the same.

Hearing aids

A hearing aid is an electronic device used to allow people with hearing difficulties to participate in normal activities such as conversation. It operates by making sounds at some frequencies louder.

All hearing aids consist of a microphone, battery, amplifier and loudspeaker. The most modern hearing aids also contain a microchip. The diagram shows the arrangement of a 'behind-the-ear' device.

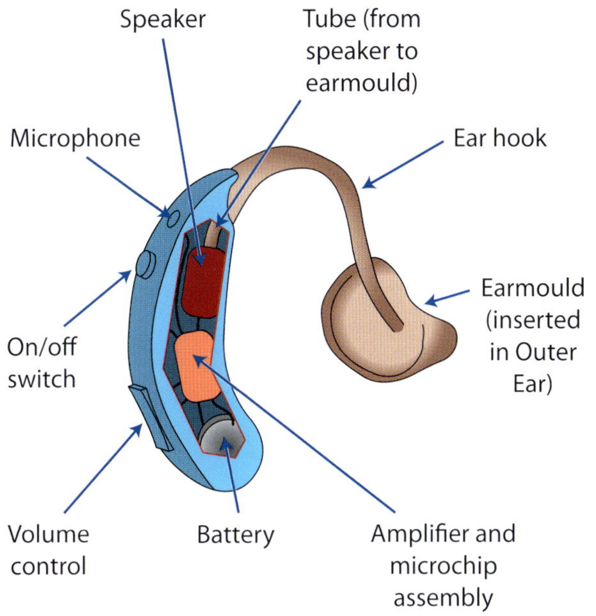

The hearing aid operates as follows:

- The microphones pick up the sound around the wearer and convert it into an electrical signal.
- This signal is passed to a microchip where it is digitised before being passed on to a digital amplifier to increase the strength of the signal.
- The amplified signal is then passed on to the speaker positioned in the ear canal.
- The battery provides the power for the microchip and the amplifier.

Questions

1. In the diagram below label the structures A to E and state their function. [10]

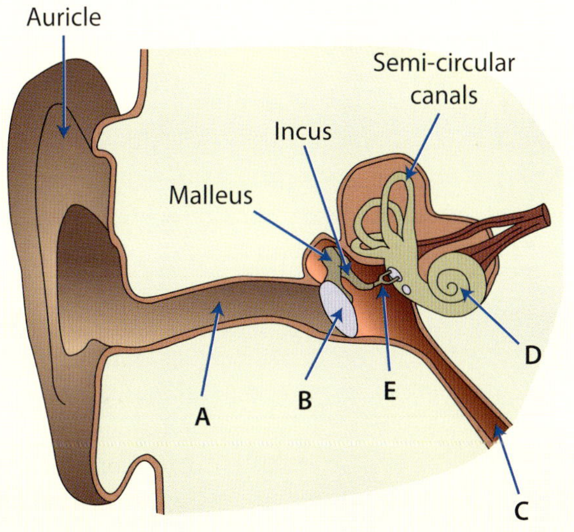

2. The semi-circular canals are structures in the inner ear which play no part in hearing.

(a) State the function of the semi-circular canals and describe how they work. [4]

(b) Why is it necessary to have three such canals? [1]

3. Copy and complete the table below by identifying the main parts of the outer, middle and inner ear. [6]

Outer ear				
Middle ear				
Inner ear				

4. Describe, in detail, the process of hearing up to the moment when signals are received by the brain. **Your quality of written communication will be assessed in this answer.** [6]

5. When sounds come from different sources their combined intensity is the sum of the intensities from the separate sources. The intensity of the sound of a ticking grandfather clock is 2.4×10^{-4} W m^{-2}. The chime from the same clock has an intensity level (dB level) of 88.8 dB.

(a) State what is meant by

(i) a sound intensity of 2.4×10^{-4} W m^{-2} and [1]

(ii) an intensity level of 88.8 dB. [1]

(b) Calculate the intensity of the chime alone and the intensity level of the clock alone. [2]

(c) Use your answer to part (b) to calculate the combined intensity of the clock and the chime. [1]

(d) Comment on your answer to part (c). [1]

6. (a) State
   (i) the threshold intensity and
   (ii) the threshold intensity level of human hearing. [2]

Over 80 years ago a scientist called Lipman found that the average threshold intensity level of hearing for almost a dozen dogs was around –25 dB but the upper frequency limit was approximately three times that of a young human with excellent hearing. (Lipman's work is now considered by some scientists to be unreliable as methods of measuring sound intensity levels have improved since his work.)

   (b) How should we interpret a negative threshold intensity level? [1]
   (c) Calculate the threshold intensity of a dog's hearing in W m^{-2}, if its threshold intensity level is –25 dB. [3]
   (d) Calculate the upper frequency limit for the dogs in the Lipman study. [1]

7. The evacuation alarm in a school produces a sound of frequency 2900 Hz. Describe, in detail, how the loudness of the alarm signal could be measured in phons. [4]

8. Study the equal loudness curves below.

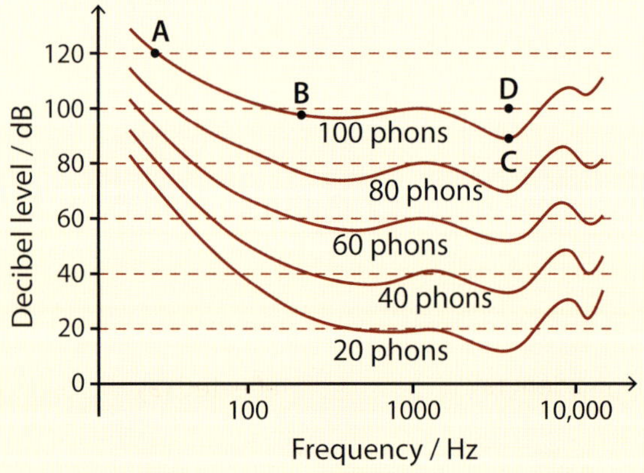

   (a) At what frequency is the sound intensity level in dB always equal to the loudness in phons? [1]
   (b) Which, if any, of the three sounds A, B or C would be perceived to be the loudest? [1]
   (c) State which of the sounds C or D would be perceived to be louder, giving a reason for your answer. [3]

13: LIGHT IN COMMUNICATION AND RADIO WAVES

Students should be able to:

10.7.1 perform an experiment to measure the critical angle of a semi-circular glass block and investigate the conditions required for total internal reflection;

10.7.2 describe how total internal reflection can be used in optical communication;

10.7.3 describe the structure of a fibre-optic cable;

10.7.4 demonstrate an understanding of the difference between single mode and multi-mode fibres;

10.7.5 contrast the uses for single mode and multi-mode fibres.

10.8.1 discover how radio signals can be created using a dipole antenna and then intercepted by a receiving antenna and decoded;

10.8.2 apply this principle to describe broadly how wireless and Bluetooth technologies work;

10.8.3 describe the main action of radio waves in radar systems;

10.8.4 demonstrate an understanding of when attenuation occurs in travelling waves and can be categorised as path loss and free space loss;

10.8.5 investigate how the Doppler Effect causes perceived frequency changes and how this can be used to calculate the relative motion of an object; and

10.8.6 interpret frequency graphs to make predictions based on the Doppler Effect.

Refraction

What is refraction?

Refraction is the bending of light when it passes from one transparent material into another.

In the following diagram, the light strikes the surface along the normal. In this case the angle of incidence is 0° (not 90° as is often mistakenly thought). In this case there is no bending, so no refraction takes place.

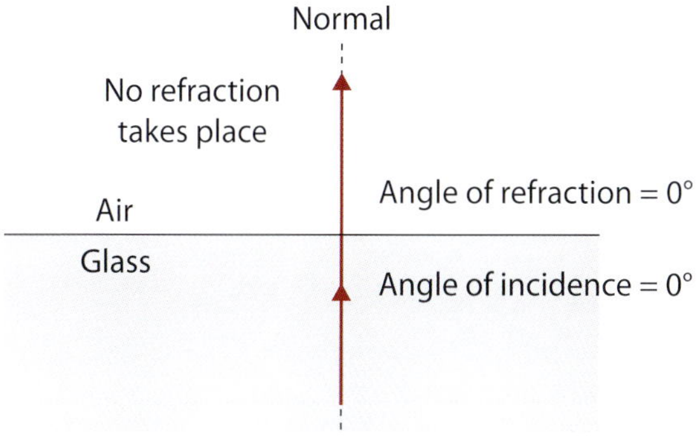

The critical angle and total internal reflection

Experimentally it is found that some reflection also occurs when there is refraction, as shown in the diagrams that follow. When the angle of incidence in the glass is small (diagram A), then the refracted ray is strong and the reflected ray is very weak. As the angle of incidence in glass increases:

- the angle of refraction in air increases;
- the refracted ray becomes weaker; and
- the reflected ray becomes stronger.

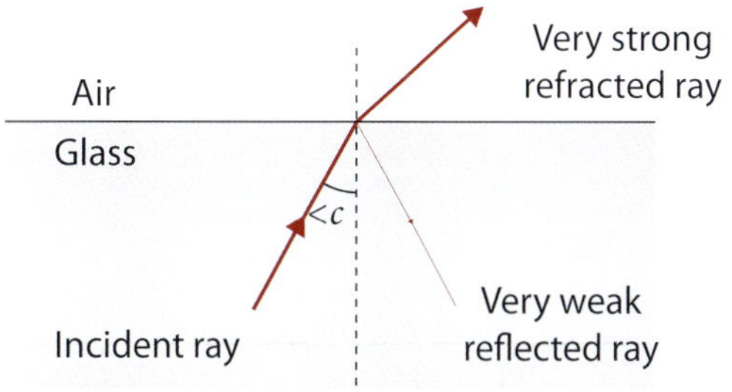

Diagram A

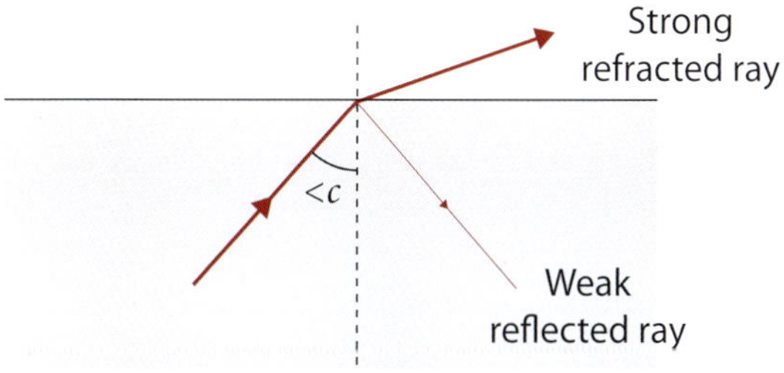

Diagram B

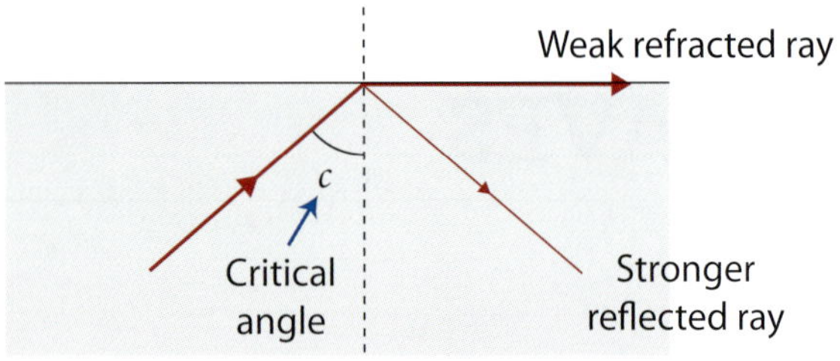

Diagram C

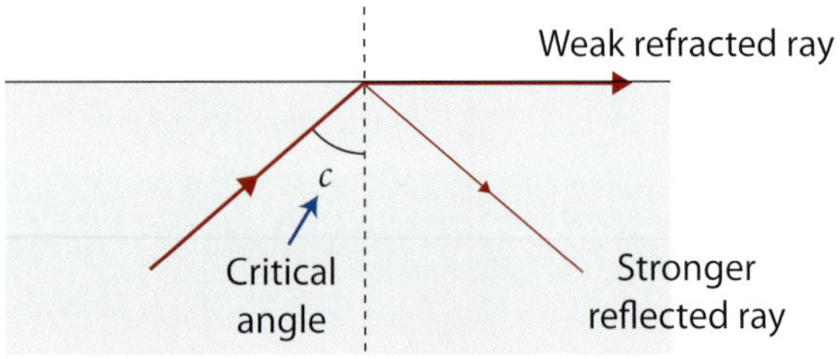

Diagram D

However, a stage is reached when the refracted ray emerges along the surface of the glass (diagram C). **The angle of incidence in the glass for which the angle of refraction in the air is 90° is called the critical angle, *c*.**

Tip: Learn the definition of critical angle. Many students lose marks needlessly because their definitions are either inaccurate or incomplete.

Different materials have different critical angles because the speed of light is different in each.

For glass, the critical angle is around 41.8°. For water it is about 48.6°.

At all angles of incidence greater than the critical angle there is no refraction at all. Instead we get **total internal reflection** (diagram D).

The refractive index

The **refractive index**, ***n***, is the ratio of the speed of light in that material to the speed of light in air. The higher the refractive index, the slower the speed of light in that material (and the lower the size of the critical angle). All transparent materials have a specific refractive index. Note that the refractive index is sometimes called the optical density.

Total internal reflection will only occur when two important conditions are met:

- the light must be travelling from a material of higher refractive index towards a material of lower refractive index; and
- the angle of incidence in the material of higher refractive index must be greater than the critical angle.

Tip: This material on critical angle and total internal reflection is essential for a thorough understanding of fibre optics.

Measuring the critical angle of a semi-circular glass block

This procedure can be used to measure the critical angle of a semi-circular glass block in the laboratory. You will need a semicircular glass block, a ray box, a power supply unit, white paper, a pencil and a protractor.

The method is as follows:

1. Place the semi-circular glass block in the centre of the sheet of white paper.
2. Draw round the outline of the block with a sharp pencil.
3. Remove the block and mark the centre, X, of the straight diameter.
4. Replace the glass block.
5. Connect the ray box to the low voltage power supply unit.
6. Switch on the power supply unit and direct a ray of light towards X, with light entering the glass from the air along the curved side as in the following diagram. Ensure that light can be seen leaving the block at X.

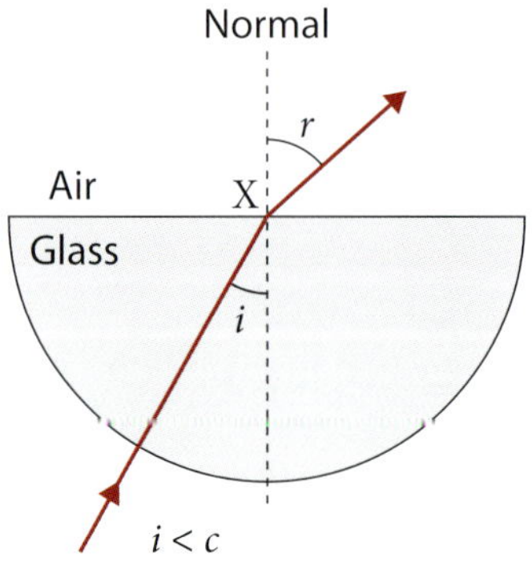

7. Continue to direct the ray towards X, but slowly move the ray box so that the angle of incidence at X increases. Observe that the emergent ray at X becomes weaker and the internally reflected ray becomes stronger.
8. Very slowly move the ray box to increase the angle of incidence at X until the refracted ray

at X just emerges along the diameter, as in the following diagram:

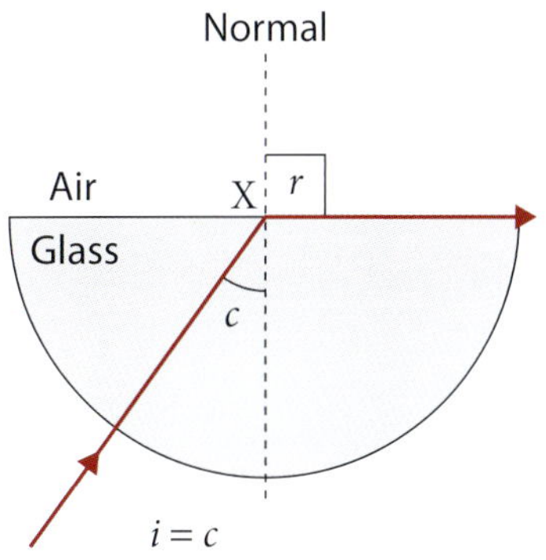

Observe that if the angle of incidence at X is now increased even slightly, the light is totally internally reflected, as in the next diagram:

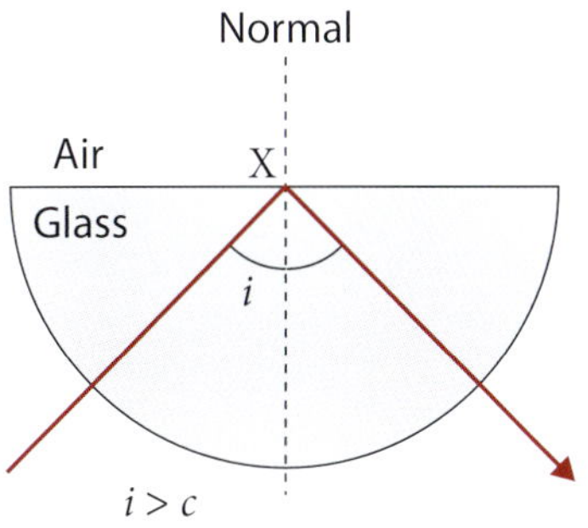

9. Use a pencil to draw two dots on the incident ray as far apart as possible.
10. Remove the glass block.
11. With a pencil and ruler, join the dots on the incident ray beyond the point of incidence until the line reaches X.
12. With a pencil and protractor, draw the normal at X, the point of emergence.
13. With the protractor, measure the critical angle at point X and record the value in a table.
14. For reliability, repeat steps 1 to 13 about three more times and find the mean value of *c*.

Fibre-optic cables

Fibre-optic cables are thin strands of glass surrounded by a cladding of lower refractive index. The whole fibre is covered by a protective plastic sheath as shown in the following diagram.

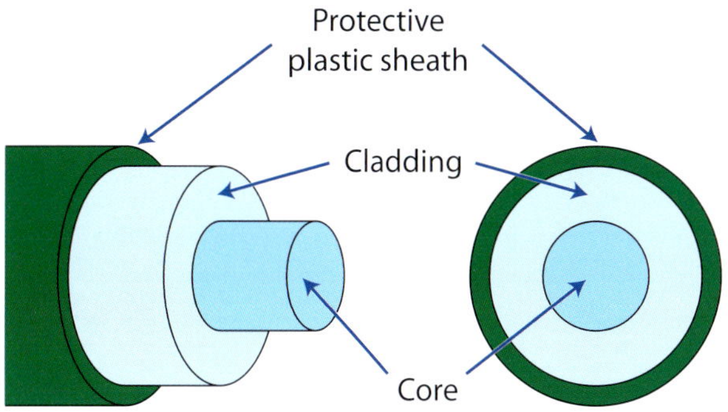

Light is confined to the fibre as long as it is incident on the core-cladding boundary at an angle greater than the critical angle. This means that the light is transmitted through the core by repeated total internal reflection, as shown below.

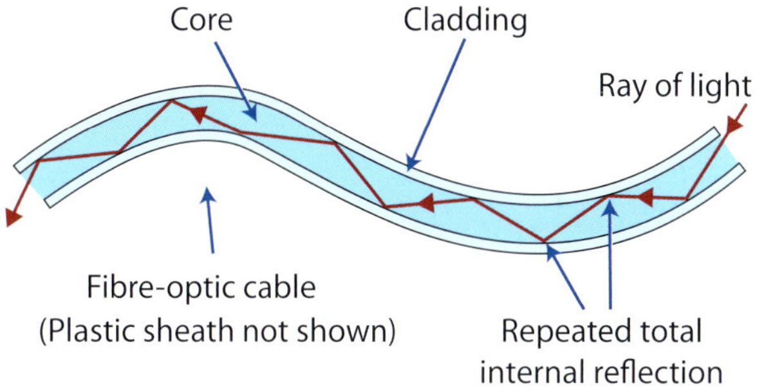

Tip: An optical fibre would work without the cladding as air also has a lower refractive index than the core glass. However, the cladding is useful as it protects the core, prevents cross talk and reduces the leakage of light.

Fibre-optic cables have undoubtedly revolutionised communications (phone and television) in the early twenty-first century. They facilitate secure, reliable ultrafast broadband and cable television.

Fibre-optic cables are also used by doctors or engineers to illuminate and observe places that are otherwise inaccessible. For example, endoscopes are used by doctors to view inside the human body (see chapter 9) and borescopes are used by engineers to inspect wear in the combustion chambers of engines.

Single mode and multi-mode fibre

A signal passing along a fibre-optic cable can take various paths depending on how much total internal reflection takes place. The shortest path is along the axis of the fibre, or very close to it. The longest path, known as the critical path, involves repeated reflections, as show in the following diagram. It takes the light slightly longer to travel along the critical path than along the axis, so the two signals arrive at the destination at slightly different times.

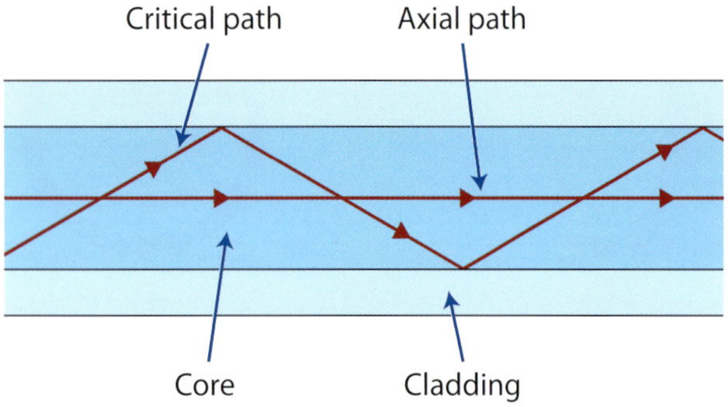

If the time taken for the signal to pass along the critical path is much longer than that along the axial path, then there is dispersion and the signal obtained will be blurred or distorted. The longer the fibre, the greater the distortion will be. This distortion is illustrated in the graphs below.

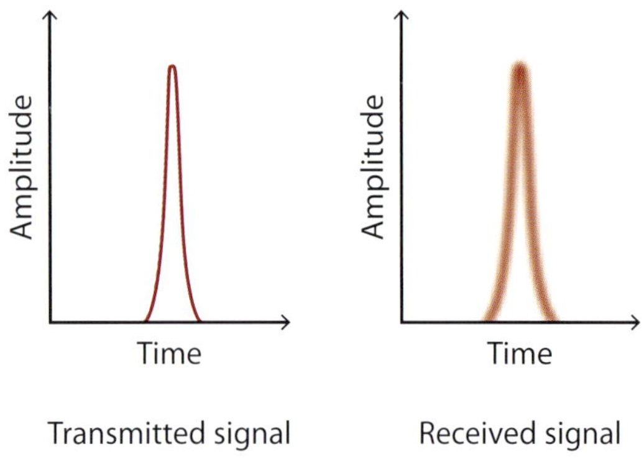

The wave pulse on the left represents one input into a fibre-optic cable. The graph on the right illustrates the output wave pulse. Observe that the amplitude has remained the same but the wave is 'stretched out' in time. This is what is meant by dispersion in the context of propagation.

The fibres used in optical communication are either step-index **single mode** or **multi-mode**.

Single mode

In a **single mode** fibre, the core is very thin. There is also a sharp decrease in the index of refraction at the cladding, which reduces dispersion. This is known as a **step-index**. There is very little difference in the distance between propagation along the axis and along the critical path. In effect, there is only one mode of propagation – along the axis or **very close** to it. With reduced dispersion, the fibre can carry light signals over long distances (many kilometres) and at high transmission speeds, without distortion. However, the main disadvantage of single-mode cables is that they are very expensive to produce. Additionally, only a single wavelength of light can be propagated at one time.

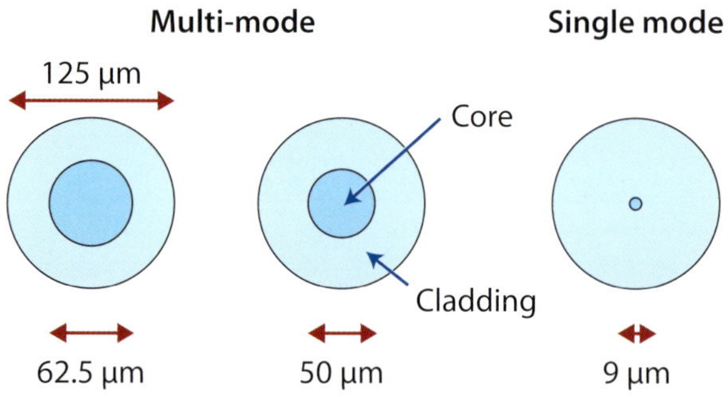

Multi-mode

In a **multi-mode** fibre, the core is thicker and the core-cladding boundary is more gradual (less well-defined). This means that there is more dispersion, which limits the transmission speed and distance over which signals can be carried. However, multi-mode fibres are much cheaper to produce than single mode cables, and so they are typically used within a building or campus where distance is less of an issue and lower transmission speeds are acceptable. They can also carry several wavelengths of light at once.

Summary

Multi-mode optical fibre	Single mode optical fibre
The core is thick (typically > 50 µm).	The core is thin (typically ~ 5 µm).
Several propagation paths are possible (by repeated reflections).	There is a single propagation path along or close to the central axis.
Overlapping signals from multiple paths cause signal distortion.	There is very little signal distortion.
It is used for short distance communication up to about 2 km (such as within a building or on a campus), for example a LAN (local area network).	It is used for long range communication (> 2 km), for example a WAN (wide area network).
It is relatively cheap (compared to single mode) to manufacture.	It is relatively expensive (compared to multi-mode) to manufacture.
It can carry several wavelengths at a time.	It can carry only one wavelength at a time.
The refractive index decreases gradually as you move away from the axis.	There is a step change of refractive index at the core–cladding junction.

Radio waves

Creating radio signals

The reader will already be familiar with two fundamental concepts:

- that radio waves are electromagnetic; and
- an electric current is a flow of electrons which produces a magnetic field.

Scientists have known for a long time that the two concepts are linked, in that causing electrons to accelerate in a conductor produces radio waves. By itself, this is not a very useful phenomenon. However, in the early twentieth century physicists developed a technique for **modulating**, or modifying, these radio waves so that they could 'carry' useful information. This technique can be used to produce a radio **transmitter**.

The simplified below diagram below shows the structure of a simple radio transmitter.

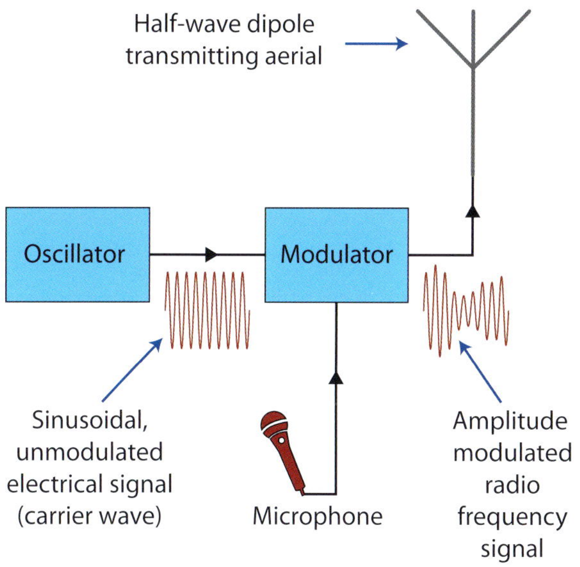

Three key components of the transmitter are as follows:

- The **oscillator** produces a sinusoidal electrical signal of a frequency which can be set by the operator. This frequency is the same as the one to which the listener will tune the radio when the signal is received. It is often called the 'carrier' signal.

Tip: A sinusoidal wave is one in which the displacement changes like a sine wave, just as you may have met in GCSE Mathematics, when studying trigonometry.

- The **modulator** adds together the signal from the oscillator and the audio frequency (AF) signal from the microphone to produce an **amplitude modulated radio frequency signal**. This signal passes up to the aerial.
- In the **aerial** (or antenna) the electrical signal is converted into a radio wave and sent into the atmosphere. The aerial is often of the **half-wave dipole** type. It is sufficient to know that two metal rods, each of a length equal to **one quarter** of the wavelength of the carrier signal, is particularly good at transmitting radio waves. The fact that its total length is about half a wavelength, gives rise to the term 'half-wave dipole'.

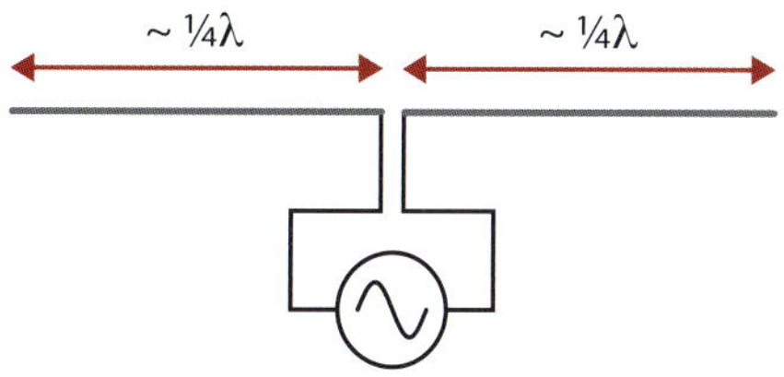

The size of aerial needed is therefore related to the wavelength of the carrier wave. For example, from the wave equation ($v = f\lambda$) we can calculate the wavelength of a 1.5 GHz carrier wave to be 20 cm. So, each dipole is of length 5 cm. This kind of aerial is so small that it can be incorporated within the radio transmitter circuitry – it does not have to be placed on a rooftop!

Receiving radio signals

The reader will recall that all electromagnetic waves are associated with oscillating electric and magnetic fields, which are at right angles to each other and to the direction of propagation of the wave, as shown below.

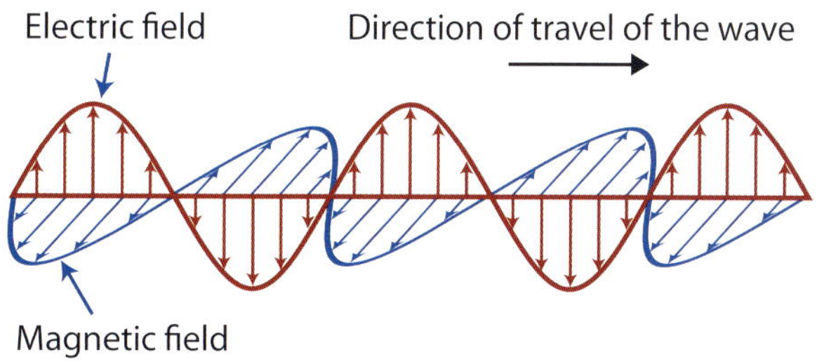

When this magnetic field encounters a metal conductor, it induces a current in it. There are then two problems to solve:

1. how to separate the desired radio signal from all the others in the air; and
2. how to separate the carrier (which has now done its work) from the useful audio frequency signal.

These two problems are solved by a **radio receiver.** The simplified below diagram below shows the structure of a simple radio receiver.

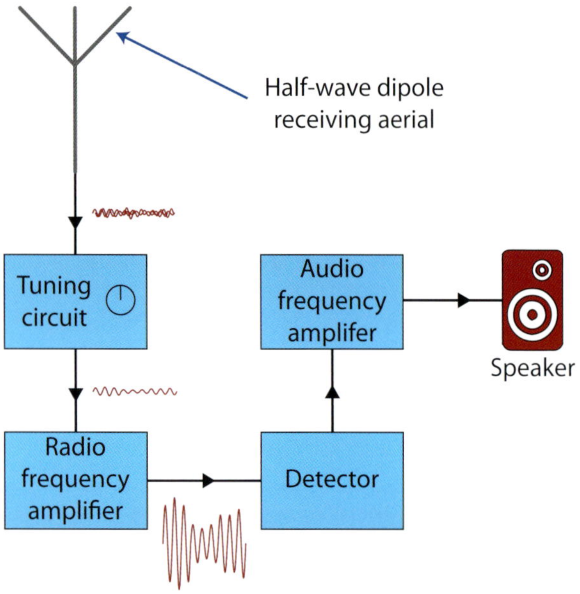

The first problem is solved by the **tuning circuit** which selects the desired signal from all the others in the receiving aerial. As we have seen, the carrier has a specific frequency, set by the oscillator in the transmitter. The tuning circuit can be set to resonate at this desired frequency, that is, it can select the signal required by knowing its carrier frequency. When a person turns the 'station select' knob on a radio, they are changing the frequency of the carrier they wish to receive. Even so, the amplitude of the signal in the tuning circuit is still very small, typically microvolts. It is therefore amplified by the **radio frequency amplifier** before being passed to the detector.

The second problem is solved by the **detector**, sometimes called a **demodulator**, which separates the useful audio frequency signal from the radio frequency carrier. At this point there is enough energy present for the user to hear sound if the signal is passed directly to an earpiece. However, if the requirement is to hear the sound from a **loudspeaker**, then the signal must be increased further using an **audio frequency amplifier**.

One the simplest pieces of radio technology that can be found in homes is a baby monitor. There is a radio transmitter, that sits in the baby's room and a portable radio receiver that the parents use to listen to the baby.

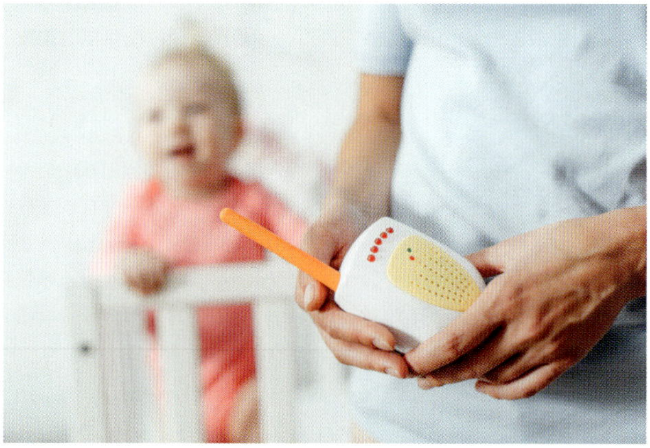

Tip: Make sure you know the names and functions of the major components of a radio transmitter and a radio receiver.

Bluetooth technologies

Radio signals can be used to carry much more than sound. They can also carry signals that can be used to switch devices on or off, transfer computer files, control mobile phones, connect to the internet and so on.

Bluetooth is a radio wave technology that is designed to enable wireless communications between two or more electronic devices over short distances. When two Bluetooth-enabled devices come within range of each other, an electronic conversation automatically takes place between them to determine whether they have data to share or one device needs to take control of the other. This occurs with no (or minimal) intervention by the user. As a result of this conversation the two devices form a radio network, over which information can be exchanged.

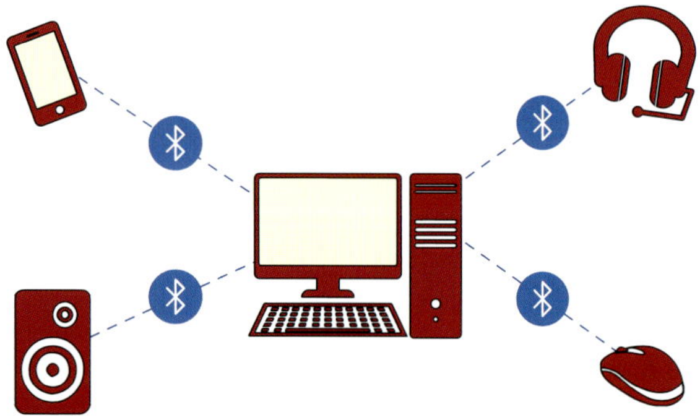

The key benefits of Bluetooth are as follows:

- It can be used to replace cables, which can be cumbersome. For example, a jogger can connect a pair of headphones to their mobile phone via Bluetooth without the need for a cable.
- It can allow even small devices to connect to a network or the internet.
- It is easy to use, and allows users to share files and other information quickly. For example, two mobile phones can exchange files via Bluetooth just by being close to each other.
- It is relatively low-cost.

Bluetooth also has a few disadvantages:

- It has limited range.
- It has relatively low bandwidth.
- Many Bluetooth devices, for example headphones, need to have their own power supply.

Every Bluetooth device has a radio receiver and a radio transmitter built within it. There are three main classes of Bluetooth device, with the power of the transmitter determining its range, as shown in the following table.

Class	Maximum output power / mW	Maximum range / m	Typical use
1	100	100	USB adapters
2	2.5	10	Mobile phones, smartcard readers
3	1	1	Bluetooth adapters

Radar

RADAR is an acronym (an abbreviation which has become a word) for **ra**dio **d**etection **a**nd **r**anging. Radar works by **transmitting** electromagnetic energy in the form of **radio** (or **micro**) **waves** from a dish or antenna toward objects, commonly referred to as **targets**, and **observing the reflected waves** (echoes) returned from them. The targets may be aircraft, ships, spacecraft, road vehicles, astronomical bodies, flying animals (birds, bats and insects) or even precipitation (rain, hail and snow). This list is by no means exhaustive. The radar antenna is part of a **transceiver**, that is, a device that both transmits radar waves towards the target and receives the echoes which come back.

The wavelengths used by radar stations lie in the range 3 cm to 30 cm, but the precise wavelength deployed depends on the application (military, marine, aviation, meteorology etc). Whatever the application, what distinguishes radar from optical and infrared sensing devices is its ability to detect faraway objects even in adverse weather conditions and to determine their range and velocity accurately. The diagram below shows the typical arrangement of a radar transceiver, and what a typical screen seen by a radar operator looks like.

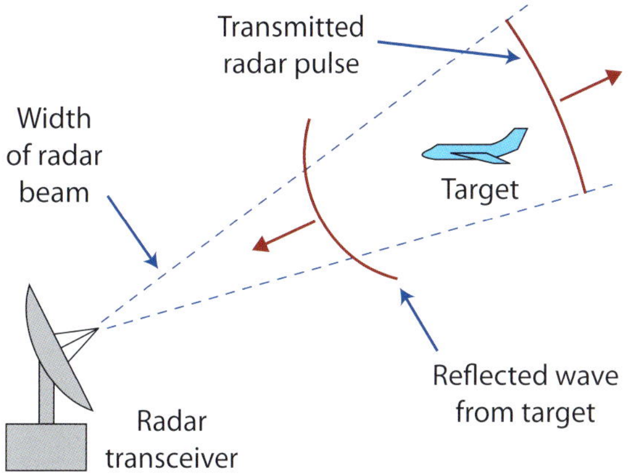

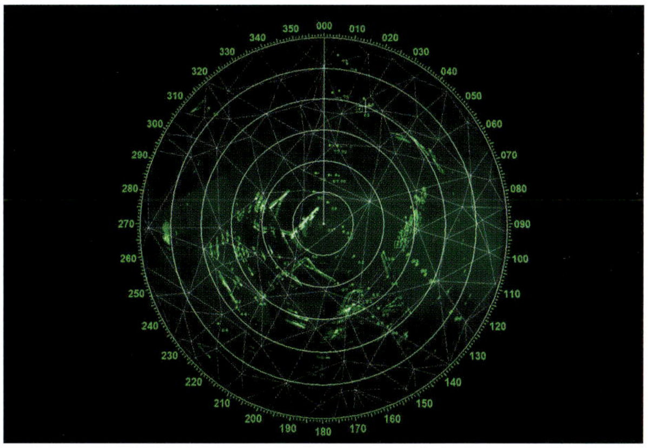

Radar waves are emitted in pulses of short duration (a few microseconds). Between these emissions the radar transmitter is effectively switched off and the station is in 'listening' mode as it receives echoes from the target. The listening time, typically a millisecond, is much longer than the duration of the emitted pulse. The reader who is also taking unit A2 3 Medical Physics will recall that a similar technique is used in ultrasound examinations of the human body. The following graph illustrates two pulse emissions with 'listening' time between them.

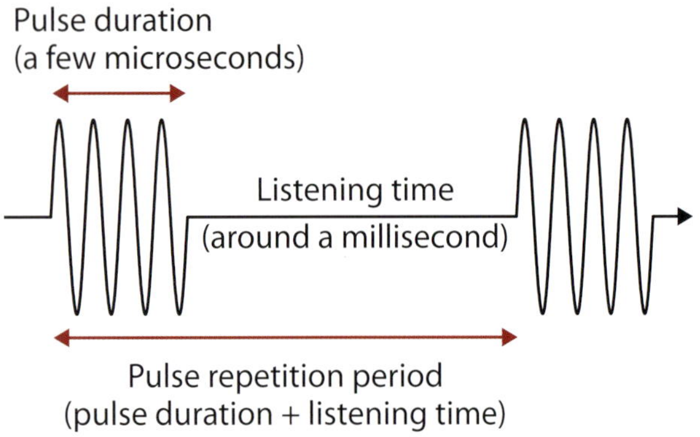

Attenuation

In the context of waves, **attenuation** is the reduction in the intensity of radiation as it propagates away from its source. There are two types of attenuation – space-loss, and path-loss.

Space-loss attenuation

Consider an electromagnetic wave travelling from a point source through space. As it does so, no energy is lost by collision with atoms in the path – there are none. But the energy is spread out more and more as the distance from the source increases, as shown below, reducing its intensity. This is the inverse-square law for radiation and is known as **space-loss attenuation**.

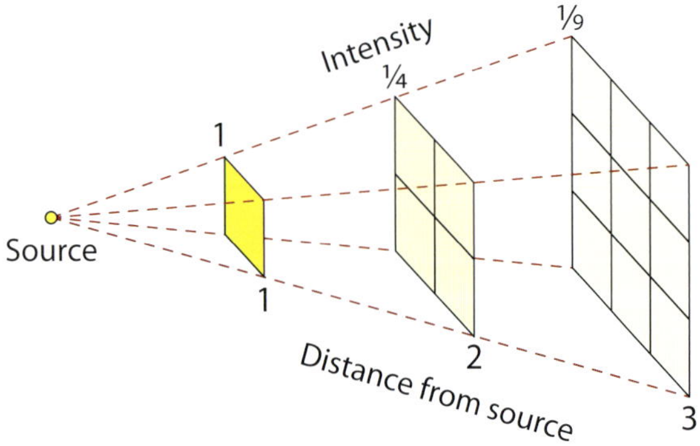

Path-loss attenuation

Path-loss attenuation is the loss of intensity in an electromagnetic wave due to the environment between the transmitter and the receiver. For example, buildings in the path of the wave absorb, reflect and diffract the waves. Environmental geography, such as whether the receiver is at the top of a mountain or deep in a valley, can have a similar effect. Such obstacles serve to reduce the intensity of the wave.

The Doppler effect

The **Doppler effect** applies to all progressive waves. You may have encountered it in GCSE sciences when considering the red-shift in the light coming from distant galaxies. Alternatively, you may have experienced it when listening to the sound of the siren coming from an ambulance as it approaches and then goes past you. However, in this section we will limit the discussion to **radar waves**.

Consider a source of radar emitting waves of frequency, f, as shown in the diagram below. Observers at points A and B will both detect the radar waves with the same frequency.

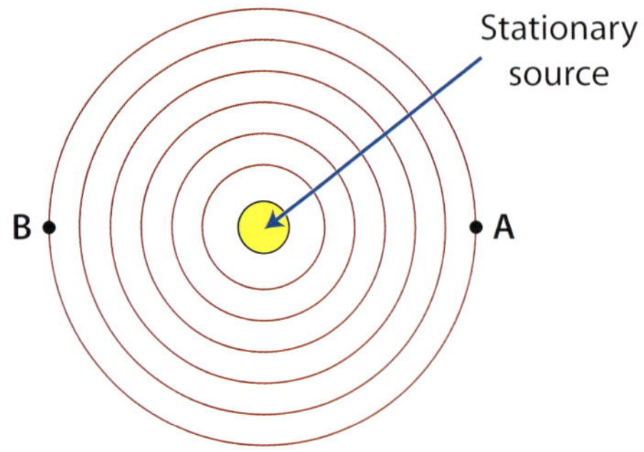

If, now, the source moves towards observer A, an increase in the frequency (and hence a decrease in the wavelength) of the waves will be detected at A. Similarly, observer B will detect a reduced frequency (and hence an increase in the wavelength). This is illustrated in the following diagram.

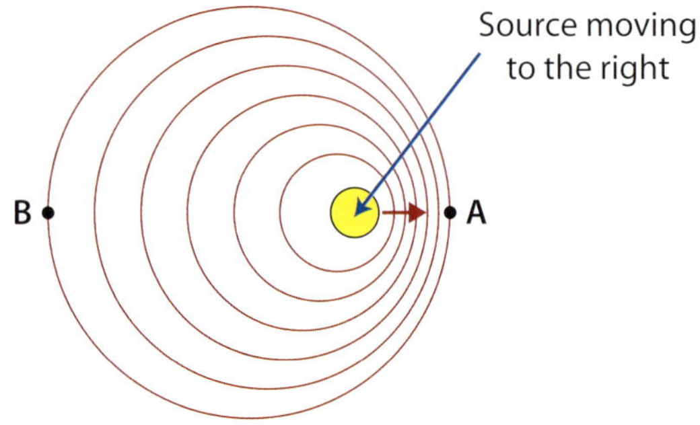

More often than not, the radar ground source is stationary. But if the emitted waves strike a moving target, the waves are reflected and the target becomes a secondary, moving source of radar waves. For the purposes of this unit, the Doppler Effect can be defined as **the changing in frequency of a signal reflected from a moving object**.

This difference in frequency between the transmitted and reflected waves can be used to determine the speed of the target. The bigger the change in frequency, the faster the object is moving.

If the frequency increases, the object is moving towards the observer and if the frequency decreases, the object is moving away from the observer.

Tip: You are sure to get a Quality of Written Communication question somewhere on your exam paper. Get as much practice as you can in answering such questions concisely and accurately.

Questions

1. (a) When light passes from air into glass, it generally bends.
   (i) What name is given to this phenomenon? [1]
   (ii) In which of the two media, air or glass, is the speed of sound greater? [1]
   (iii) Under what circumstance will light passing from air into glass not bend? [1]
   (b) What do you understand by the term 'critical angle' for a glass-air boundary? [1]
   (c) What are the two conditions required for total internal reflection? [2]

2. Describe, in detail, how you would measure the critical angle of glass using a semicircular glass block.
   Your quality of written communication will be assessed in this answer. [6]

3. (a) Draw a labelled diagram of a fibre-optic cable, showing the propagation by total internal reflection. Indicate on your diagram the medium in which the speed of light is greatest. [3]
   (b) In what way is the design of a single mode optical fibre different from that of a multi-mode fibre? [1]
   (c) What is a step-index optical fibre? [2]
   (d) Describe one advantage and one disadvantage of a single mode fibre-optic cable. [2]

4. (a) What is meant by dispersion in fibre-optic technology? [2]
   (b) Describe two ways in which a systems designer might reduce the dispersion caused by a multi-mode fibre. [2]

5. (a) Which type of electromagnetic wave is used in radar systems? [1]
   (b) What do you understand by the Doppler effect in the context of radar systems? [1]
   (c) How are radar waves used to detect aircraft in flight about 50 km from an airport? [3]
   (d) How can the Doppler effect be used to determine the relative motion of these aircraft? [4]

   Ultrasound waves are used to detect moving submarines, radar waves are used to detect moving aircraft.
   (e) Give two reasons why ultrasound waves are unsuitable for detecting moving aircraft. [2]

6. (a) What are the four main components of a radio transmitter? [4]
   (b) (i) A radio transmitter operates on a frequency of 300 MHz using a half-wave dipole aerial consisting of two metal rods. If the speed of radio waves is 3×10^8 m s^{-1}, calculate the length of each of the metal rods. [3]
   (ii) State the frequency of the carrier wave for such a transmitter. [1]
   (c) Radio waves are electromagnetic. What does 'electromagnetic' mean? [2]

7. (a) State three different applications of Bluetooth devices. [3]
   (b) Why is it necessary for Bluetooth devices to have both a radio transmitter and a radio receiver? [1]
   (c) All Bluetooth devices are in one of three different classes. In what way are these classes different? [1]

8. A train's whistle is continuously sounded as the train approaches and passes through a station. The frequency of the sound emitted is 680 Hz and its speed is 340 m s^{-1}. An observer on the station's platform listens carefully to the sound. Describe, in detail, how the wavelength and intensity of the sound observed by the person on the platform change as the train approaches and passes through the station. [6]

14: THE EYE

Students should be able to:

10.6.1 label a diagram of the eye, including the lens, cornea, pupil, iris, ciliary muscles, retina, macula, fovea, optic nerve, aqueous humour and vitreous humour;

10.6.2 describe the functions of each of the constituent parts of the eye in 10.6.1;

10.6.3 demonstrate an understanding of the function of rod and cone cells;

10.6.4 appreciate why two eyes allow stereoscopic vision and three-dimensional sight;

10.6.5 describe accommodation to focus on near and distant objects;

10.6.6 use the lens equation to calculate the optical power of a converging lens and state the unit of power as the dioptre;

10.6.7 carry out experiments to find the optical power of a lens;

10.6.8 given the lens power, use the lens equation to find either the object or image distance; and

10.6.9 practically determine the normal near point for human vision, state that the normal near point is 25 cm from the eye and use this in calculations to correct long sight.

Human vision

The diagram below shows the main parts of the human eye. When light enters the eye, it is focused on the retina and an electrical signal is sent via the optic nerve to the brain which interprets the image. This allows us to see.

The main parts of the eye

The main parts of the eye are as follows:

- The **cornea** is the curved, transparent outer covering of the eye. Most of the light refraction required to produce a focused image on the retina actually occurs in the cornea.
- The **pupil** looks like a black dot in the middle of the eye. This black area is actually a hole that takes in light so the eye can focus on the objects in front of it.
- The **iris** is the area of the eye that contains the pigment which gives the eye its colour. The iris can grow and shrink, closing or widening the pupil and hence controlling the amount of light reaching the retina. If it is too bright, the iris will shrink the pupil, if it is too dull it will enlarge the pupil.

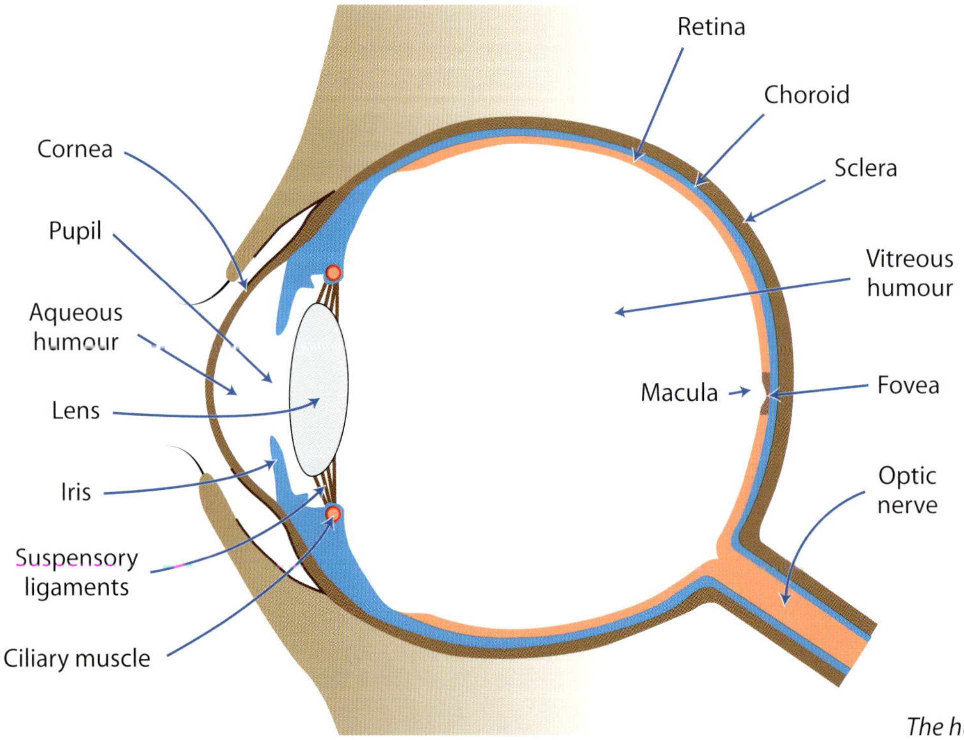

The human eye

- The **lens** sits directly behind the pupil. It is clear and has curved surfaces that focus the light taken in via the pupil. It can change shape so that an image can be sharply focused on the retina.
- The **ciliary muscles** hold and control the movement of the lens using suspensory ligaments. When these muscles contract, the suspensory ligaments pull the lens thicker. When they relax, the suspensory ligaments slacken, allowing the lens to spring back to a thinner more relaxed state, as required.
- The light focused by the lens falls on the **retina**, at the rear of the eye, producing a sharp, real, inverted and diminished image. The retina itself is made of **rods** and **cones** arranged in layers (see next section) which then produce electrical pulses. The retina is connected to the optic nerve that will transmit the signal produced by the rods and cones to the brain so that it can be interpreted.
- The **macula** is located near the centre of the retina. It contains a very high concentration of cones and is responsible for fine detail and colour vision.
- The **fovea** is a tiny pit in the macula that receives light directly and contains only cones. It provides the most finely-detailed area of vision.
- The **optic nerve** is a bundle of nerve fibres that travel from the retina to the brain. Each fibre encodes the image data recorded by the retina in the form of neural signals that can be read by the brain.
- The **aqueous humour** is a clear fluid filling the space in front of the eyeball. It contains water, vitamins and nutrients. It nourishes the lens and provides shape to the eye.
- The **vitreous humour** is transparent gelatinous tissue filling the eyeball behind the lens giving the eye its spherical shape. It takes in nutrients from the aqueous humour and the retinal blood vessels so the eye can remain healthy.

Photoreceptors

Cells which respond to light are called **photoreceptors**. There are two types of photoreceptors in the retina: **rods** and **cones**. They get their names from their shape.

Rods

Rods are responsible for vision at low light levels (twilight vision or scotopic vision) and help us to see moving objects. They are not involved in distinguishing different colours, and are unable to discern fine structures. There are around 120 million of them in the eye, concentrated on the outer edges of the retina and hence give us our peripheral vision.

Cones

Cones are active at higher light levels (photopic vision) and are responsible for our colour vision and our ability to discern fine structures. There are 6 to 7 million of them in the eye, concentrated in and around the fovea, the small pit in the back of the eye that helps with the sharpness or detail of images. There are no rods in the fovea. Cones require much more light to trigger them, which is why at night, although the rods may trigger, everything appears to be in shades of grey.

Tip: Remember – rods are responsible for peripheral vision and the ability to see in dim light; cones are responsible for colour vision and our ability to see fine structures.

Humans normally have three different types of cones. The first responds most to light of longer (red) wavelengths; peaking at about 560 nm; the second responds most to light of medium (green) wavelength, peaking at 530 nm and the third responds most to light of short (blue) wavelength, peaking at 420 nm. This means that different colours in the light reaching the retina stimulate different cone cells and the resulting mix is then processed by the brain to produce a colour image.

Summary

The table on the next page summarises the key differences between rods and cones.

Accommodation

Accommodation is the ability of the eye to produce a sharp image on the retina, depending on whether the object is distant or close to the eye. The human eye has a lens which can **alter its focal length**, using the ciliary muscles. When the lens is thick it gives a short focal length (high power) for focusing on near objects. When the lens is thin it gives a long focal length (low power) for focusing on distant objects. When the eye is focused on very distant objects, it is said to be relaxed.

	Rods	Cones
Intensity of light	More sensitive to light and function well in dim light.	Less sensitive to light and function well in bright light.
Light wavelengths	Only one type of rod is found in the retina. It can absorb all wavelengths of visible light.	Three types of cones are found in the retina. One type is sensitive to red light, one type to blue light and one type to green light.
Ratio of receptor cells to neurones and how this affects vision	The impulses from a group of rod cells pass to a single nerve fibre in the optic nerve – this explains why they function well in dim light, but do not resolve fine structures.	The impulses from a single cone cell pass to a single nerve fibre in the optic nerve – this explains why they can see fine structures.

Summary of the key differences between rods and cones

Stereoscopic vision and three-dimensional sight

Stereoscopic vision is the ability of our brain to process the images from both eyes to create a single image with a perception of depth. Each eye captures a slightly different image. This difference is known as **retinal disparity**. The brain processes these two images in a way that lets us see slightly around solid objects without needing to move our heads. It does this by pairing up the similarities in the two images and then factoring the differences into our perception of a scene, giving us three-dimensional sight. This allows us to judge how far away different objects are.

Lenses

A lens consists of a piece of glass or other transparent material with one or two curved surfaces. Lenses can be classified as **converging** (convex) or **diverging** (concave). The effect of these two types of lens on a parallel beam of light is shown below.

Converging or convex lens

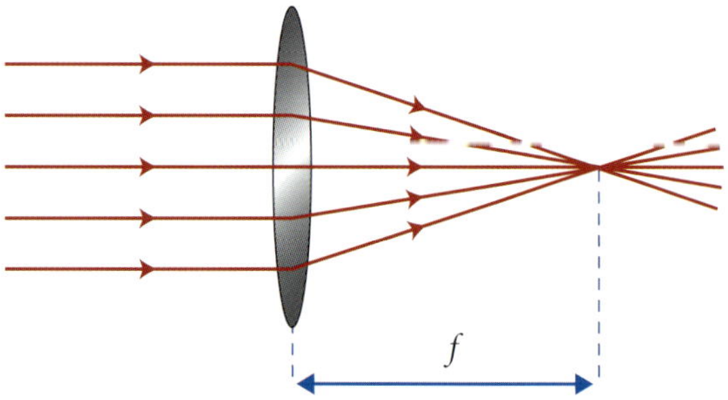

When parallel rays of light pass through a converging lens they are refracted so that they pass through the **focal point** or **principal focus** of the lens. This type of principal focus is described as **real**.

Diverging or concave lens

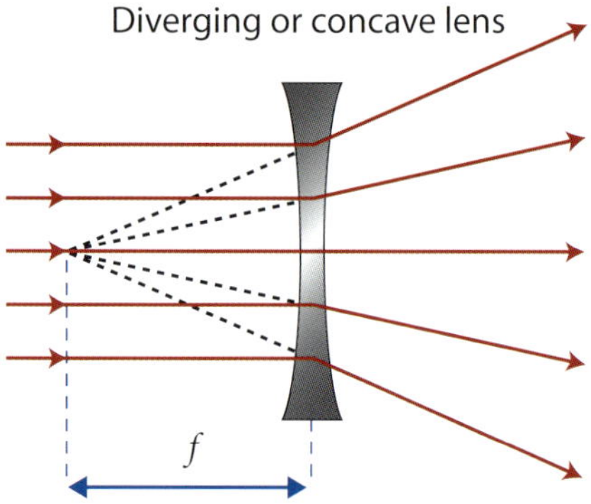

In the case of a diverging lens, the parallel rays are refracted so that they spread out (diverge) from the focal point or principal focus of the concave lens. This type of principal focus is described as **virtual**.

The distance from the centre of a lens to the focal point F is the **focal length**, *f*.

Power of a lens

The **power** of a lens is defined by the equation:

$$P = \frac{1}{f}$$

where P = power (m^{-1}, or dioptres, symbol D)
f = the focal length (m)

A diverging lens has a negative power, while a converging lens has a positive power. For example, a converging lens of focal length 25 cm has a power of +4 D, while a diverging lens of focal length 50 cm has a power of −2 D.

Tip: A common mistake when finding the power of a lens is to forget to change the unit for focal length from centimetres to metres.

Experiment to measure the power of a lens

This is a prescribed experiment which LHS students must be able to describe for their examination.

Method

The apparatus should be set up as shown in the diagram, and includes:

- a convex lens in a lens folder;
- a metre stick taped to the bench;
- a white screen in a holder; and
- an illuminated object (lamphouse with grid).

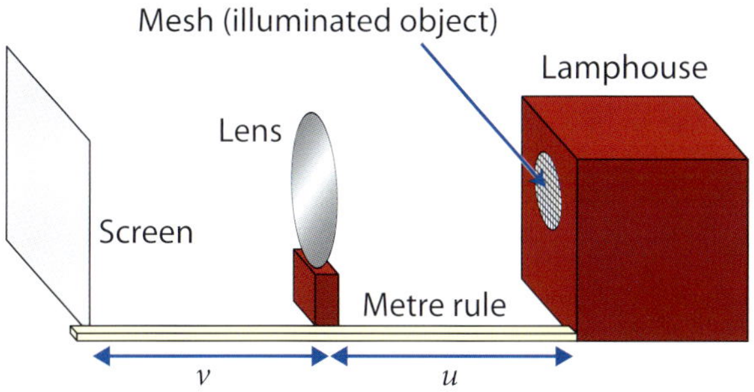

The method is as follows:

1. Place the lens, illuminated object and screen beside the metre stick as shown.
2. Start with the screen and lens close to one end of the stick and the illuminated object close to the other.
3. Slowly move the lens away from the illuminated object towards the screen until a sharp, inverted image of the lamphouse grid is seen on the screen.
4. Using the metre stick, measure and record the object distance from the lens (u) and the image distance from the lens (v).
5. Repeat steps 2 to 4 to obtain a total of 6 values of u along with corresponding values of v.

Typical results for a lens of power +5 D are shown in the following table:

Object distance u / m	0.30	0.35	0.40	0.45	0.50	0.55
Image distance v / m	0.60	0.47	0.40	0.36	0.33	0.31

Using the lens equation to find the power of the lens

There is a mathematical relationship, known as the **lens equation**, which LHS students need to remember and be able to use. This equation is:

$$P = \frac{1}{f} = \frac{1}{u} + \frac{1}{v}$$ where P = power (D)
f = focal length (m)
u = object distance (m)
v = image distance (m)

Rearranging this equation gives:

$$\frac{1}{v} = \frac{1}{f} + (-1)\frac{1}{u}$$

Comparing this with the equation of a straight line, $y = c + mx$, shows that a graph of $\frac{1}{v}$ (vertical axis) against $\frac{1}{u}$ (horizontal axis) will give a straight line of gradient −1 and an intercept on the vertical axis of $\frac{1}{f}$. The graph intercepts the horizontal axis at the point where $\frac{1}{v} = 0$. Hence, the intercept on the horizontal axis is also $\frac{1}{f}$. The graph plotted should therefore be extended to cross both axes and the average intercept found.

The average intercept is the power in dioptres, provided the units on both axes are m^{-1}. The reciprocal of this average intercept is taken as the focal length.

The results shown in the earlier table have been used to plot the graph below. The two intercepts are both 5, giving a value for f of 0.20 m. This verifies that the power of the lens, P = +5 D. Note that the graph also serves as verification of the lens equation.

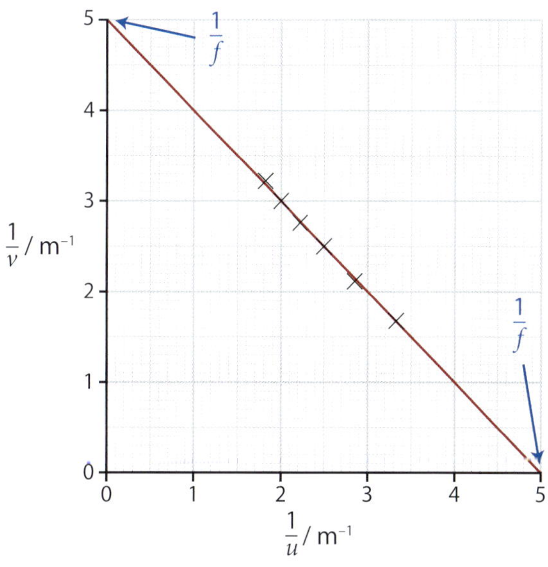

Alternative methods to find lens power

The experimental method described above to find the power of a converging lens is by far the best and most accurate. However, once the table of values of u and v have been found there are different ways to proceed, all of which have appeared in LHS mark schemes.

The non-graphical way is to calculate the mean value of $\left(\frac{1}{u} + \frac{1}{v}\right)$ directly from the table. This mean value is the power, P of the lens. Remember to take the reciprocal of the power if you are required to find the focal length, f.

There are two other graphical methods. The first is to plot the product uv (y-axis) against $u + v$ (x-axis). This graph is a straight line through the origin and its gradient is equal to the focal length, f, as shown below.

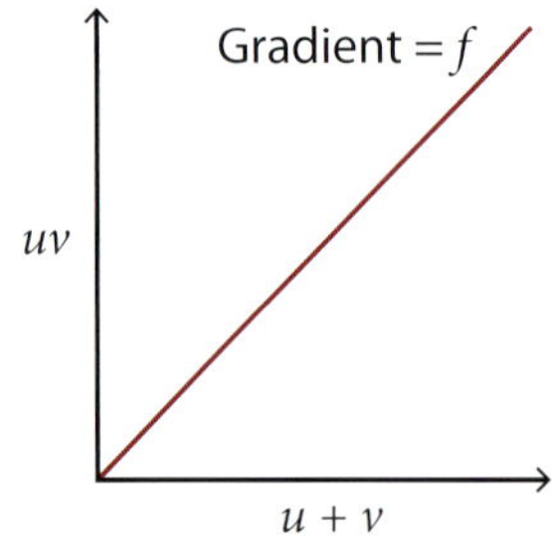

The second method is to plot the graph of u (y-axis) against v (x-axis) and then plot the straight line graph of $u = v$ on the same axes. These graphs will intersect at the point ($2f$, $2f$). Halving the x-coordinate will therefore yield the value of the focal length, f.

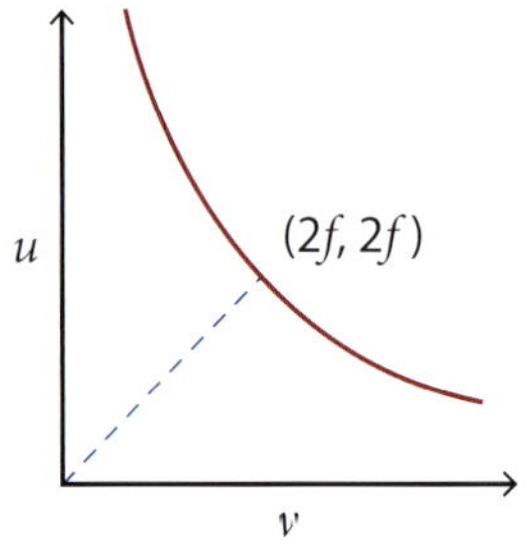

Using the lens equation in calculations

As we have seen, the lens equation is:

$$P = \frac{1}{f} = \frac{1}{u} + \frac{1}{v}$$

However, using the lens equation correctly requires knowledge of the **real-is-positive** sign convention. In this convention, v is taken to be a **positive** number if the image is **real** and a **negative** number if the image is **virtual**.

Tip: Remember, a real image is one which can be projected onto a screen; a virtual image is one which cannot be projected onto a screen.

A converging (convex) lens produces a virtual, erect image when the object is placed at a distance from the lens which is less than the focal length. For all other positions of the object the image is real and inverted (upside down). This can be summarised as:

- If $u < f$, the image is virtual and erect; object and image are on the same side of the lens.
- If $u > f$, the image is real and inverted, object and image are on opposite sides of the lens.

This concept is important and should be remembered.

Worked example

A converging lens produces a real image 60 cm away from the lens when the object is 20 cm from the lens.

(a) Calculate the focal length of the lens and its optical power.

(b) At what distance is the object from the lens when the image produced is 60 cm away from the lens and is virtual?

(c) An object placed 90 cm from the same lens produces an image. Calculate the distance between the object and the image and state whether the image is real or virtual, erect or inverted.

Answer

(a) Since the image is real, v is positive. So:

$$\frac{1}{f} = \frac{1}{u} + \frac{1}{v}$$

$$= \frac{1}{20} + \frac{1}{60}$$

$$= \frac{4}{60} = \frac{1}{15}$$

$$f = \frac{15}{1} = 15 \text{ cm} = 0.15 \text{ m}$$

$$P = \frac{1}{0.15}$$

$$= +6.67 \text{ D}$$

(b) Since the image is virtual, v is negative. In this case $v = -60$ cm. So:

$$\frac{1}{f} = \frac{1}{u} + \frac{1}{v}$$

$$\frac{1}{15} = \frac{1}{u} + \left(\frac{1}{-60}\right)$$

$$\frac{1}{u} = \frac{1}{15} + \frac{1}{60}$$

$$= \frac{5}{60} = \frac{1}{12}$$

$$u = \frac{12}{1} = 12 \text{ cm}$$

So the object is 12 cm from the lens. (Note that this is consistent with the rule that $u < f$ when the image is virtual.)

(c) Since $u > f$, the image is real and inverted (and on the opposite side of the lens to the object). So:

$$\frac{1}{f} = \frac{1}{u} + \frac{1}{v}$$

$$\frac{1}{15} = \frac{1}{90} + \frac{1}{v}$$

$$\frac{1}{v} = \frac{1}{15} - \frac{1}{90}$$

$$= \frac{5}{90} = \frac{1}{18}$$

$$v = 18 \text{ cm}$$

So the distance between object and image

$= u + v$

$= 90 + 18$

$= 108$ cm

Tip: When using the lens equation, remember that if the image is virtual, the value of v is negative.

Long-sightedness

Normal vision

As we have seen, the human eye can alter its focal length to see objects clearly at different distances, an ability known as accommodation.

The farthest point which can be seen clearly by the unaided eye is called the **far point**. For a normal eye, this is at infinity. Light from the far point reaches the eye as parallel rays. The rays are refracted by the eye so that they meet on the retina forming a sharp image of the distant object, as shown:

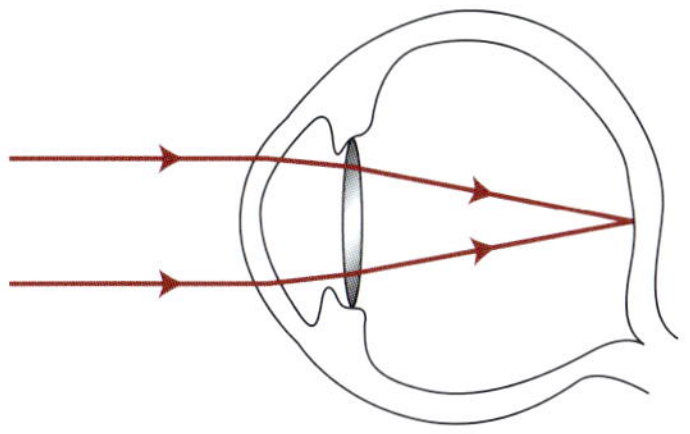

The nearest point which can be seen clearly by the unaided eye is called the **near point**. It is usually 25 cm from the eye. Although the normal eye can focus for a short time on objects closer than 25 cm, the eye muscles will quickly become strained. The following diagram shows rays being refracted from the near point to meet on the retina.

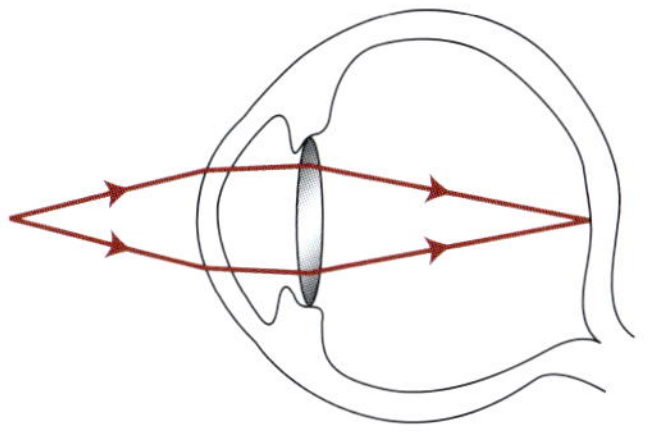

Long sight (hypermetropia)

A person is said to have long sight (hypermetropia) if their near point is further away than 25 cm. The eyeball is too short, **so the light is brought to a focus behind** the retina. A long-sighted eye has no difficulty focusing on far away objects but cannot produce enough converging power to create a focused image of nearby objects, as shown below.

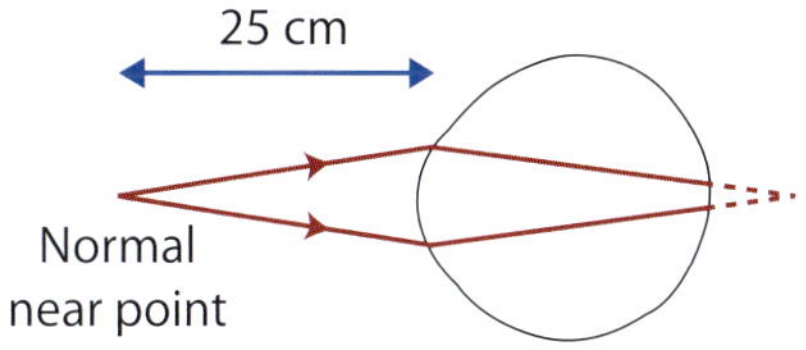

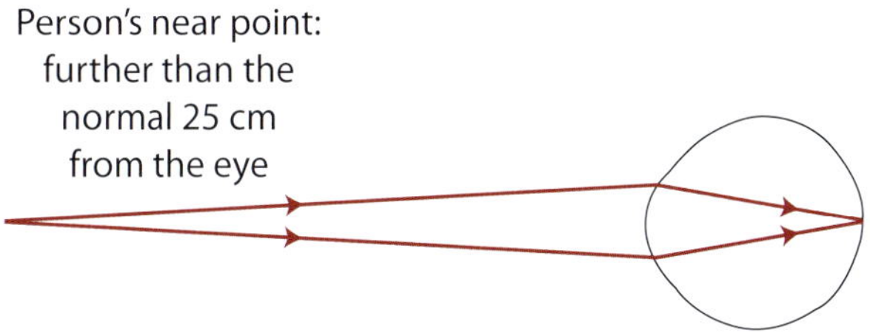

When not wearing their glasses, people with long sight tend to hold a book or newspaper as far from their eyes as their arms will reach in order to read it!

Correcting long sight

A long sighted person needs glasses with a **converging** (convex) lens to view objects close to the eye. Given the near point of someone with long sight, LHS students must be able to calculate the power of the correcting lens. This is illustrated in the following worked example.

Worked example

A patient with long sight has a near point of 75 cm. What is the focal length and power of the lens required to correct this defect of vision?

Answer

Suppose an object is placed at a distance of 25 cm from the eye, the normal near point. We have to find the power of the converging lens which will give a **virtual** image of this object at the patient's near point. This means that for the patient, the light now appears (hence 'virtual') to be coming from the near point, 75 cm from the eye. Remember that converging lenses give a virtual image only when $u < f$.

$$\frac{1}{f} = \frac{1}{u} + \frac{1}{v}$$

$$\frac{1}{f} = \frac{1}{25} + \frac{1}{(-75)}$$

(v is negative because the image is virtual)

$$\frac{1}{f} = 0.02666 \text{ cm}^{-1}$$

$f = 37.5$ cm (consistent with $u < f$)

When finding the power, remember that f must be in metres. So:

$f = 0.375$ m

Then using:

$$P = \frac{1}{f}$$

$$= \frac{1}{0.375}$$

$$= +2.67 \text{ D}$$

Note that this lens corrects the patient's long sight – but when wearing these glasses, distant objects will now appear blurred. This problem can be overcome by the use of bifocals – where the top part of the lens is plain glass for distance vision, the bottom is a converging lens for close-up vision.

Determining the position of the near point

While the normal near point is 25 cm from the eye, this figure varies from person to person – it is, for example, smaller for young people and those suffering from short sight, and larger for older people and those suffering from long sight. The following diagram shows one way in which the near point might be found.

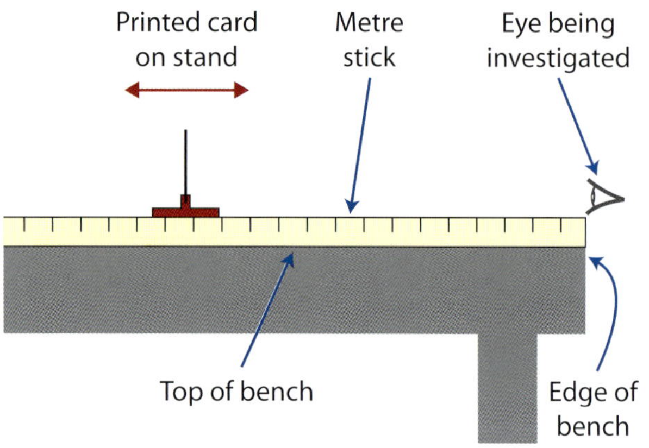

The method is as follows:

1. The person whose eye is being investigated looks over a metre stick at eye level.
2. A printed card is moved, beside the metre stick, from 1 m distance towards the person's eye.
3. When the image on the card can no longer be seen without strain, the distance, d_1, to the eye is measured.
4. The card is then moved from a point very close to the eye and the person indicates when the image on the card can just be seen without strain. The distance, d_2, to the card from the eye is measured.
5. Steps 2 to 4 are repeated about 6 times. The mean value of the measured distances from the card to the eye is then taken as the near point.

Questions

1. (a) Below is a line drawing of the human eye. Copy the table and in the appropriate places write the name and function of each of the parts A – F.

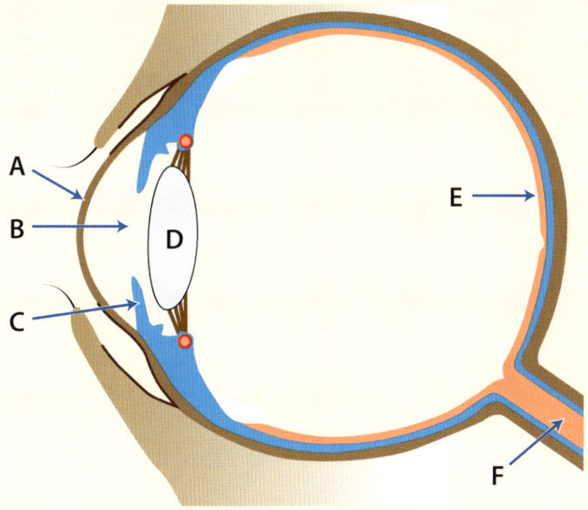

Part	Name	Function
A		
B		
C		
D		
E		
F		

(b) Rods and cones are different types of cells found in the retina of the human eye. Copy the table below, placing a tick (√) in the appropriate box to show whether the statement refers to the rods or the cones. One has already been done for you.

Statement	Rods	Cones
There are more than 120 million of these cells in the retina.	√	
They are used for our peripheral vision and are concentrated in the outer edges of the retina.		
They are responsible for straight-ahead vision.		
They allow us to see colour.		
They are only found in the fovea.		
They cannot discern sharp images or perceive fine detail.		
They are responsible for sensing motion.		
They cells are needed for the perception of light and darkness and adapting to night-time vision.		

2. (a) (i) Describe the major changes in the eye when we view a distant object moving to a point which is very close to us. [3]

(ii) What name is given to the phenomenon described in part (i)? [1]

(b) (i) What is stereoscopic vision? [1]

(ii) What aspect of human anatomy allows us to have stereoscopic vision? [1]

3. (a) (i) What is long sight? [1]

(ii) Copy and complete the diagram below to show what happens to the rays of light coming from a person's normal near point and entering this long-sighted eye.

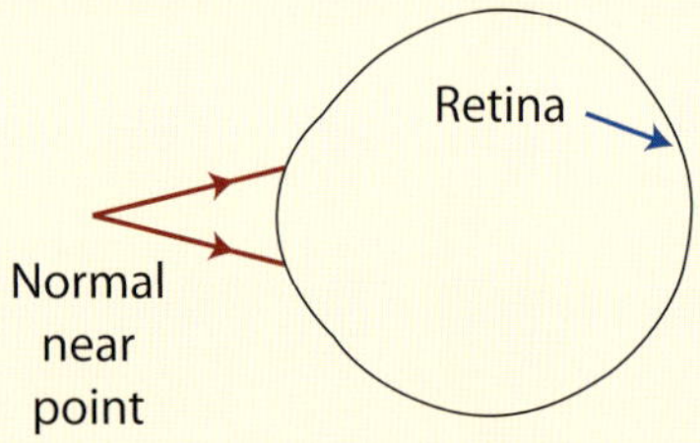

[3]

(b) To correct a defect in his vision, a student must wear glasses containing a lens of optical power +2.5 D.

(i) From what defect of vision is this person suffering? [1]

With the glasses prescribed this student's near point is 25 cm from his eye.

(ii) Calculate the position of the student's near point without glasses. [4]

4. (a) In what way is the **shape** of the lens in the human eye different when viewing distant objects compared to when it is viewing close-up objects? [1]

(b) The distance between the centre of the lens in the human eye and the retina is approximately 2 cm.

(i) What is the optical power of the lens in the eye required to focus on an object 25 cm away? [2]

A certain woman's near point is 2.0 m from her eyes.

(ii) Show that the maximum power of her unaided eye is +50.5 D. [1]

(iii) Hence find the power of the converging lens in her glasses if her long sight is to be corrected. [1]

Unit A2 5:
Genetics, Gene Technology and Stem Cells

15: DNA AND THE GENETIC CODE

Students should be able to:

11.1.1 recall that DNA is an information-carrying molecule and that its sequence of bases determines the structure of proteins, including enzymes;

11.1.2 describe the double helix structure of DNA, which enables it to act as a stable information-carrying molecule, in terms of:
- the components of DNA nucleotides – deoxyribose, phosphate and the bases adenine, cytosine, guanine and thymine;
- two sugar-phosphate backbones held together by hydrogen bonds between base pairs; and
- specific base pairing;

11.1.3 provide evidence for the structure of DNA via:
- chemical analysis;
- Chargaff's work on base equivalence;
- Franklin and Wilkins' work on X-ray crystallography; and
- Watson and Crick's work on modelling;

11.1.4 describe and explain the structure and function of ribonucleic acid (RNA), including ribosomal, transfer and messenger RNA and compare with that of DNA;

11.1.5 describe genes and polypeptides;

11.1.6 explain how a gene occupies a fixed position, called a locus, on a particular strand of DNA;

11.1.7 recall that genes are sections of DNA that contain coded information as a specific sequence of bases;

11.1.8 recall that genes code for polypeptides which determine the nature and development of organisms;

11.1.9 demonstrate an understanding of how the base sequence of a gene can change as a result of a mutation, including base deletion, insertion and substitution, producing one or more alleles of the same gene;

11.1.10 recall that a sequence of three bases, called a triplet, codes for a specific amino acid;

11.1.11 demonstrate an understanding that the base sequence of a gene determines the amino acid sequence in a polypeptide;

11.2.1 describe a mechanism for the exact copying or replication of DNA;

11.2.2 explain briefly the three theories of replication of DNA that existed:
- dispersive;
- conservative; and
- semi-conservative;

11.2.3 describe and explain in detail the semi-conservative hypothesis derived by Meselson and Stahl in 1958, including:
- the unwinding of the double helix;
- the breakage of hydrogen bonds between complementary bases in the polynucleotide strands;
- the role of DNA helicase in unwinding DNA and breaking its hydrogen bonds;
- the attraction of new DNA nucleotides to exposed bases on template strands and base pairing;
- the role of DNA polymerase in the condensation reaction that joins adjacent nucleotides; and
- comparison with the dispersive and conservative model.

The structure and function of DNA

Nucleotides and base pairing

Deoxyribose nucleic acid (DNA) is an information-carrying linear molecule which is formed of a long chain of **nucleotides**. Each **nucleotide** consists of three components:

- **deoxyribose** (a sugar);
- a **phosphate**;
- a nitrogenous **base**.

The three components are bonded together as shown in the following diagram to produce a nucleotide.

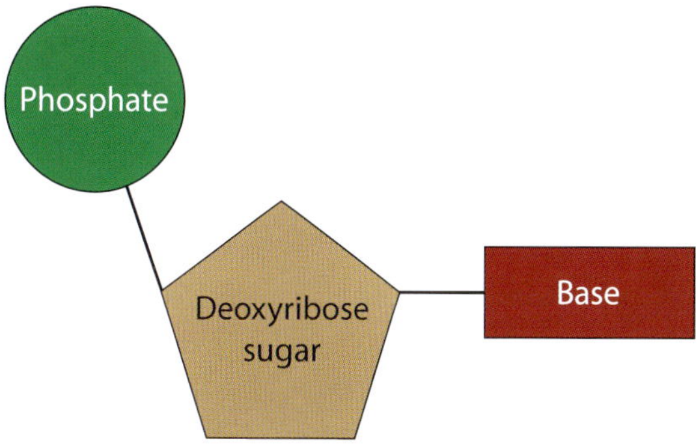

A nucleotide

Tip: Remember that each nucleotide consists of one phosphate, one deoxyribose sugar and one base.

The nucleotides are linked together as shown in the following diagram. Phosphodiester bonds link adjacent nucleotides together to form a long chain or strand which acts as the backbone of the DNA.

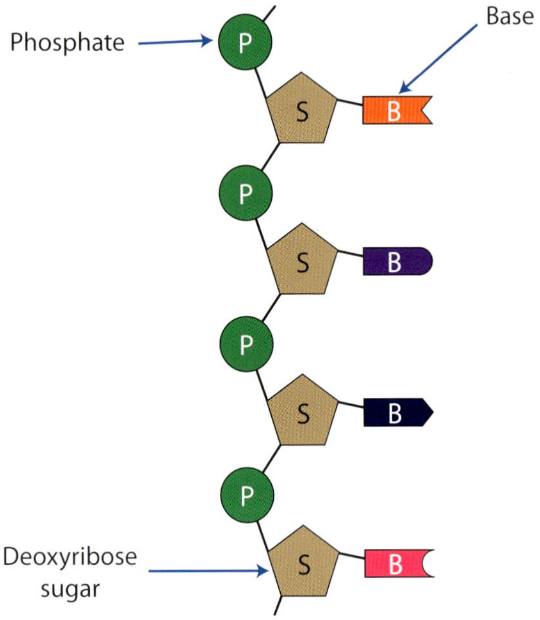

Linking nucleotides together to form a DNA backbone

Although the phosphate and the deoxyribose (sugar) components of DNA are unchanged throughout the DNA molecule, there are four different types of base, these being **adenine**, **guanine**, **cytosine** and **thymine**, giving four different types of nucleotide. The names of these bases are often shortened to the letters A, G, C and T.

Furthermore, the bases on adjacent (backbone) strands combine together in a process known as complementary **base pairing**. The nature of base pairing ensures that:

- **adenine** only pairs with **thymine** (by two hydrogen bonds);
- **guanine** only pairs with **cytosine** (by three hydrogen bonds).

Base pairing allows two side-by-side sugar-phosphate backbones to link together through hydrogen bonds linking complementary bases together. In terms of chemical structure, adenine and guanine are **purines** (containing two rings of atoms) and thymine and cytosine are **pyrimidines** (containing a single ring of atoms). This means that paired bases in DNA will contain one purine and one pyrimidine.

A molecule of DNA consists of two anti-parallel strands joined together by hydrogen bases – the strands are described as **anti-parallel** as they run in opposite directions, as can be seen by the shape of the deoxyribose sugars in the following diagram.

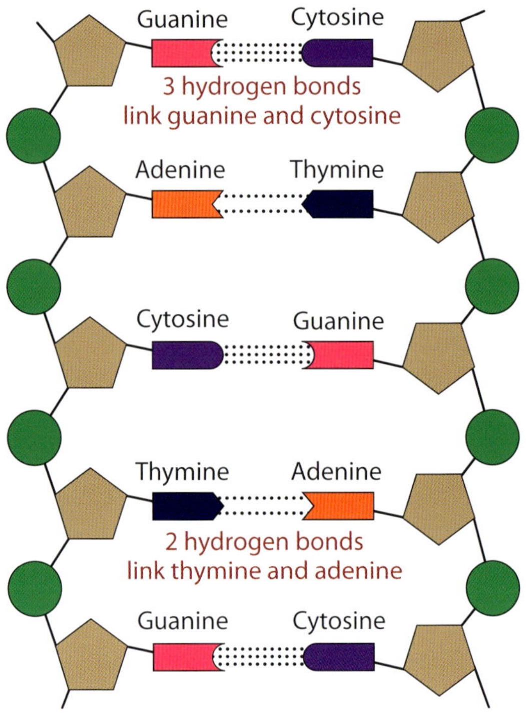

A short section of DNA

Tip: The diagram shows that only A – T and C – G base combinations are possible, and that the DNA molecule consists of two long, sugar-phosphate backbones linked together by hydrogen bonds formed between complementary bases.

The DNA molecule is organised as a **double helix**, with each of the strands being wound round each other like a twisted ladder, linked and held together by the bases. The organisation of the DNA is very regular, with a set number of base pairs for each turn of the helix as shown in the diagram on the next page.

DNA as an information-carrying molecule

The fact that DNA has four different types of base is important in its role as an information-carrying molecule. It is the **sequence of bases**, along one strand, that **determines the structure** of **polypeptides** and **proteins**. Proteins are very important in living organisms and they include structural proteins such as found in muscle and functional proteins such as enzymes and antibodies.

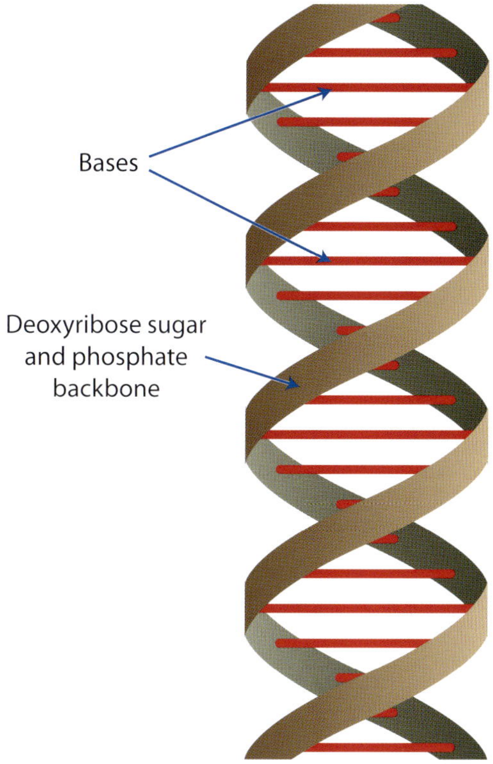

The Double Helix

Tip: Remember that it is the **sequence** of bases, (e.g. T,T,G,C,T,A etc) along **one** strand that is important in DNA's information-carrying role and that this sequence determines the type and structure of polypeptides and proteins formed within each cell, which in turn determine the nature and development of organisms.

Tip: The bases form the 'genetic' code in DNA, but it is also important to remember that it is the hydrogen bonds between bases that hold the two sugar-phosphate backbones together.

Worked example

(a) Name the three components of a nucleotide.
(b) Name the type of bond which links the bases of adjacent DNA strands together.
(c) Using examples, explain what is meant by the term 'specific base pairing'.

Answer

(a) Deoxyribose (sugar), phosphate and a base.
(b) Hydrogen.
(c) That only thymine can combine with adenine and only cytosine can combine with guanine (or converse) (linking the two strands of DNA together).

Key players in working out the structure of DNA

It took many years for scientists to work out the structure of DNA and, as with many scientific breakthroughs, knowledge came in small steps until a final understanding was achieved.

By 1950 scientists had worked out that DNA was the molecule that determined how organisms developed, yet its structure was still unknown. **Chemical analysis** had shown that the DNA molecule contained deoxyribose sugar, phosphate and nitrogen bases. In 1950 Erwin **Chargaff** worked out that a DNA molecule contained an **equal number of units** (equal amounts) of adenine and thymine and the same with cytosine and guanine (i.e. **base equivalence**). He also concluded that the **relative amounts of the four bases varied between species**.

Tip: The two conclusions in the previous paragraph are often referred to as 'Chargaff's rules'.

Rosalind **Franklin** and Maurice **Wilkins** were able to build on Chargaff's work using **X-ray crystallography** (X-ray diffraction). By firing beams of X-rays into DNA molecules and analysing the pattern produced by the beams they were able to work out some details of DNA's three-dimensional structure. Franklin and Wilkins work was able to show that DNA had a **helical structure** with **phosphate on the outside**.

The final part of the DNA structure jigsaw was pieced together by James **Watson** and Francis **Crick** in 1953. Building on the work of the earlier discoveries, and by using large, complex **models** in their laboratory in Cambridge, they were able to work out the structure of DNA, including how the different bases link together to hold the two backbones in place. It was Watson and Crick who appreciated that DNA was formed of a **'double' helix**, i.e. **two** intertwined backbones, rather than a single coiled strand.

Polypeptides, proteins and genes

A **polypeptide** is a sequence of amino acids linked together by peptide bonds. **Proteins** are molecules formed of one or more polypeptides – for example, haemoglobin is a protein formed of four polypeptides, two each of two different types.

Amino acids are the building blocks of polypeptides and proteins. The structure of a generalised amino acid is represented by the following diagram.

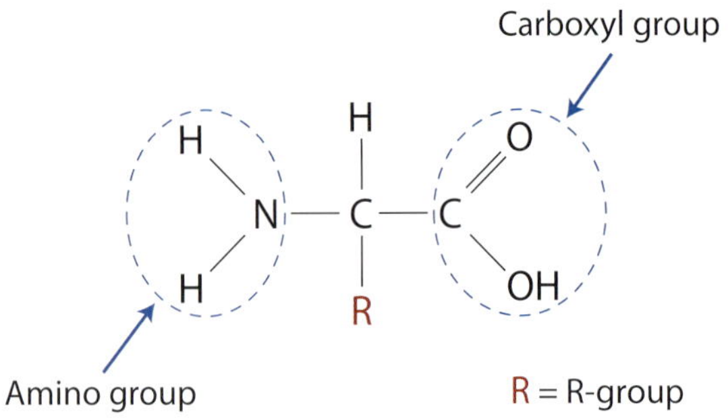

A generalised amino acid

The R-group is different in each amino acid. Three examples are shown in the following diagram.

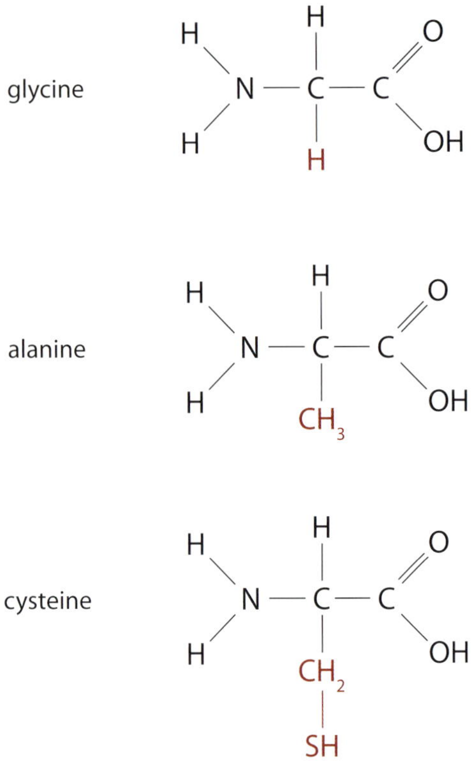

Some amino acids

The diagram below shows how the amino acids are linked together in a polypeptide. The NH_2 (amino group) and COOH (carboxyl group) are at the ends of the polypeptide as they each can only bond with one other amino acid.

There are twenty different types of amino acid and so polypeptides (and proteins) differ in the number of amino acids, the types of amino acid present and the sequence in which these amino acids are linked together by peptide bonds.

Tip: You should remember that polypeptides differ from each other in many ways including:
- the number of amino acids they have;
- the types of amino acid they have;
- the sequence in which the amino acids are arranged.

Each polypeptide in a cell is coded for by a **gene**. A gene is a section of DNA which codes for a particular polypeptide; it is the **linear sequence** of nitrogenous **bases** along one of the two backbone strands, the **template strand**, that forms the **DNA code**.

Not all genes are the same size – a gene which codes for a long polypeptide will be much longer than a gene that codes for a shorter polypeptide (you will see why later). Additionally, the position of a gene along a length of DNA is fixed, relative to other genes. A gene's position is referred to its **locus**.

How does the DNA code work?

We have already noted that it is the bases along one side (strand) of the DNA molecule that forms the genetic code. Each sequence of three bases along this coding strand codes for a particular amino acid and the sequence of three bases that code for an amino acid is called a **base triplet**. DNA is therefore a (very) long sequence of base triplets arranged in order, coding for amino acids in a very specific sequence.

Tip: It is very important that the amino acids are arranged in sequence – this is the primary structure of the polypeptide – as this will allow the polypeptide to fold and twist and form bonds in the correct position to become its functioning, finished form.

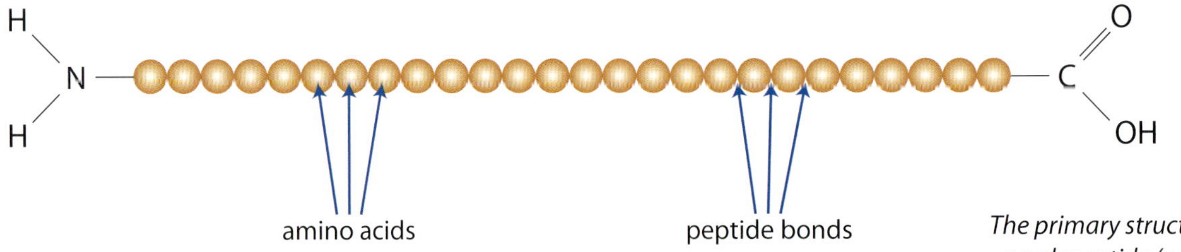

The primary structure of a polypeptide (protein)

The following diagram represents a very short section of DNA with four base triplets. It is important to note that only the coding (or template) strand of DNA in this section is shown.

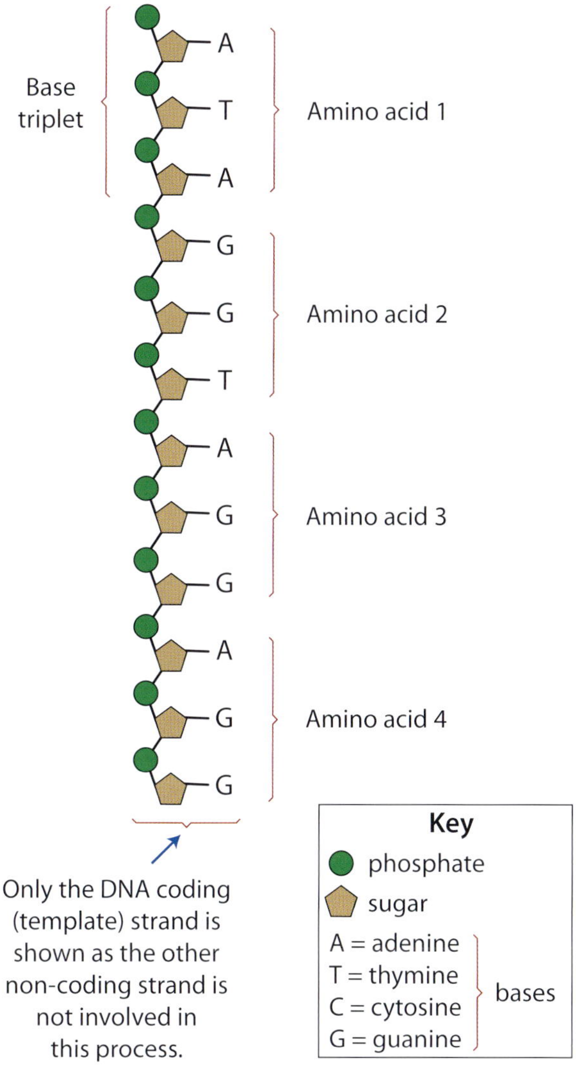

Base triplets and coding for amino acids

Note that the third base triplet and the fourth base triplet in the diagram are the same. This means that the amino acids coded for by these triplets will be the same. As there are only twenty different types of amino acid, obviously a large polypeptide (containing well over 100 amino acids) will contain many of the same type of amino acid.

Tip: The diagram above shows that only one strand (the coding or template strand) actually codes for amino acids. The other strand provides stability and is important in DNA replication (see later).

Tip: Only some of the DNA is coding (around 2%), i.e. has bases that code for amino acids. The other 98% is non-coding – some contain 'switches' that regulate gene activity by switching genes on or off, and some other parts have no known function.

Mutations

Although DNA is a very stable molecule, permanent changes to it do occur and these changes are called **mutations**. There are many different types of mutation, affecting from as little as one base to whole chromosomes.

Base substitution

The simplest type of mutation involves a **base substitution**, in which **one base replaces** (substitutes) for **another base**. An example of a base substitution is shown in the following diagram, in which a G base replaces a C base in the third base triplet shown.

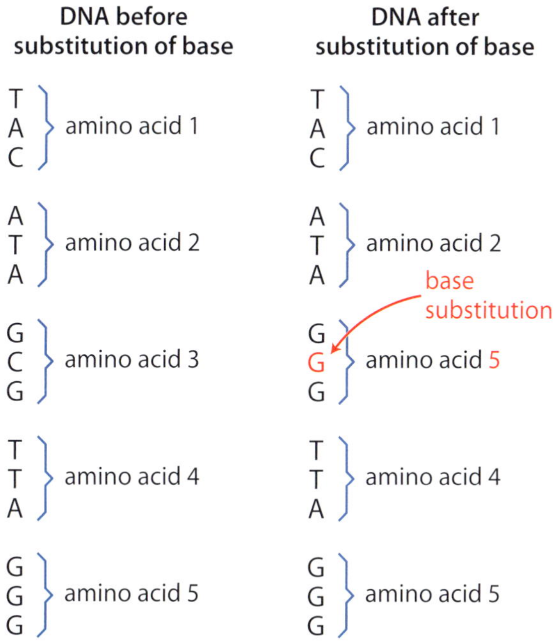

A mutation involving the replacement of a single base

Note that in this example the change of a single base results in a different amino acid being produced at that point in the sequence. This may, or may not, have a significant effect on the polypeptide being produced.

Base deletion

In a mutation involving a **base deletion, one base is removed** (deleted) from the DNA sequence (gene). The result of this can be very significant, as base deletions cause '**frameshift**' mutations due to the DNA sequence being read in 'threes'. A base deletion results in the base triplet templates being changed throughout the gene from the point of deletion on, meaning that all the amino acids produced from that point in the gene may change as shown in the diagram below.

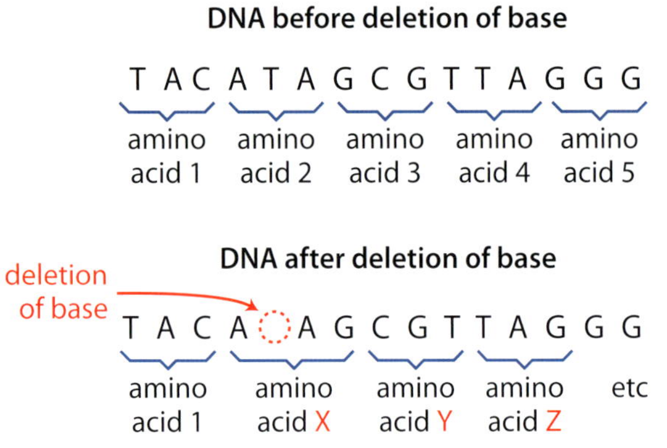

A base mutation involving the loss of a single base'

Base insertion

In a mutation involving a **base insertion, one base is added** (inserted) into the DNA sequence (gene). As with base deletions, this can have significant consequences as it also results in a frameshift mutation with all the amino acids produced from that point in the gene on being affected.

Mutations change the base sequence in a gene – the different forms of a gene (produced by mutation) are referred to as **alleles**.

Tip: Remember that the loss or addition of a base (**deletion** and **insertion** respectively) will have a much greater effect than a base substitution. This is because, with bases being read in threes (base triplets), the 'reading frame' is adjusted so that **all** base triplets and amino acids are affected beyond the point of mutation. With a base substitution only affecting one base triplet, and other triplets being unaffected, this will have a much smaller affect.

Tip: Remember that **mutations are permanent changes** to the DNA and these changes can pass to any offspring.

Worked example

(a) The partially-completed table below shows the percentages of the different types of bases in a chromosome.

Bases	adenine	guanine	cytosine	thymine
% of each base		22		

(i) Copy and complete the table to calculate the percentages of the other three bases.

(ii) State one similarity and one difference that would be expected for these percentages in a different chromosome.

(b) (i) Describe what is meant by the term base triplet.

(ii) Explain the consequence of a mutation leading to a different base being present in a base triplet.

Answer

(a) (i)

Bases	adenine	guanine	cytosine	thymine
% of each base	28	22	22	28

If 22% of the bases are guanine, 22% must be cytosine (as these two bases are complementary). Therefore, 44% of the bases are G and C. The remaining 56% must be equally split between adenine and thymine.

(ii) The number of adenine and thymine bases would be the same as each other and this would also apply to cytosine and guanine bases. (While the number of A and T bases would be the same as would the number of C and G bases), the relative proportion of the number of A and T bases to the number of C and G bases would not be the same in different chromosomes.

(b) (i) A base triplet is a sequence of three bases on the coding/template strand of DNA which codes for a particular amino acid.

(ii) A different amino acid would be coded for leading to a polypeptide which differs by one amino acid from the polypeptide normally produced.

Different types of nucleic acid

DNA belongs to a group of molecules called **nucleic acids**. The other major type of nucleic acid is **ribose nucleic acid (RNA)**, and unlike with DNA, there are several forms of RNA.

RNA has many **similarities** with DNA, including that it consists of a backbone of alternating phosphates and sugars, with four different types of bases.

However, there are important **differences**, including that RNA exists in **single strand** form, the sugar is **ribose** (rather than deoxyribose) and the base **uracil** is used rather than thymine. Furthermore, there are three different types of RNA as outlined below.

Messenger RNA (mRNA)

Chromosomes (and therefore DNA) occur in the nucleus, but polypeptide and protein synthesis takes place in the cytoplasm of cells. Therefore, there must be some way that the genetic code is able to get from the nucleus to the cytoplasm. In reality, the code is copied from the DNA into **messenger RNA (mRNA)** in the nucleus – a process called **transcription** – and it is the mRNA which travels from the nucleus to the cytoplasm carrying the code.

Transcription is summarised in the diagram below. As the mRNA is formed on the basis of 'base pairing' with the DNA **template strand** (although the two complementary bases do not remain linked together), the mRNA 'code' is not an exact copy of the DNA template strand; it is a **complementary** copy instead.

When the mRNA reaches the cytoplasm, it links to a **ribosome**, another structure important in protein synthesis.

Tip: Note, in the diagram, that the base **uracil** is used in mRNA where you would expect thymine to be and that the mRNA has the sugar **ribose** and is **single-stranded**.

Tip: The mRNA coding for a particular polypeptide is much shorter that the length of the DNA in an entire chromosome (making it easier for it to move out of the nucleus) – the length of mRNA corresponds to the length of that gene in the DNA. Using mRNA as the messenger also protects the DNA as the cytoplasm (site of protein synthesis) is more volatile than the nucleus.

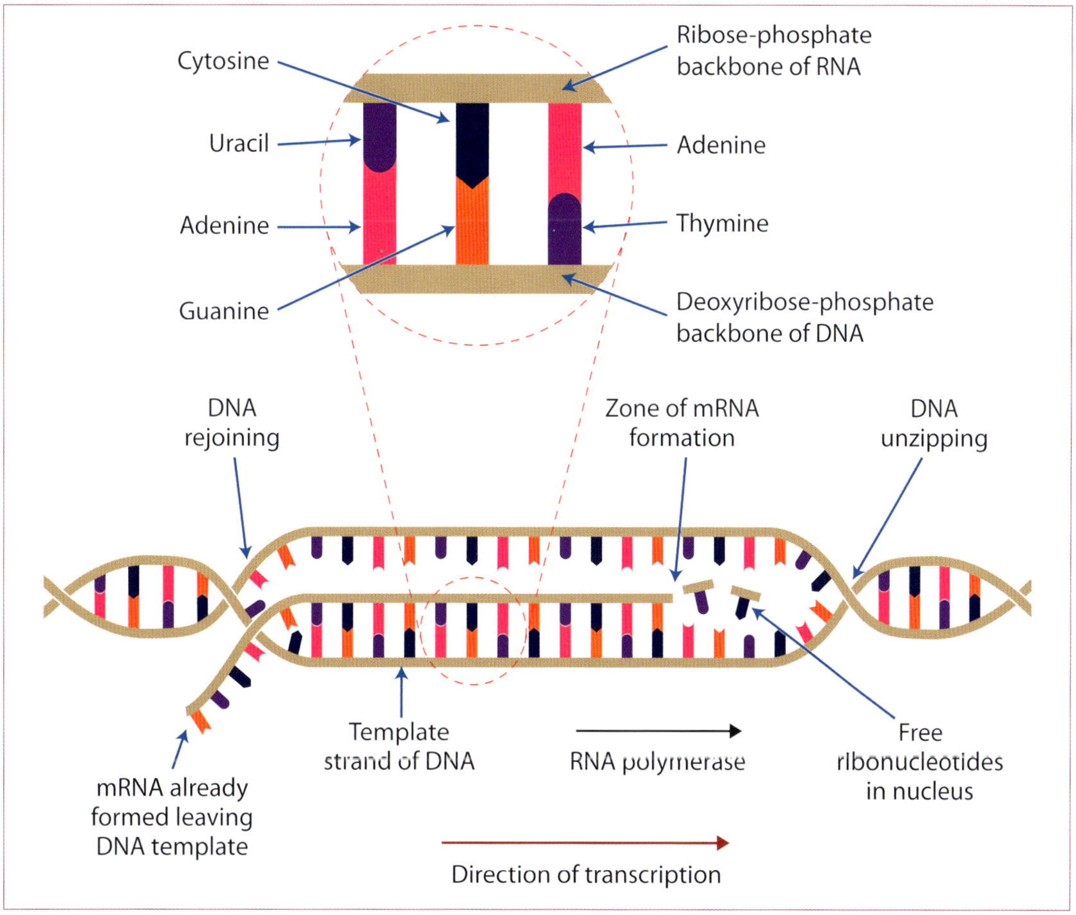

Transcription – the formation of mRNA

Tip: The role of the mRNA is to carry the base code in a gene from the DNA in the nucleus to the cytoplasm where protein synthesis takes place.

Tip: Chromosomes are the cellular structures that contain DNA. Each chromosome consists of the DNA and proteins that support the DNA.

Transfer RNA (tRNA)

Transfer RNA (tRNA) is also made in the nucleus, but it has an important role in the build-up of polypeptides in the cytoplasm. It is a much smaller molecule (containing 70 to 80 nucleotides) than DNA or mRNA and it is 'clover shaped', as shown in the diagram on the right.

The role of the tRNA is to **bring amino acids into the correct position on the mRNA**. Remember that a triplet of bases on DNA codes for an amino acid. The same principle applies to the mRNA. The sequence of three bases which codes for an amino acid on mRNA is referred to as a **codon**. There are 20 different types of amino acids and therefore there are 20 different types of tRNA molecule, each only able to link to one type of amino acid.

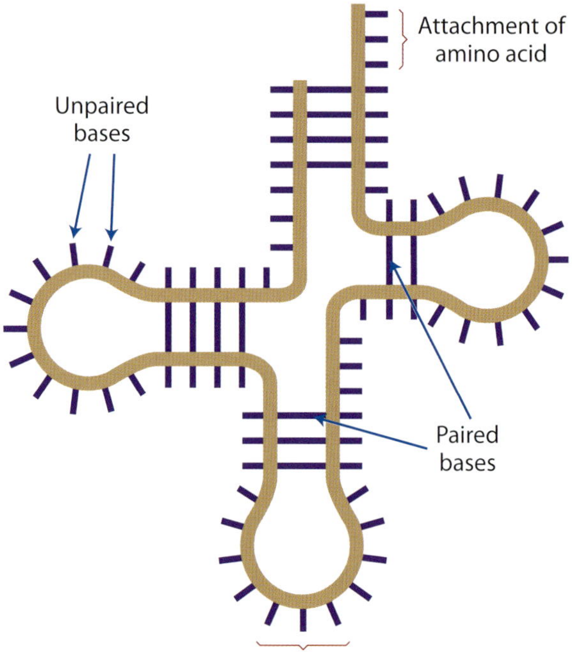

A tRNA molecule

But how is the tRNA able to link to the correct position (**codon**) on the mRNA? The diagrams above and below show that at one end of the tRNA molecule there is a set of three bases (called an **anticodon**), and that the tRNA (and amino acid) will be linked up in

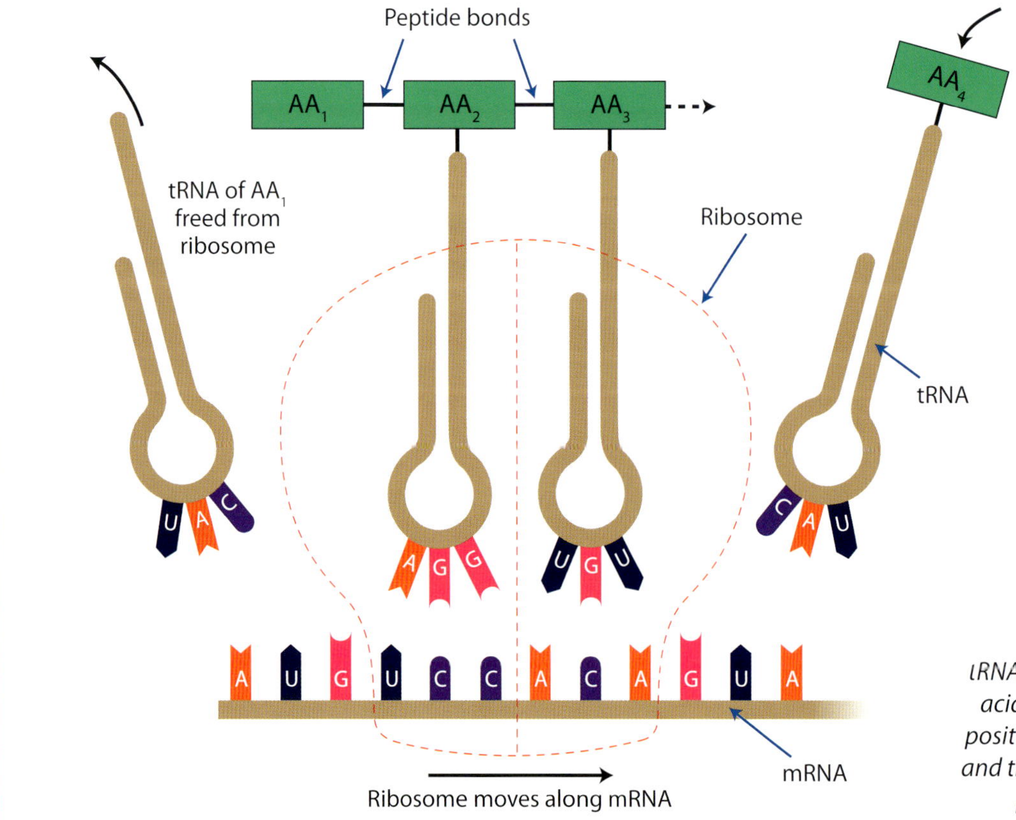

tRNA bringing amino acids to the correct position on the mRNA and the formation of a polypeptide

the correct sequence through base pairing between the anticodon on the tRNA and the codon on the mRNA. The diagram on the previous page also shows that the amino acids are bonded together (by **peptide bonds**) in the correct sequence as the ribosome moves along the mRNA, essentially 'zipping' them together.

Tip: Note, in the diagram, that A-U base combinations exist rather than A-T (as with DNA).

Note that as an amino acid is linked to the growing polypeptide sequence, the tRNA molecule which brought that amino acid to its correct position on the mRNA is freed and returns to the cytoplasm to repeat the process, as required.

Tip: Remember that the tRNA has the function of bringing the appropriate amino acids to the correct codon (position) on the mRNA and lining them up in such a way that they will be linked together in the correct sequence.

The building up of polypeptides and proteins in the cytoplasm involving mRNA, tRNA and ribosomes is called **translation**.

Ribosomal RNA (rRNA)

The ribosomes referred to above are largely formed of a third type of RNA, called **ribosomal RNA (rRNA)**. rRNA is formed in the nucleus and combines with protein to form a ribosome – the rRNA makes up over half of a ribosome. The ribosome is initially in two sections (a large and a small sub-unit) which join together and lock around the start of the mRNA molecule at the start of the translation process. As the ribosome moves along the mRNA it bonds the amino acids together to form a polypeptide.

Summary

The differences between RNA and DNA are summarised in the table at the bottom of the page.

The process of DNA replication

For DNA to be a stable information-carrying molecule it is essential that it is able to **replicate** or **copy** accurately. Essentially, the DNA in chromosomes must remain unchanged as cells divide by mitosis as an organism develops and grows. A mature animal or plant may contain many billions of cells and the DNA in these cells will have replicated each time cells divide as the organism grows by producing new cells.

Historically, there have been three theories to try to explain the process of DNA replication – these being **dispersive**, **conservative** and **semi-conservative** replication. These three methods are outlined in the following table.

Method of replication	Description of method of replication
Dispersive	The DNA breaks into short fragments with new nucleotides filling the gaps.
Conservative	The double-stranded DNA remains intact and is copied to produce a second identical DNA molecule (much like how a photocopier works by replicating exactly what is being copied, without changing the original).
Semi-conservative	The double-stranded DNA unzips and each strand acts as a template, allowing matching complementary strands to be build up by base pairing.

Feature	DNA	RNA
Relative size	Much longer in length than RNA – millions of nucleotides. Often measured in number of base pairs. The DNA in a chromosome can be over 200 million base pairs in length.	Much shorter in length than DNA (70 – 3000 nucleotides).
Polynucleotide arrangement	Double-stranded	Single-stranded
Pentose sugar	Deoxyribose	Ribose
Nitrogenous bases	Adenine (A), guanine (G), cytosine (C) and thymine (T)	Adenine (A), guanine (G), cytosine (C) and uracil (U)
Location	Nucleus	Throughout cell (made in nucleus but mainly present at sites of protein synthesis).

Semi-conservative replication

Scientists eventually worked out that DNA in fact replicated by the **semi-conservative method** as outlined in the table. In this process the enzyme **DNA helicase** 'unzips' (unwinds) the two strands of the DNA by breaking the **hydrogen bonds** between the bases. This allows **each** of the **original strands** to become a **template** for the formation of two DNA molecules. Free DNA nucleotides are attracted to the exposed bases on each of the (two) template strands and link together in the correct sequence as a consequence of following **base pairing** rules. The nucleotides on each newly formed strand are joined together by **DNA polymerase** which catalyses phosphodiester bonds (a **condensation reaction**) between adjacent deoxyribose and phosphate groups on the strand.

The process of DNA replication by the semi-conservative theory is summarised in the diagram below.

Tip: Remember that in the semi-conservative model of DNA replication both strands of the original DNA act as a template (not the same as in polypeptide/protein synthesis – where only one strand acts as a template).

The Meselson and Stahl experiment

It was a ground-breaking biological investigation, carried out by two scientists named **Meselson** and **Stahl** in 1958, that showed that the semi-conservative model was the one that explained DNA replication. In their investigation, Meselson and Stahl cultured the bacterium *Escherichia coli* using the 'heavy' isotope of nitrogen ^{15}N. The ^{15}N was incorporated into the bases of the DNA in all the bacteria over time, as older bacteria (containing the normal ^{14}N) died and were replaced.

The bacteria (with ^{15}N bases) were then transferred to a medium containing the lighter (normal) ^{14}N. Following the transfer, the bacterial DNA was extracted and analysed at intervals. Key stages were:

- bacteria growing in ^{14}N (before transfer to the ^{15}N)
- bacteria growing in ^{15}N
- one generation after transfer to ^{14}N
- two generations after transfer to ^{14}N

Density-gradient centrifugation was used to separate the bacterial DNA following sampling at the stages listed above. DNA containing the 'lighter' ^{14}N accumulated in a zone near the top of the centrifuge tube, whereas DNA consisting of 'heavy' ^{15}N formed a zone near the bottom of the centrifuge tube.

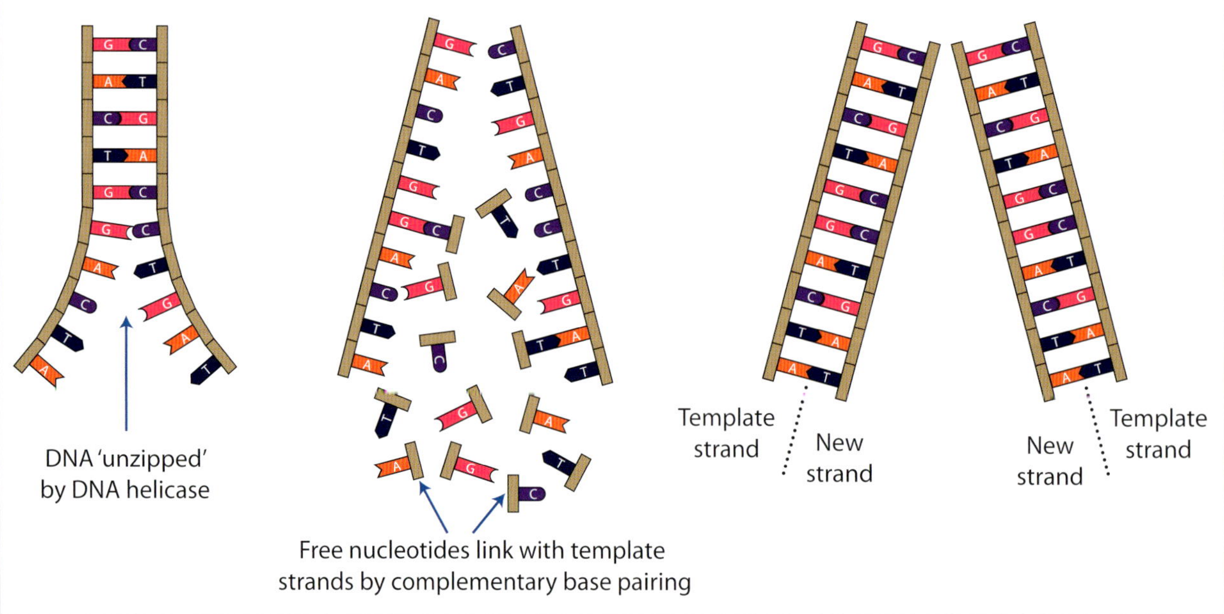

Diagram of semi-conservative DNA replication

Meselson and Stahl's results are represented by the following diagram.

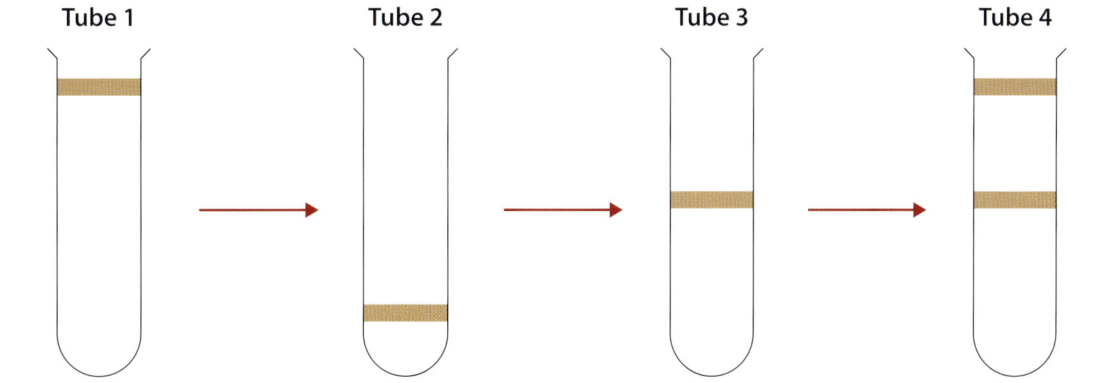

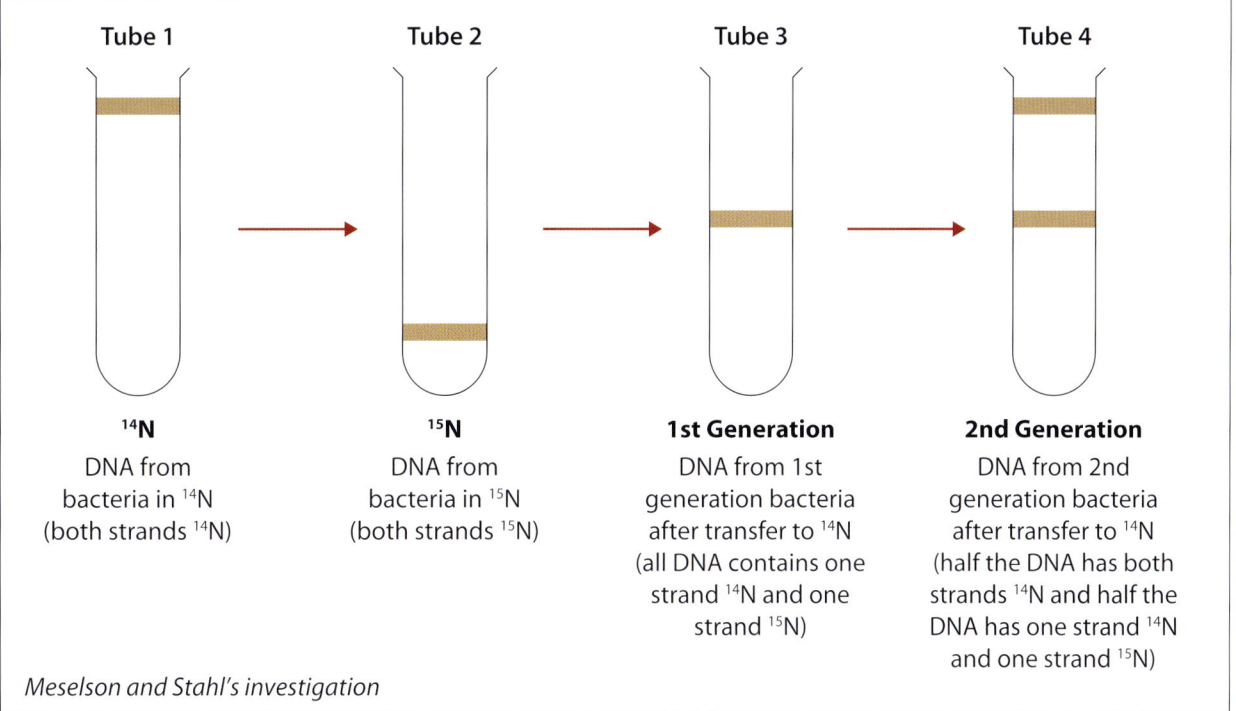

Meselson and Stahl's investigation

Explanation of Meselson and Stahl's results

After one generation the intermediate position of the DNA can be explained by all the DNA consisting of one strand which has (nitrogenous) bases containing ^{15}N and one strand having bases containing ^{14}N.

After two generations about half the DNA consisted of 'mixed' DNA of both ^{14}N and ^{15}N but the other half was DNA that contained only ^{14}N.

These results can only be explained by the semi-conservative model. After one generation, the new generation of bacteria had DNA that contained one parental strand (with ^{15}N bases) and one strand formed using ^{14}N from the medium in which the parental bacteria had been transferred. In the second generation, each strand from the 'mixed' DNA of the first-generation bacteria acted as a template to produce bacteria, half of which contained 'mixed' DNA and the other half only DNA with ^{14}N.

Tip: In the third (and any further) generations the same pattern would be evident as with the second generation. However, there would be proportionally fewer bacteria containing the 'mixed' DNA and much more containing only the 'lighter' DNA. Therefore, the lighter band (zone) in the centrifuge tube would get denser as the mixed band would get relatively lighter.

Tip: Remember it is the bases in DNA that contains nitrogen, not the sugar or phosphate groups.

Questions

1. The diagram below represents the coding strand of part of a DNA molecule.

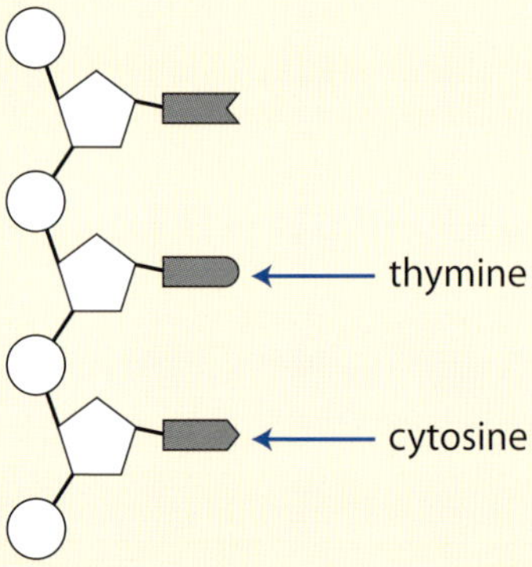

(a) Name the DNA base not represented in the diagram. [1]
(b) How many phosphate groups are shown in the diagram? [1]
(c) Name the type of bond which links adjacent bases. [1]

2. A number of scientific researchers were involved in working out the structure of DNA with the later scientists building on the knowledge of earlier workers. The table below summarises the main workers and their methodologies. Copy and complete the table.

Researcher(s)	Methodology
Franklin and Wilkins	
	modelling
	base equivalence

3. (a) The table below describes some features of DNA and mRNA molecules.

	DNA	mRNA
Length	45 – 250 million base pairs	70 – 3000 nucleotides
Bases	adenine, guanine, thymine, cytosine	

(i) The length of a DNA section is commonly measured in number of base pairs. Explain why the length of an mRNA molecule cannot be measured in this way. [2]
(ii) Name the bases found in a mRNA molecule. [1]
(iii) Explain the large difference in length between DNA and mRNA. [2]

(b) Describe the function of a transfer RNA (tRNA) molecule. [2]

4. (a) Name the scientists who worked out that the structure of DNA formed a double helix. [1]
(b) The semi-conservative theory explains how DNA replicates.
(i) Summarise the 'semi-conservative' theory of DNA replication. [2]
(ii) Describe the roles of DNA helicase and DNA polymerase in this process. [4]

(c) Meselson and Stahl were the scientists who developed the experiment to confirm that DNA replication was by 'semi-conservative replication. They grew *Escherichia coli* using the 'heavy' isotope of nitrogen (^{15}N) so that all the bacteria in the colony had ^{15}N rather than the 'normal' and lighter ^{14}N. After being cultivated in ^{15}N, the bacteria were then transferred to and grown in a ^{14}N culture medium. At intervals, some bacteria were removed, and the DNA analysed following centrifugation. The centrifugation separates the DNA based on density with the lighter DNA forming a band higher up the tube. Results of this investigation are represented by the diagram below.

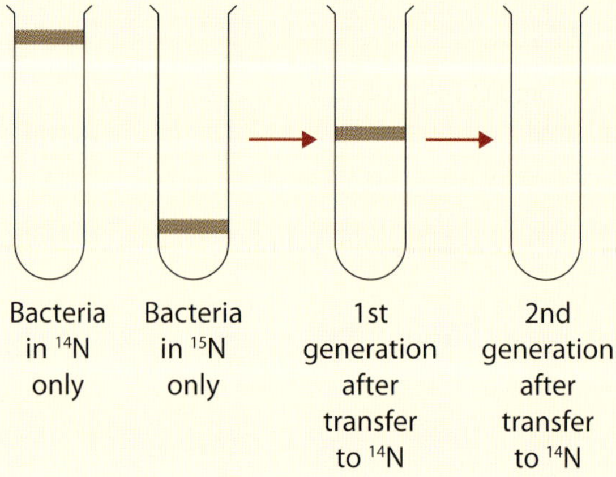

In terms of DNA banding, describe and explain the results you would get in the fourth test tube. [4]

16: MEIOSIS AND GENETICS

Students should be able to:

11.3.1 demonstrate an understanding of the importance of meiosis in producing cells that are genetically different, including:
- the formation of haploid cells;
- independent assortment of homologous chromosomes in metaphase I;
- genetic recombination by crossing over (chiasma formation) in prophase 1;
- that gametes are genetically different as a result of different combinations of maternal and paternal chromosomes; and
- how random fertilisation of haploid cells further increases genetic variation.

11.1.12 explain genotype as the genetic constitution of an organism;

11.1.13 explain phenotype as the expression of this genetic constitution and its interaction with the environment;

11.1.14 demonstrate an understanding of and describe how alleles may be dominant, recessive or codominant;

11.1.15 show, for a diploid organism, that alleles at a specific locus may be either homozygous or heterozygous;

11.1.16 use fully labelled genetic diagrams to interpret, or predict, the results of:
- monohybrid and dihybrid crosses involving dominant, recessive and codominant alleles;
- crosses involving sex linkage, autosomal linkage, multiple alleles and epistasis;

11.1.17 make use of the chi-squared test to compare the goodness of fit of observed phenotypic ratios with expected ratios;

11.1.18 predict the probability of offspring with a particular genotype using a Punnett Square Diagram;

Meiosis

When cells divide and increase in number (as during growth) they do this in a way that maintains constancy of chromosome number, and therefore each new cell formed has the same DNA as the parent cell which produced it. This constancy is achieved through the process of mitosis. For example, there are 46 chromosomes in the first human cell following conception and there are 46 chromosomes in the cells of the resulting adult.

Tip: In chapter 15 we covered the topic of DNA replication. DNA replication (i.e. doubling the amount of DNA) takes place just before mitosis so that each new daughter cell can receive the same DNA as was in the parent cell.

However, in organisms which reproduce sexually through producing gametes (for example sperm and eggs), it is important that gametes have half the number of chromosomes compared to normal cells, so that when the gametes combine in fertilisation the normal chromosome number is maintained in the zygote (first cell of new individual). The process of halving the chromosome number during gamete formation is called **meiosis**.

In humans and other mammals, chromosomes are arranged in pairs referred to as **homologous pairs**. One of the chromosomes in a pair is paternal (coming from the father's gamete) and the other maternal (coming from the mother's gamete). **Genes** are sections of DNA (chromosomes) and each gene occurs at the same position (**locus**) on each chromosome in a homologous pair. However, some genes exist in more than one form, called **alleles**, meaning that at the same locus for a homologous pair, the two alleles (genes) could be different, as shown in the following diagram.

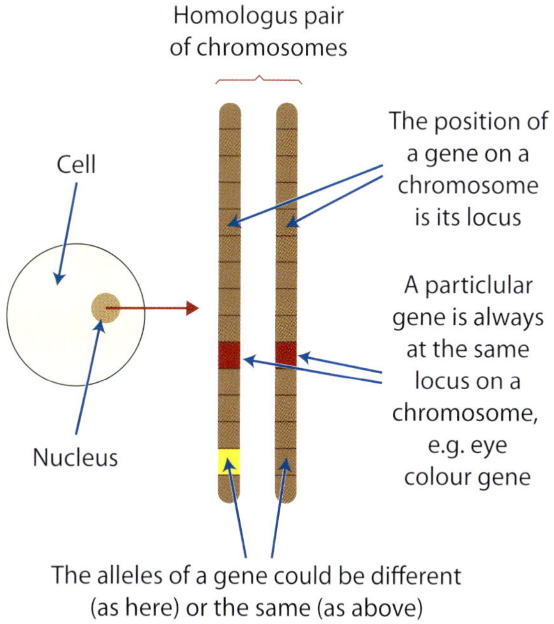

A homologous pair of chromosomes

Organisms which have chromosomes organised as homologous pairs are described as **diploid** (diploid can be represented as **2n**). During meiosis, the chromosome number is halved, but it is not just a random halving – in meiosis, only one chromosome from **each** homologous pair goes into a gamete. Gametes (or cells with only one chromosome from each homologous pair) are referred to as **haploid** and are represented as **n**.

> **Tip:** Meiosis is also referred to as **reduction division** – you should be able to work out why!

The process of meiosis

Meiosis only takes place where gametes are formed, for example in humans in the testes and the ovaries. It involves two divisions, **meiosis I** and **meiosis II**, with each division having four distinct stages, referred to as **prophase**, **metaphase**, **anaphase** and **telophase**.

Meiosis I

During **meiosis I**, the chromosomes are separated into two sets, with each set containing one chromosome from each homologous pair. The four stages of meiosis I are described in the following diagrams and accompanying text.

Prophase I

By this stage, the homologous chromosomes are arranged as pairs called **bivalents**. The other main features of prophase I are:

- each chromosome (and therefore the DNA) has now **replicated** – the two chromosomes originating from each chromosome are now referred to as **chromatids** and are held together by a **centromere** (acting like a belt);
- each **chromosome (chromatid) condenses** (and packs more tightly together) and this makes them **more visible** when viewed using a microscope;
- the **nuclear membrane breaks down** and the nucleus is no longer distinct;
- a **spindle** consisting of **microtubules** (proteins with contractile properties) begins to form.

The diagram at the top of the page represents a cell in prophase I. (For clarity, only four homologous pairs are shown.)

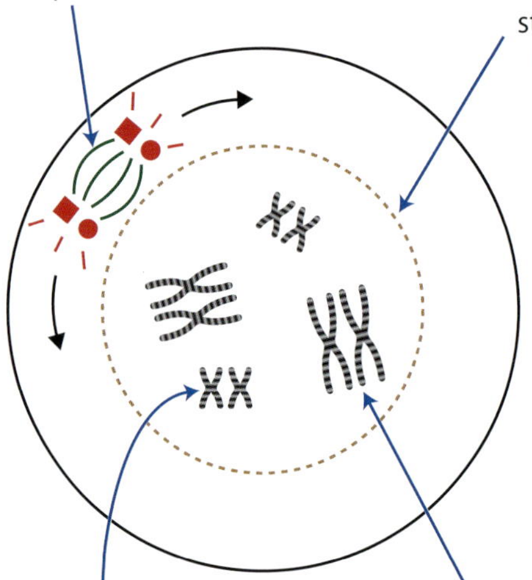

Prophase I

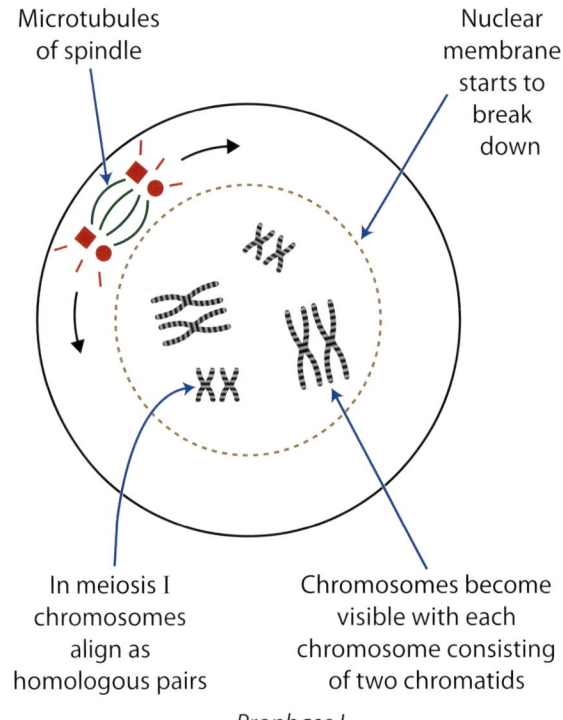

> **Tip:** The diagram shows that the centromere holds the two chromatids of each chromosome together (not the two chromosomes in a homologous pair).

Metaphase I

Bivalents (pairs of homologous chromosomes, with each chromosome split into two chromatids) align along the 'equator' of the cell. The spindle fibres attach to the centromeres of each chromosome as shown in the following diagram.

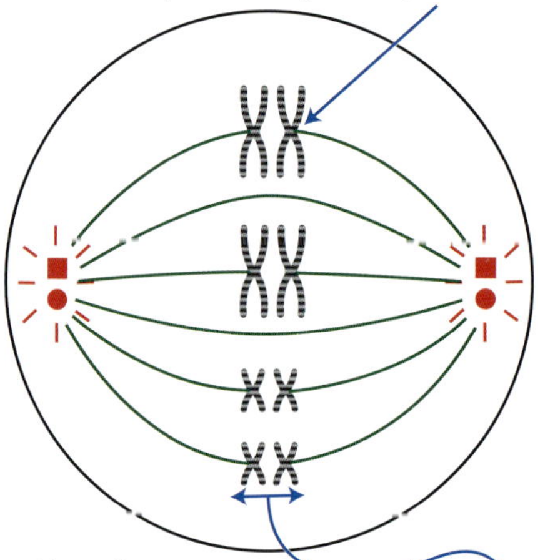

Metaphase I

Anaphase I

As the microtubules of the spindle **contract** they pull **chromosomes** (each consisting of two chromatids) to opposite ends of the cell. With the two chromosomes of each bivalent (homologous pair) pulled to opposite ends of the cell, and separated, this ensures that only one chromosome from each homologous pair will end up in a daughter cell (gamete). Anaphase I is represented by the following diagram.

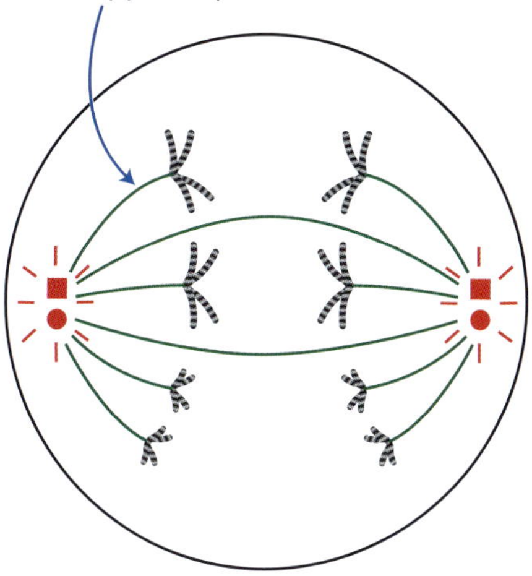

Anaphase I

Tip: You should remember that it is the separation of homologous **chromosomes** in anaphase I that results in gametes (daughter cells produced in meiosis) being haploid.

Tip: The diagram shows that while homologous chromosomes are being separated, each chromosome still consists of two chromatids.

Tip: The diagram also shows that the spindle fibres attach to the centromere (the point where the 2 chromatids of each chromosome are attached. As the chromosomes/chromatids are pulled from their centre (due to the centromeres being in the middle of the chromosomes in this example), the ends of the chromosomes/chromatids lag behind.

Telophase I

Once the chromosomes (still consisting of two chromatids) have been pulled to opposite ends of the cell, the nuclear membrane reforms, the spindle dissolves, and the chromosomes lengthen to become invisible again, as shown in the following diagram.

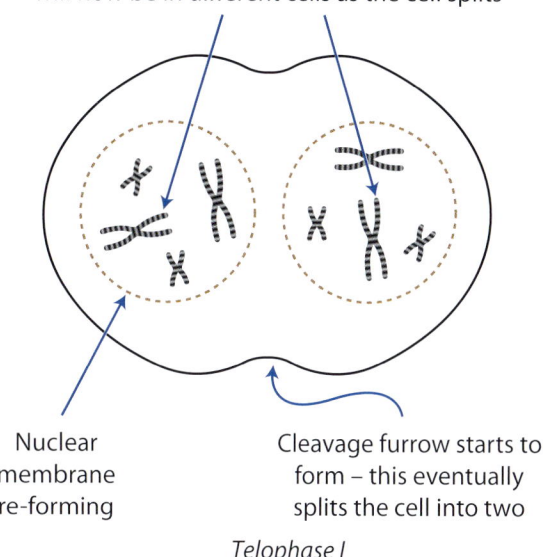

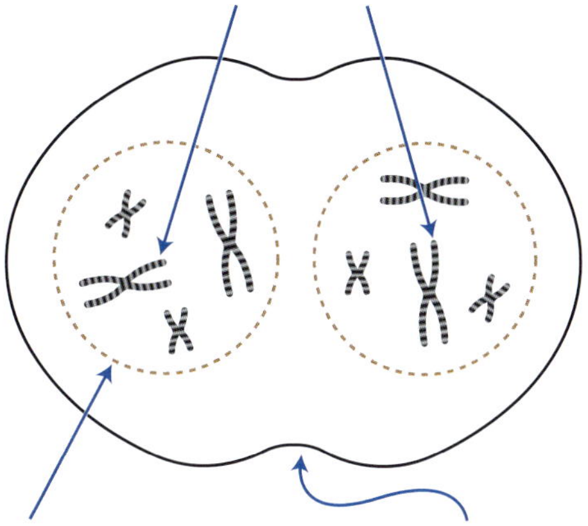

Telophase I

Following telophase I, the cell divides into two in a process called **cytokinesis**. In summary, this division produces two new cells, each with one chromosome from each homologous pair (although each chromosome is split longitudinally into two chromatids).

Meiosis II

At the end of meiosis I, two daughter cells are produced each with the haploid (in humans = 23) number of chromosomes. However, in these two cells, each of the chromosomes consists of two chromatids. Meiosis II is essentially a stage during which each of these cells split again with one chromatid from each chromosome going to one of the daughter cells and the other chromatid going to the other daughter cell. Following telophase II, cytokinesis occurs again to produce **four haploid cells** (gametes) in **total**. Meiosis II is summarised in the following diagram.

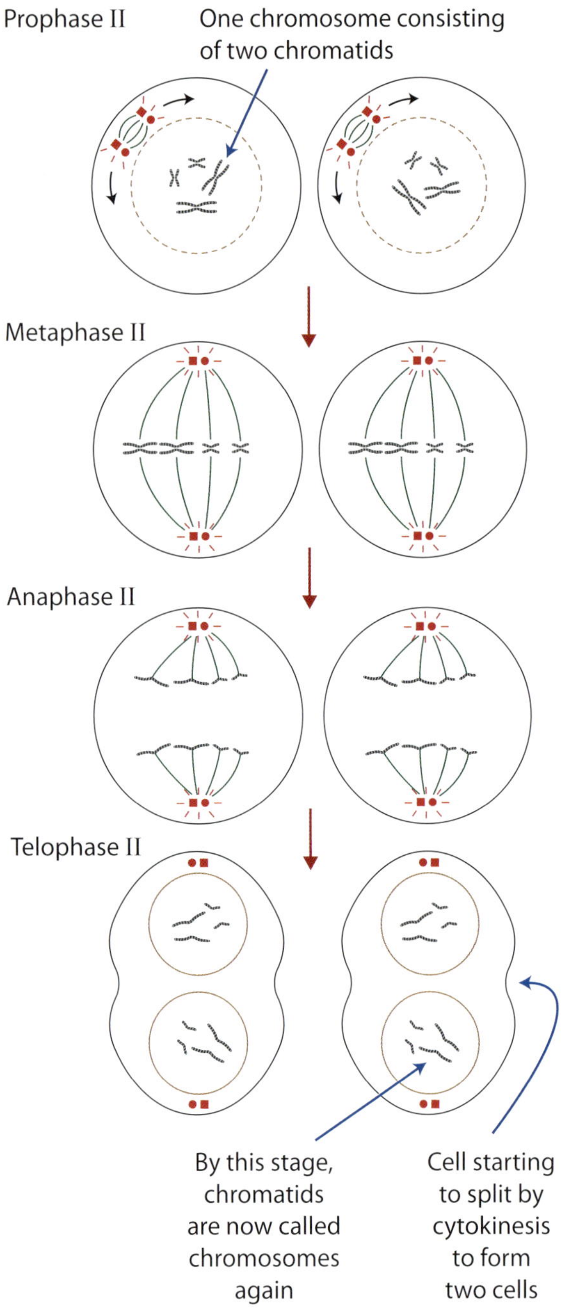

Meiosis II

Tip: Note that the diagram has two columns showing that meiosis II occurs in each of the two daughter cells from meiosis I, forming four gametes in total from each original cell.

Tip: Chromatid is a term used to explain the process of meiosis as it would be very difficult to explain without distinguishing between chromosomes before and after splitting otherwise.

Tip: A key feature of meiosis is that it not only halves the chromosome number in daughter cells, but it also ensures that each daughter cell (gamete) has one chromosome from each homologous pair. The importance of this will be explained later.

Meiosis and genetic variation

Although meiosis is necessary to ensure constancy of chromosome number in sexually reproducing organisms, it is also very important in producing **variation**. Variation in meiosis is produced as a result of two specific processes, **independent assortment** and **crossing over**.

Independent assortment

In meiosis, only one chromosome from a homologous pair can enter a gamete. However, for any one gamete it can be **either of the two chromosomes from a homologous pair**.

The chromosome (maternal or paternal) of a homologous pair which actually enters a particular gamete is dependent on the random nature of how the bivalent (homologous pair) lines up at the cell 'equator' at the start of **metaphase I**. The way **one chromosome pair** lines up (i.e. which of the two chromosomes in a pair is closer to a particular pole or edge of the cell) **is totally independent of how any other pair aligns** – this is the principle of **independent assortment**.

Tip: If you refer back to the diagram of metaphase I, this means that it is purely chance which chromosome in a homologous pair is on the left or right (and therefore will be pulled to the left or right side of the cell during anaphase I).

Tip: All the gametes are genetically different as they contain different combinations of maternal and paternal chromosomes (even though they have only one chromosome from each homologous pair).

With 23 homologous pairs of chromosomes in humans, there are therefore millions of possible chromosome combinations for any one gamete.

Crossing over

As noted before, by the start of prophase I, homologous pairs of chromosomes are aligned very closely together and have each replicated (to give four chromatids per homologous pair) to form bivalents.

Sometimes two non-sister chromatids (originating from the different chromosomes in a homologous pair) break and exchange sections of chromosome (DNA) with each other. This happens during **prophase I** and is called **crossing over**. The points where the chromosomes cross over are called **chiasmata** (singular **chiasma**).

Crossing over is very significant because of two key facts:

- the two **chromosomes** of a homologous pair have **identical genes** but some **alleles may differ** between the chromosomes;
- the two **chromatids** of each chromosome are identical (before crossing over) – they possess the **same genes *and* the same alleles**.

The diagram below shows how crossing over can lead to genetic change.

As a consequence of crossing over (and shown in the below diagram):

- the two chromatids of the same chromosome may no longer be genetically identical;
- some chromatids may contain unique sequences of alleles that did not exist in either parental chromosome.

Tip: Crossing over works because, while sequences of alleles may change as a result, the position (locus) of genes (for example a gene for eye colour) will not be altered.

The following diagram shows how meiosis can produce four gametes from a parental cell and how each of the gametes differ from each other.

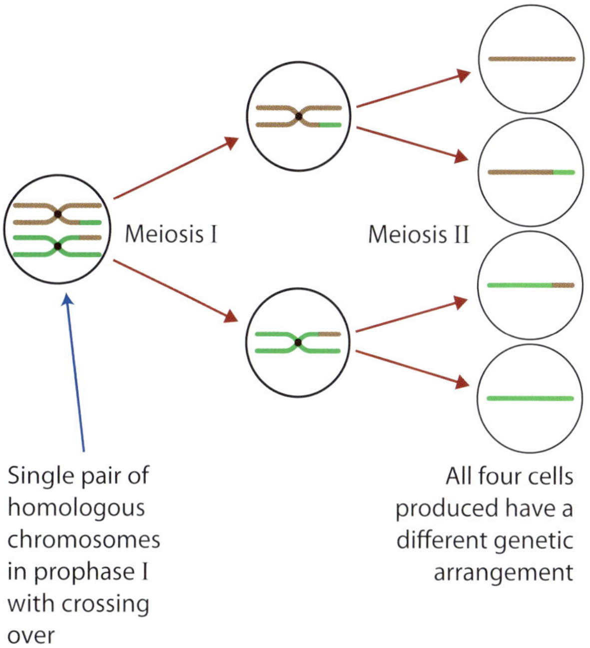
Meiosis I
Meiosis II
Single pair of homologous chromosomes in prophase I with crossing over
All four cells produced have a different genetic arrangement

Meiosis and crossing over produces variation in gametes'

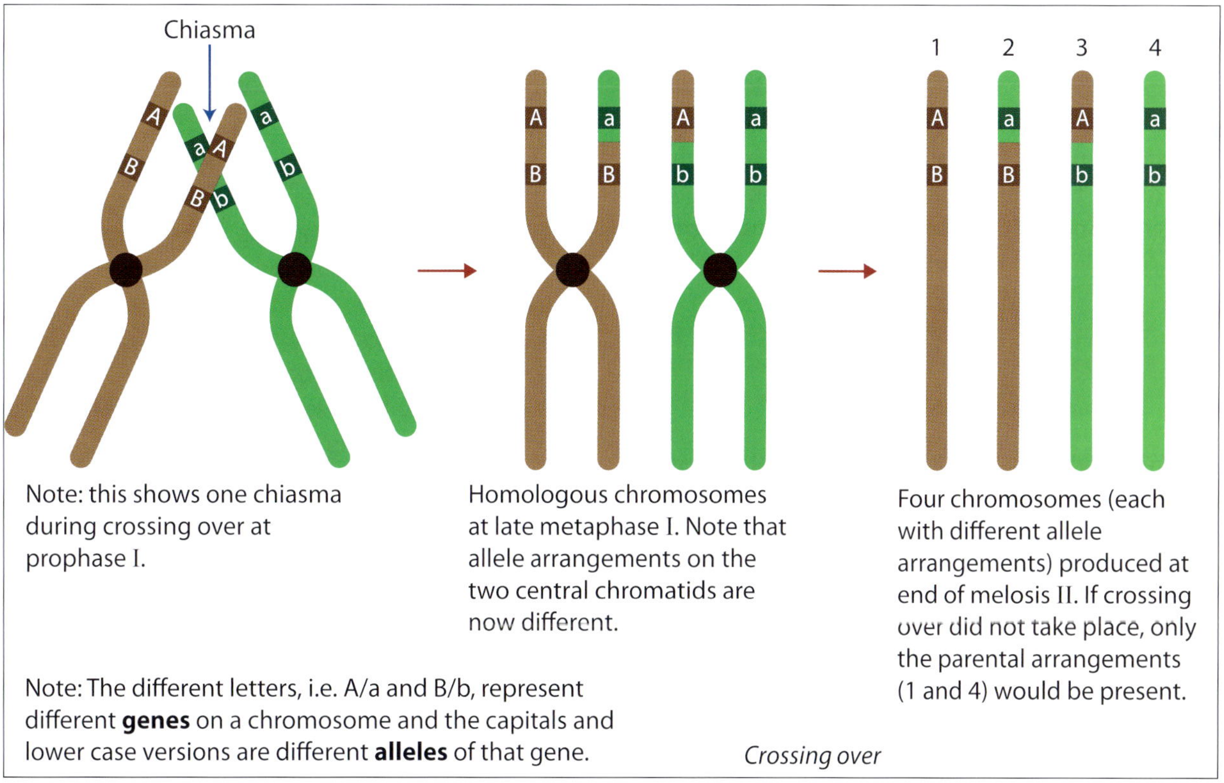
Chiasma
A
B
a
b
1
2
3
4
Note: this shows one chiasma during crossing over at prophase I.
Homologous chromosomes at late metaphase I. Note that allele arrangements on the two central chromatids are now different.
Four chromosomes (each with different allele arrangements) produced at end of meiosis II. If crossing over did not take place, only the parental arrangements (1 and 4) would be present.
Note: The different letters, i.e. A/a and B/b, represent different **genes** on a chromosome and the capitals and lower case versions are different **alleles** of that gene.

Crossing over

Tip: The diagrams show crossing over at one position (chiasma). In reality, crossing over can take place many times along the length of one bivalent.

The concepts of independent assortment and crossing over show why gametes vary so much. However, it is important to remember too that **cross-fertilisation** also contributes to variation, i.e. that any one male gamete (out of millions of different possibilities) can combine with any one female gamete (also out of millions of different possibilities).

Tip: The random fertilisation (cross-fertilisation) of haploid cells (gametes) further increases genetic variation above and beyond that contributed by crossing over and independent assortment.

Genetics

Genes and chromosomes

As chromosomes occur in homologous pairs, each chromosome in a pair will carry the same gene (for example for flower colour in plants) but the gene for flower colour may have different forms (alleles) in the two chromosomes (for example one allele may be for purple flower colour and the other for white flower colour). If the alleles are the same, that gene is said to be **homozygous**, but if they are different, the gene is said to be **heterozygous** as shown in the following diagram.

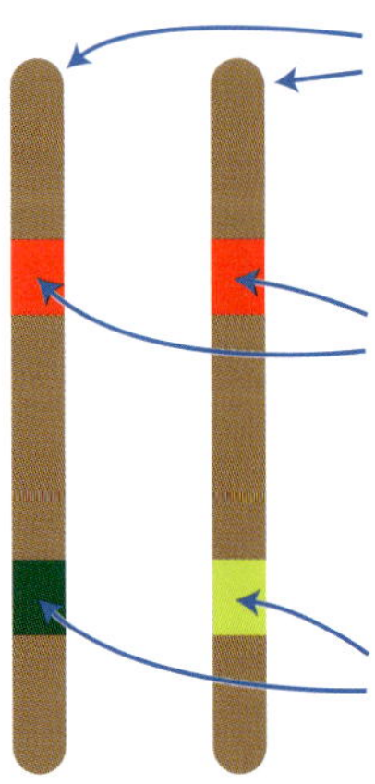

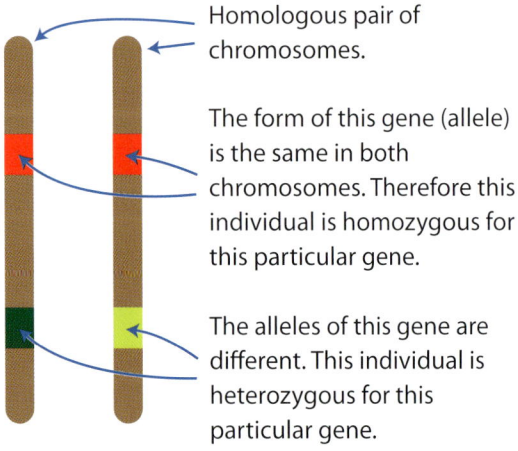

A homologous pair of chromosomes with the positions of two genes shown

Tip: For most genes in humans (out of around 20,000) the gene on one homologous chromosome is exactly the same as the gene on the partner homologous chromosome. However, when they are different (as noted in the diagram), the different alleles are due to a mutation affecting the gene on one of the homologous chromosomes in an ancestor sometime in the past.

Some important genetic terms are defined in the following table.

Term	Definition
gene	short section of a chromosome that codes for a particular polypeptide / protein / characteristic
allele	a particular form of a gene
homozygous	both alleles of a gene are the same on homologous chromosomes
heterozygous	the alleles of the (same) gene are different on homologous chromosomes
gene locus	the position of the gene on the chromosome

Tip: Remember that only diploid organisms (i.e. those with homologous chromosome pairs) can be homozygous or heterozygous as two alleles of the same gene are needed.

Monohybrid inheritance

Monohybrid inheritance describes the way in which a particular characteristic, for example flower colour in peas, is passed through the generations. In **monohybrid inheritance**, one gene consisting of two alleles is usually responsible for controlling the trait (characteristic).

Some key points about monohybrid crosses are as follows:

- when gametes are being formed, only one of the two alleles pass into a gamete (this is consistent with our understanding of meiosis, as if only one chromosome enters a gamete only one allele of a particular gene can too);
- it is totally random which of the two alleles pass into a gamete;
- there is an equal chance of any one gamete from one parent combining with any one gamete from the other parent;

- traditionally, characteristics, such as flower colour, are given symbols. For example, purple could be represented as P and white flower colour as p – we'll see later why a P is used and why there is one capital and one lower case;
- in each individual, there are two alleles for a monohybrid characteristic – the two symbols reflecting the alleles present refer to the **genotype**;
- the outward appearance, for example purple flowers, is referred to as the **phenotype**.

Let us consider one example of a monohybrid cross in detail – pea plants. Pea plants can be of the 'common' tall variety or a much shorter, low-growing variety. The height characteristic is controlled by one gene so is an example of monohybrid inheritance.

In a particular genetic cross, a homozygous tall pea plant was crossed with a short low-growing pea plant. All the offspring were tall. This can be explained by the allele for tall being **dominant** over the allele for short (which is described as being **recessive**). The recessive allele will only be shown in the phenotype if the genotype is homozygous recessive; i.e. there is no dominant allele present. We will use the symbols **T** for the tall allele and **t** for the short allele.

Tip: In symbols, make the dominant allele a capital, for example T, and the recessive allele lower case, for example t. The letter used also usually reflects the dominant allele feature, i.e. **T** for tall.

When two of the first set of offspring (normally referred to as the F_1 generation) are crossed, the ratio of tall to short in the next generation (F_2) is 3 tall to 1 short. These ratios can be explained by the diagram below.

Tip: Although a 3 : 1 ratio is shown in the diagram, offspring numbers seldom work out as exact ratios, especially if small numbers are involved.

Tip: A heterozygous genotype shows the dominant phenotype.

Tip: Two heterozygous parents, (in this case Tt × Tt) will give a 3 : 1 offspring ratio.

Tip: When working out genetic crosses, it is traditional to place a circle around the gametes – this stops them being mixed up with genotypes. (Shaded boxes are used in this book for greater clarity.)

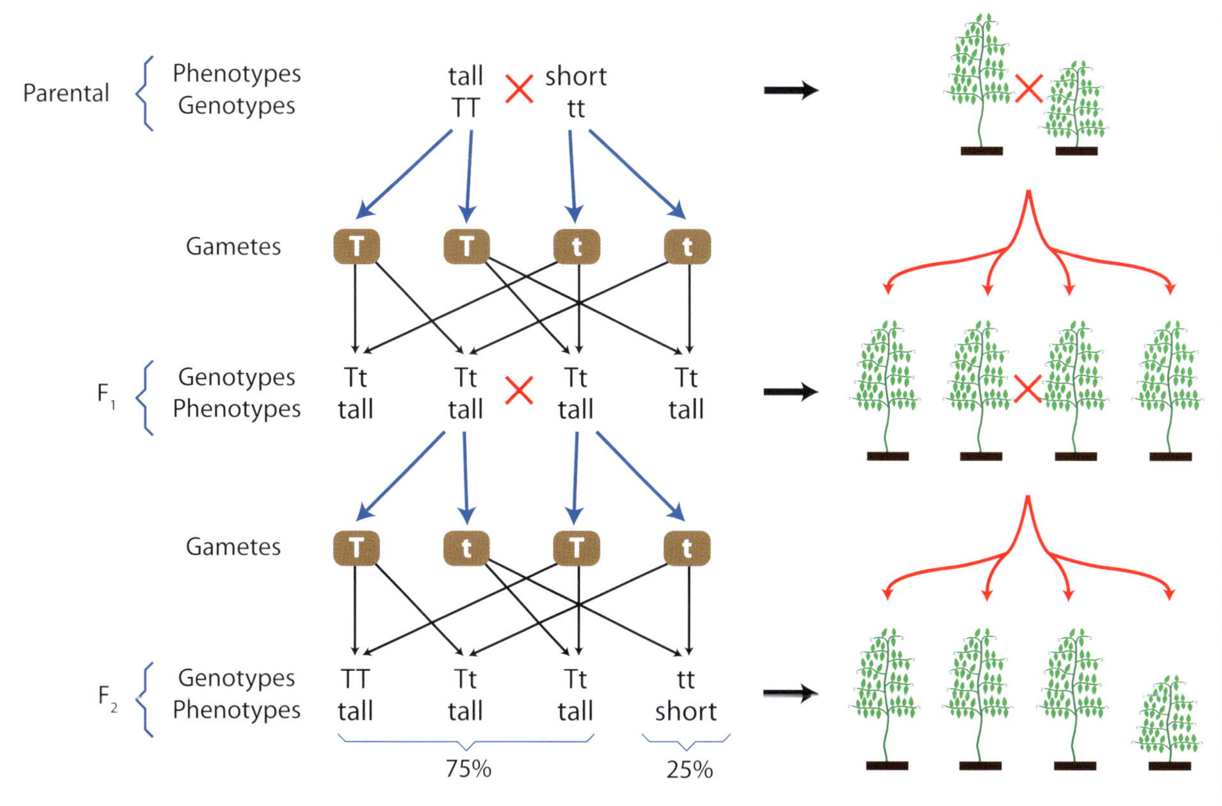

Explaining the 3:1 monohybrid ratio

The following table gives definitions of some of the genetic terms used above.

Term	Definition	Example(s) in cross above
genotype	the genetic constitution of an organism (in this example, the two alleles for a particular characteristic [trait])	TT or Tt or tt
phenotype	the outward appearance of an individual in terms of the trait under consideration (which may also be affected by the environment*)	tall or short
dominant	in the heterozygous condition, the dominant allele will mask the non-dominant (recessive) allele	the F_1 offspring are all tall even though they are heterozygous and possess a t
recessive	the recessive allele will only show itself in the phenotype if there are two recessive alleles (i.e. the recessive allele is masked by the dominant allele)	only the tt genotype in the F_2 generation gives a short phenotype

*phenotype is also influenced by the environment as well as genotype – for example, a pea plant will only grow tall if it gets enough light and water.

Another common ratio in offspring in monohybrid crosses is the 1 : 1 ratio. In this example, the parental cross is heterozygote × homozygous recessive. In the example of height in peas, the parental genotypes to give this ratio are Tt × tt. You should be able to work out how this gives a 1 : 1 ratio.

Codominance

In **codominance**, the two possible alleles of a particular gene are different, but neither has a dominant or masking effect over the other. Due to the absence of dominance, the phenotype of the heterozygote is different to the phenotypes of both homozygous genotypes.

Snapdragon plants show codominance for flower colour. Flowers can be red, pink or white, with the heterozygote genotype giving the pink colour. The genotypes and phenotypes for snapdragon flower colour are shown in the following table.

Genotype	Phenotype
C^RC^R	red flowers
C^RC^W	pink flowers
C^WC^W	white flowers

Tip: The genotypes are represented as shown in the table rather than using the 'typical' capital and lower case symbols which would confuse in terms of dominance and recessiveness as this situation does not apply with codominance.

The following diagram shows the expected outcome when two plants with pink flowers are crossed.

Parental
- Phenotypes: pink flowers × pink flowers
- Genotypes: C^RC^W C^RC^W

Gametes: C^R C^W C^R C^W

Punnett square

	C^R	C^W
C^R	C^RC^R	C^RC^W
C^W	C^RC^W	C^WC^W

Offspring

Genotypes	C^RC^R	C^RC^W	C^WC^W
Phenotypes	red flowers	pink flowers	white flowers
	1 :	2 :	1
	(25%)	(50%)	(25%)

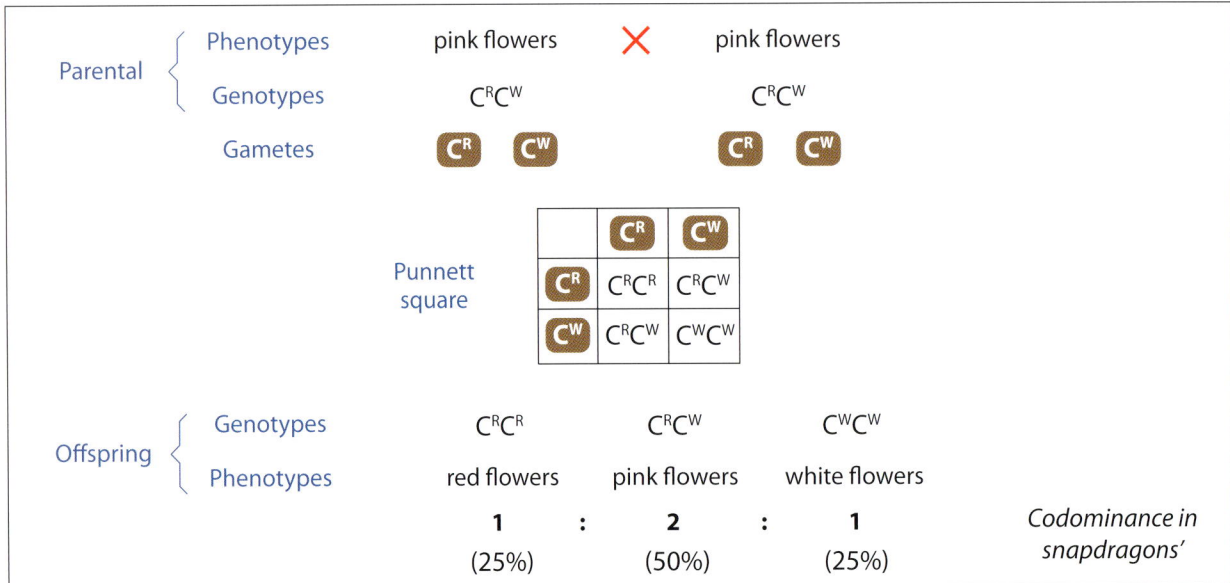

Codominance in snapdragons'

The cross above is completed in a 'box' called a **Punnett square**. The gametes are added to 'cells' along the top and side and the offspring genotypes are then worked out from these. Genetic crosses are typically presented in Punnett squares.

It is important to be aware of the concept of **probability** in genetics. In a question you could be asked to give the probability of a certain genetic outcome – for example, what is the probability of the offspring (children) of two parents having a certain genetic disease? Answers can usually be given as percentages or expressed as 1 in 4 or similar or even shown as ratios, for example 1 : 3.

Multiple alleles

In examples of monohybrid inheritance which we have looked at so far, there have only been two possible types of alleles at a particular gene locus. Sometimes there are three or more possible types of alleles at a locus. Inheritance involving three or more alleles at a particular gene locus is an example of **multiple alleles**.

There are many examples of multiple alleles in inheritance, with many being further complicated by codominance or a hierarchy of dominance across the range of alleles. Take, for example, the inheritance of human **blood groups**. There are four blood groups in the ABO system and each person is one of blood group A, B, AB or O. Allele A is codominant with B, and both A and B are dominant to O. Taking this into account, the possible genotypes of each blood group are shown in the following table.

Blood group	Possible genotypes
A	I^AI^A and I^AI^O
B	I^BI^B and I^BI^O
AB	I^AI^B
O	I^OI^O

Tip: When using symbols for multiple alleles, the gene is often represented by the letter (in this example, I) and the alleles by the superscript (in this example, ^{A}, ^{B} or ^{O}).

There are a range of possible crosses and outcomes with the different blood groups. However, the only possible cross which can produce offspring showing the range of the four blood groups is a cross between a parent heterozygous for blood group A and a parent heterozygous for blood group B as shown in the diagram below.

Sex-linkage

Humans have 46 chromosomes and 23 homologous pairs. 22 of these pairs are described as **autosomes** with the remaining pair being the **sex chromosomes**. There are two types of sex chromosomes; **X** chromosomes and **Y** chromosomes. **Females** have two X chromosomes and the genotype **XX** whereas **males** have an X and a Y and the genotype **XY**.

All the genetic traits covered so far in this chapter are independent of the sex of the individuals. However, for some characteristics there is a close

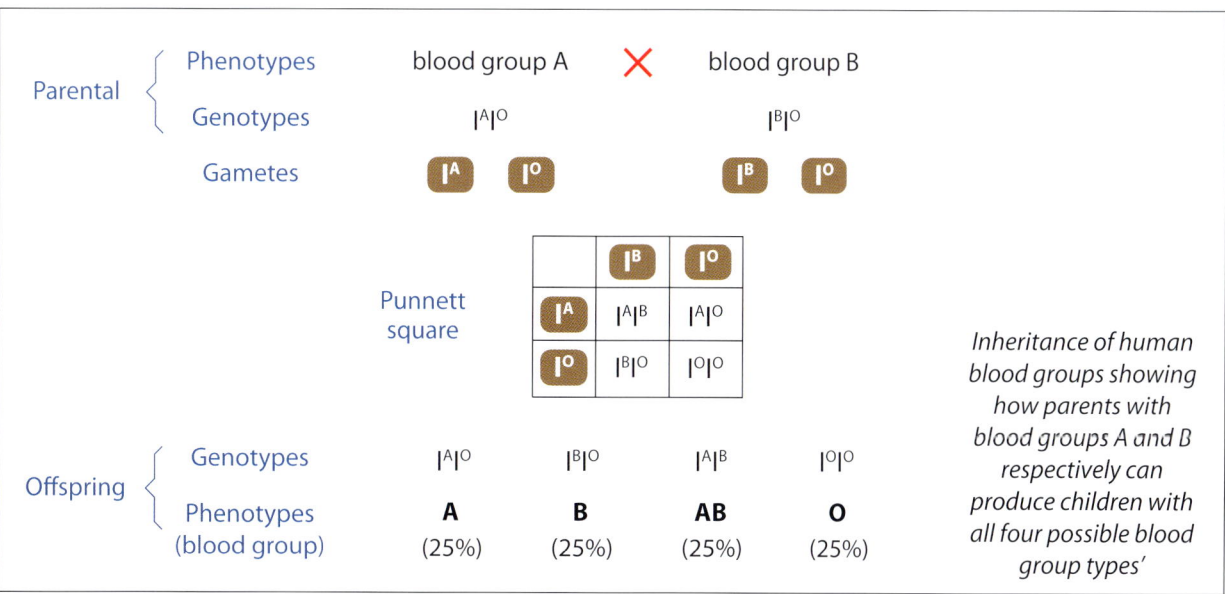

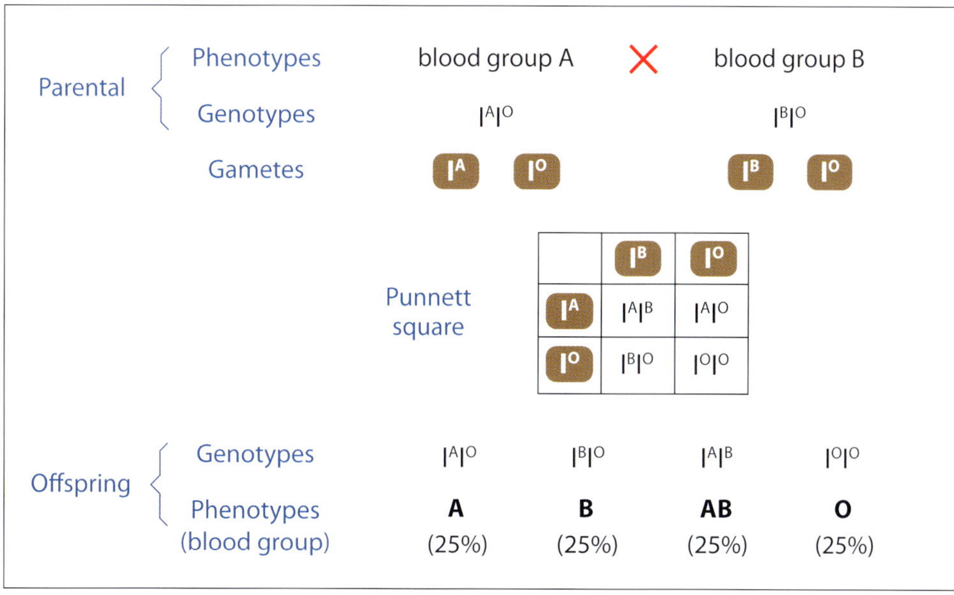

Inheritance of human blood groups showing how parents with blood groups A and B respectively can produce children with all four possible blood group types'

correlation between the trait and the sex of the individual, i.e. the traits are said to be **sex-linked**.

In humans, the Y sex chromosome is essentially 'genetically empty'. Therefore, the X chromosome has large sections (and many genes) that are non-homologous, meaning there are no corresponding genes on the Y chromosome.

The non-homologous nature of the X chromosome (in males) explains the sex-linked nature of several human conditions. **Red-green colour blindness** and **haemophilia** almost always occur in **males**. Each of these conditions can be caused by the presence of a single recessive allele on the X chromosome.

While females can carry the recessive allele for a sex-linked condition on an X chromosome, it is nearly always masked by the dominant (normal) allele on their other X chromosome – they can be carriers but very rarely have the trait as they would need to have a recessive allele on **both** X chromosomes. However, as explained above, males only need to have one recessive allele on their X chromosome as there is no allele on the Y chromosome to mask it.

The following diagram shows why sex-linked conditions such as haemophilia are nearly always restricted to males.

Tip: Note that for crosses involving sex-linkage, it is important to identify the sex chromosomes with the alleles on the X chromosomes shown as superscripts.

Tip: It is possible (although very rare) for females to have a recessive sex-linked condition such as haemophilia or colour blindness. To have a recessive allele on each of their chromosomes, their father would have to show the condition (have the recessive allele on his X chromosome) and their mother would need to be a carrier (or have the condition.)

Tip: Sex-linked alleles can also be dominant; if dominant there would be no carriers – if the allele is present (in the male or the female) the condition would appear.

Dihybrid inheritance – the inheritance of alleles at two gene loci

Dihybrid refers to analysing the **inheritance of the alleles of two different genes together**. However, the same principles which apply to monohybrid inheritance also apply to dihybrid inheritance. These include:

- only one allele of each gene can enter a gamete;
- if the inheritance of two genes is being considered at the same time (i.e. dihybrid), then each gamete will have two alleles – one from each gene.

For example, if we consider plant height and seed shape in peas – again, tall is dominant to short and

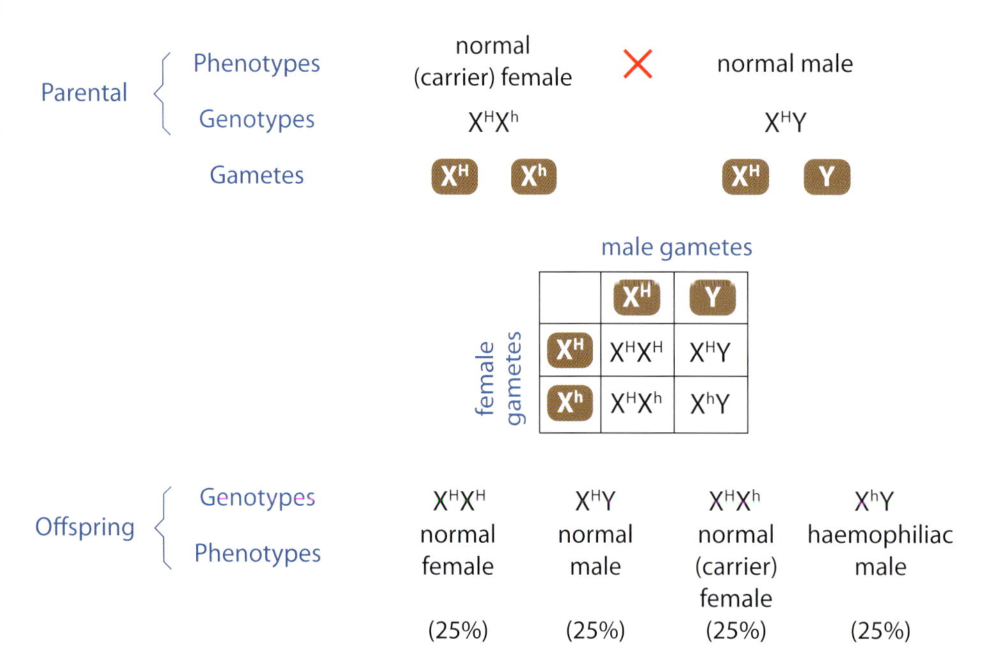

The inheritance of haemophilia from a normal male and a female carrier.

round seed shape is dominant to wrinkled seed shape. Appropriate symbols to use are T (tall) or t (short) for height and R (round) and r (wrinkled) for seed shape.

If we cross two pea plants, one of which is homozygous dominant for each of tall height and producing round seeds and one of which is homozygous recessive for both short height and wrinkled seeds we can only get heterozygous offspring that are tall and produce round seeds as shown in the following diagram.

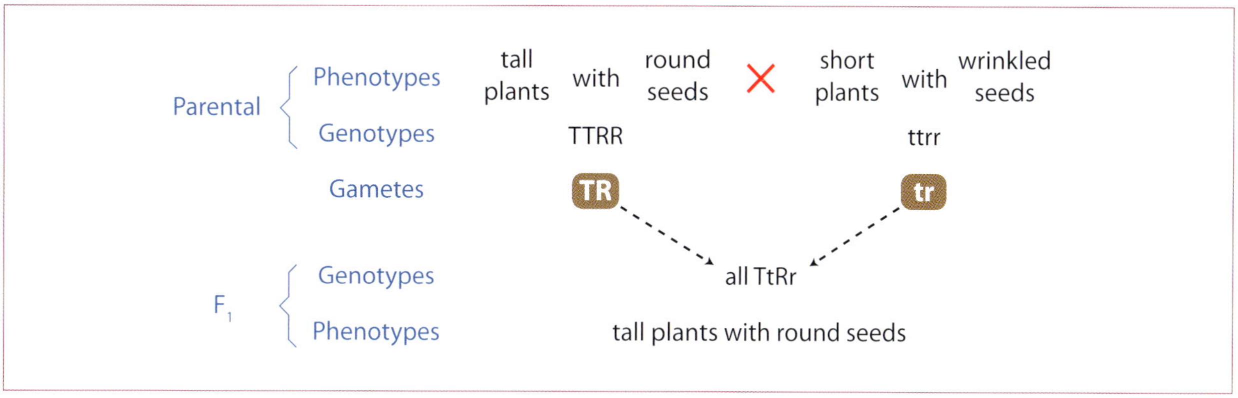

Dihybrid inheritance'

If two of the offspring of the above cross are crossed then a 9 : 3 : 3 : 1 ratio as shown in the next diagram is achieved.

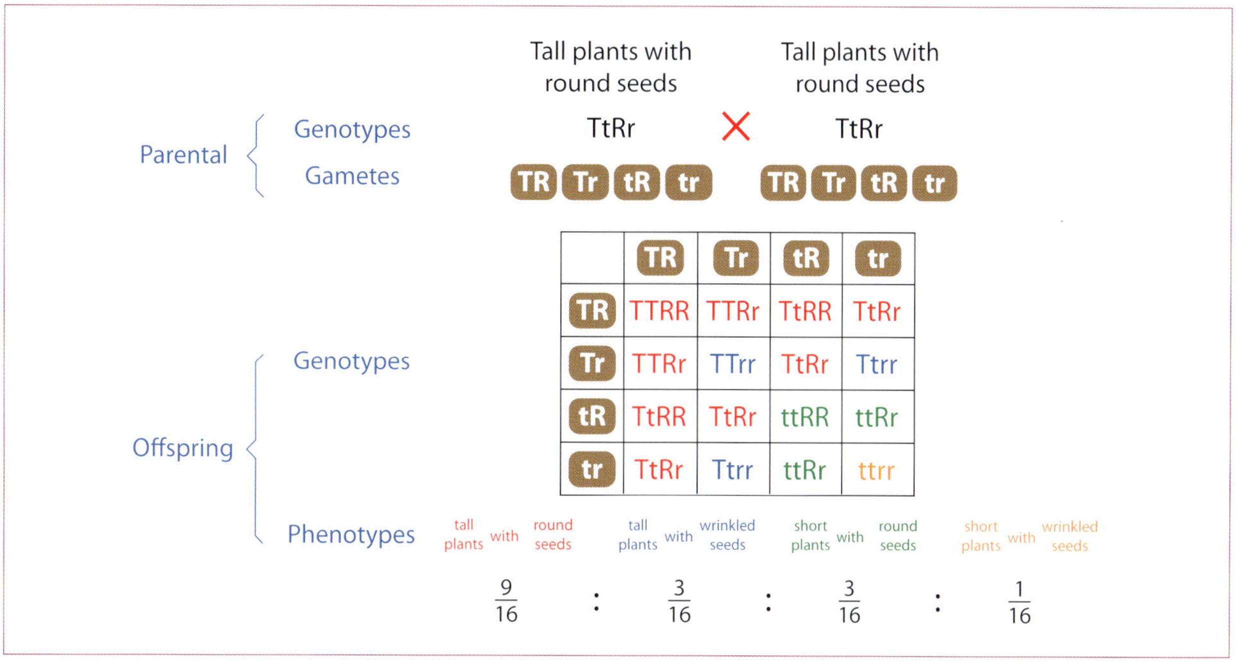

	TR	Tr	tR	tr
TR	TTRR	TTRr	TtRR	TtRr
Tr	TTRr	TTrr	TtRr	Ttrr
tR	TtRR	TtRr	ttRR	ttRr
tr	TtRr	Ttrr	ttRr	ttrr

$\frac{9}{16}$: $\frac{3}{16}$: $\frac{3}{16}$: $\frac{1}{16}$

Dihybrid inheritance giving a 9 : 3 : 3 : 1 ratio

Tip: In the above cross, each of the parents can produce four possible types of gametes. Due to independent assortment during meiosis (in the formation of gametes) there will be approximately equal numbers of each gamete type. That is, in the formation of gametes, the segregation of the alleles of one gene (into any one gamete) is independent to the segregation of the alleles of any other gene.

Worked example

Using the examples covered above, work out the offspring genotypes and phenotypes for a cross between a plant which is heterozygous for both height and seed shape and one that only has recessive alleles for both genes. In your answer show the probabilities for each offspring phenotype.

Answer

Parental
- Phenotypes: tall plants with round seeds × short plants with wrinkled seeds
- Genotypes: TtRr × ttrr
- Gametes: TR, Tr, tR, tr × tr

F_1
- Genotypes:

	TR	Tr	tR	tr
tr	TrRr	Ttrr	ttRr	ttrr

- Phenotypes: tall plants with round seeds 25% · tall plants with wrinkled seeds 25% · short plants with round seeds 25% · short plants with wrinkled seeds 25%

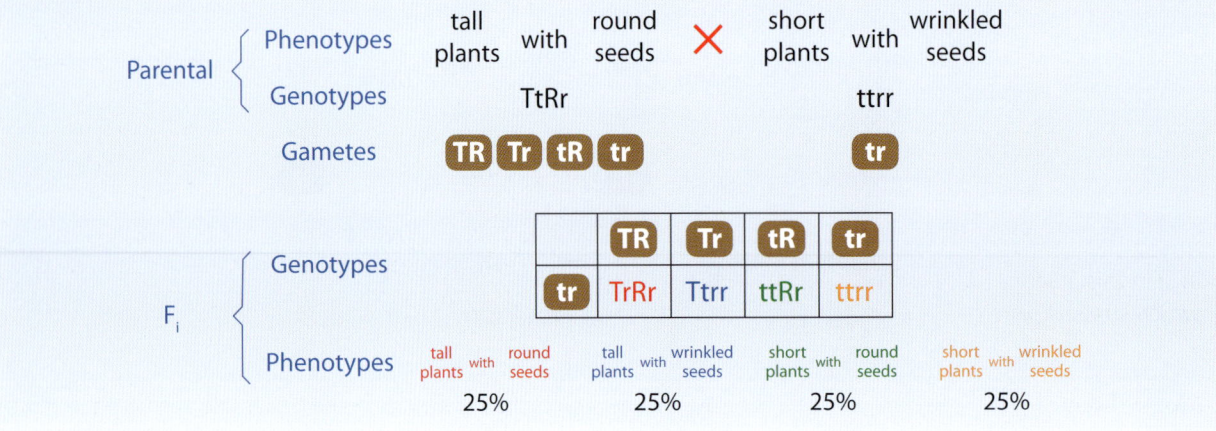

Tip: When using a Punnett square, the number of rows (and columns) used should depend on the number of **different** types of gametes for each parent (in addition to the first column and row used for gametes) as shown in the diagram above.

Epistasis

This is the form of **gene interaction** where one **gene** interferes with the expression of another **gene** or influences it in some way.

Tip: With epistasis it is important to remember that it is a **gene** interfering with the expression of another **gene** and not the alleles within one gene as with dominant and recessive alleles.

Comb type in the domestic chicken is an example of epistasis where the phenotype is dependent on the genotype of two different, independently inherited, genes. The two genes responsible for comb formation are designated P and R. The four phenotypes possible for comb type, their possible genotypes and an explanation of the link between genotype and phenotype are listed in the table below.

The diagram at the top of the next page shows how a cross between a particular chicken with a pea comb and a particular chicken with a rose comb can produce progeny (offspring) showing all four possible phenotypes.

Comb type	Possible genotypes	Explanation
Walnut	PPRR, PpRR, PPRr, PpRr (i.e. P_R_)	At least one dominant P and one dominant R allele present.
Pea	PPrr, Pprr (i.e. P_rr)	At least one dominant P allele but no dominant R allele.
Rose	ppRR, ppRr (i.e. ppR_)	At least one dominant R allele but no dominant P allele.
Single	pprr	Both genes homozygous recessive (no dominant alleles at all).

Parental: Phenotypes — pea comb × rose comb
Parental: Genotypes — Pprr, ppRr
Gametes — Pr, pr; pR, pr

F_1 Genotypes

	pR	pr
Pr	PpRr	Pprr
pr	ppRr	pprr

F_1 Phenotypes — walnut (25%), pea (25%), rose (25%), single (25%)

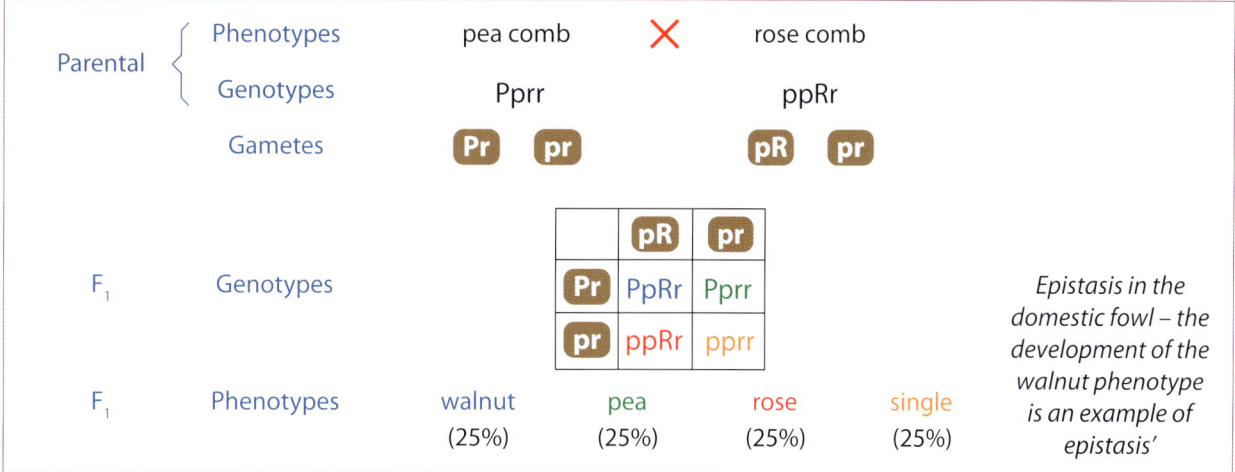

Epistasis in the domestic fowl – the development of the walnut phenotype is an example of epistasis'

Tip: In this example, it is the walnut phenotype which shows epistasis.

Tip: In this cross, reference was made to it being between 'particular' chickens with pea and rose combs. It was worded like this as a pea of genotype PPrr and a rose of genotype ppRR would not give all four phenotypes.

Flower colour in sweet pea is another example of epistasis. In this example, there are two genes (C and P) responsible for flower colour. If **each of the two** independently assorted genes has **at least one dominant allele** present (C-P-) then purple flowers will result.

However, if only one (or neither) of the genes is present in its dominant state (C-pp or ccP- or ccpp) then the flowers are white. The ratio of offspring produced when crossing two double heterozygotes is shown in the diagram below.

The ratio shown (**9 : 7**) is a variation on the normal 9 : 3 : 3 : 1 dihybrid theme as is the situation with other crosses involving epistasis where two genes are independently inherited.

In another example of epistasis, an allele at one locus could **mask** an allele (or alleles) at another locus (i.e. particular alleles of different genes). For example, squash can be yellow, green or white with colour controlled by two genes (1 and 2) with alleles (W and w) and (Y and y) respectively. If there is at least one dominant W allele present (W- for gene 1) the squash will be white, irrespective of the genotype of gene 2.

Parental: Phenotypes — purple flowers × purple flowers
Parental: Genotypes — CcPp, CcPp
Gametes — CP, Cp, cP, cp; CP, Cp, cP, cp

F_1 Genotypes

	CP	Cp	cP	cp
CP	CCPP	CCPp	CcPP	CcPp
Cp	CCPp	CCpp	CcPp	Ccpp
cP	CcPP	CcPp	ccPP	ccPp
cp	CcPp	Ccpp	ccPp	ccpp

F_1 Phenotypes — purple (coloured) flowers : white flowers

9 : 7

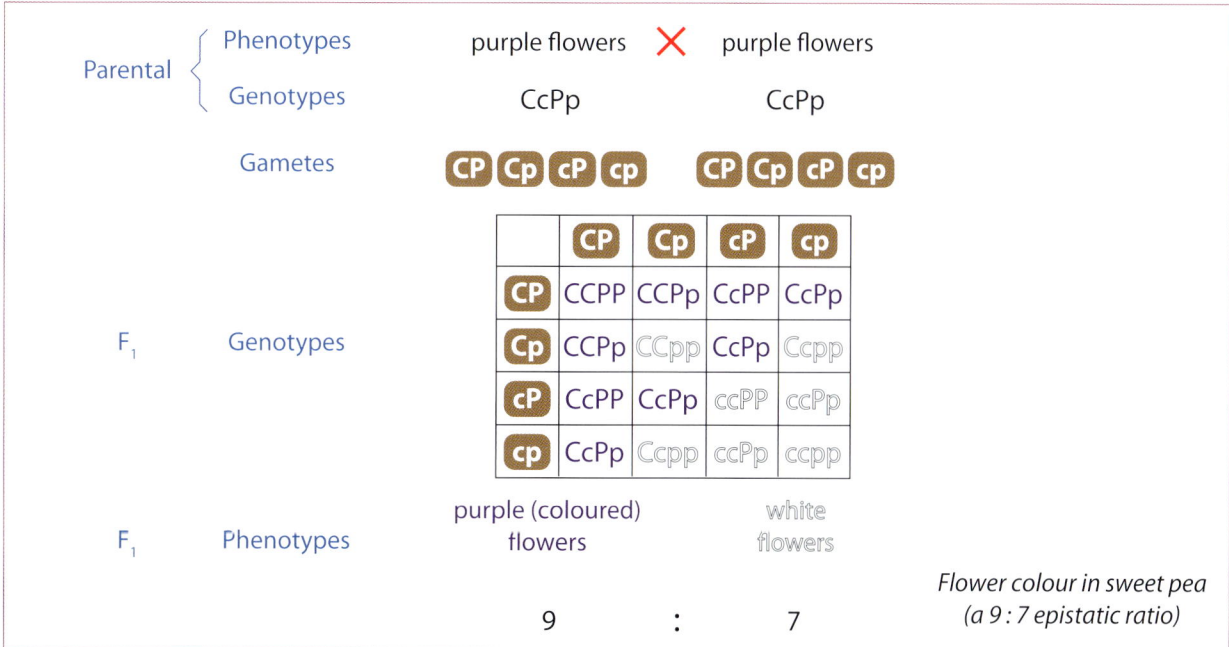

Flower colour in sweet pea (a 9 : 7 epistatic ratio)

If gene 1 has only recessive alleles (ww) then the squash fruit will be coloured, but the actual colour produced depends on gene 2. Genotypes of wwY- give a yellow colour and wwyy gives a green colour. A cross between two plants producing white squashes, but both heterozygous for each gene, produces an offspring phenotypic ratio of 12 : 3 : 1 as shown in the following diagram. In this example, gene 1, if homozygous dominant or heterozygous, masks the effect of gene 2.

Parental: Phenotypes — white × white
Parental: Genotypes — WwYy, WwYy

Gametes: WY Wy wY wy   WY Wy wY wy

F_1 Genotypes

	WY	Wy	wY	wy
WY	WWYY	WWYy	WwYY	WwYy
Wy	WWYy	WWyy	WwYy	Wwyy
wY	WwYY	WwYy	wwYY	wwYy
wy	WwYy	Wwyy	wwYy	wwyy

F_1 Phenotypes: white : yellow : green

12 : 3 : 1

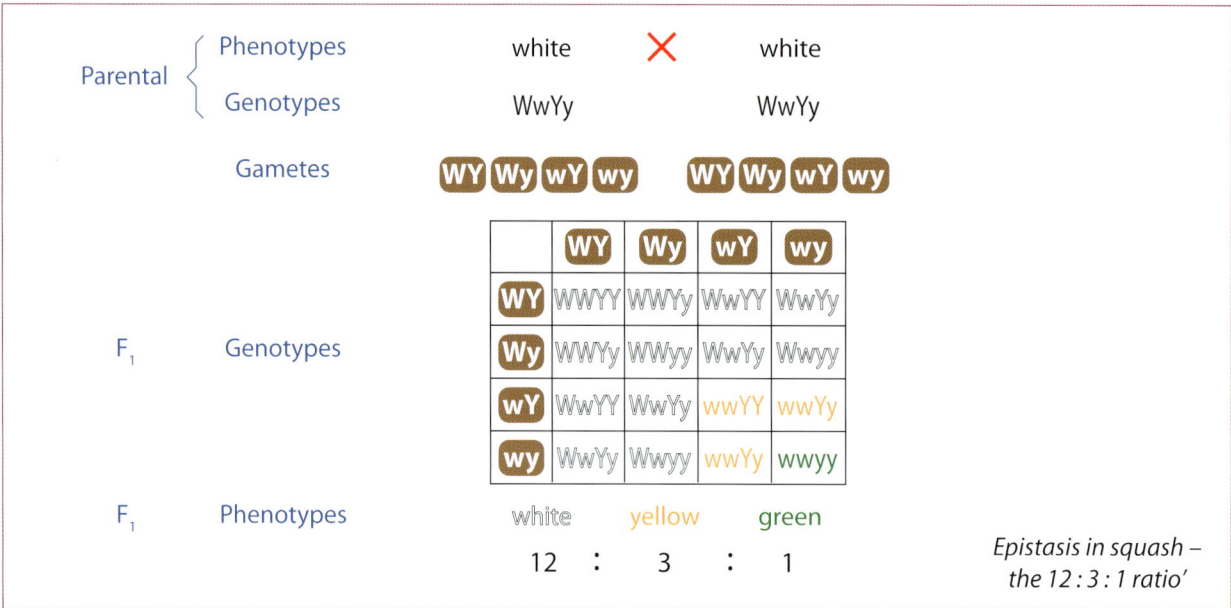

Epistasis in squash – the 12 : 3 : 1 ratio'

In other examples of epistasis, such as wheat kernel colour, two or more genes can substitute for each other (sometimes referred to as duplication). This means that a cross between two double heterozygotes (AaBb) will give a 15 : 1 ratio.

Tip: Note that again in this example, a cross between two double heterozygotes produces a variation of the typical 9 : 3 : 3 : 1 ratio.

The following worked example gives another case of this.

Worked example

In wheat plants, two genes A and B, can each produce coloured kernels (seeds or grains) from a colourless precursor if a dominant allele is present from **either** of these genes. The genes A and B can therefore substitute for each other.

Two wheat plants were crossed, one heterozygous for both A and B genes and the other doubly recessive. Using a Punnett square, work out the genotypes and phenotypes of the offspring produced and the ratio of the different phenotypes.

Answer

Parental
- Phenotypes: coloured kernels × colourless kernels
- Genotypes: AaBb × aabb
- Gametes: AB Ab aB ab × ab

	AB	Ab	aB	ab
ab	AaBb	Aabb	aaBb	aabb

Genotypes	AaBb	Aabb	aaBb	aabb
Phenotypes	coloured	coloured	coloured	colourless

Ratio 3 : 1

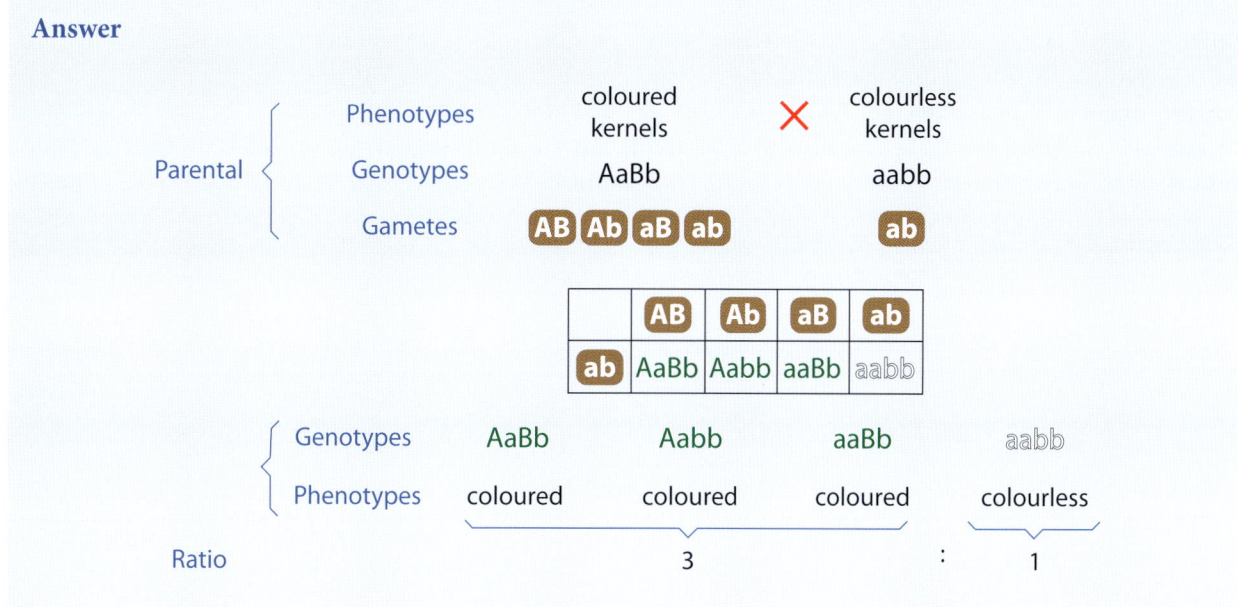

Tip: In this example of epistasis by substitution, the only genotype which results in no colour is the double recessive aabb.

Linkage

In each of the dihybrid examples we have covered so far in this chapter, it has either been stated that the genes were independently inherited or this was assumed. If two genes are independently inherited then they are on chromosomes from **separate** homologous pairs. This means that the chromosomes (and therefore the genes on them) can be independently assorted during metaphase I of meiosis.

However, if two genes are on the **same chromosome** (as they will be if on the same homologous pair) they are said to be **linked**. If they are linked they tend to be inherited together and the outcome appears more like a monohybrid cross.

Tip: Do not confuse 'linkage' in this context with sex-linkage where the linkage refers to the linking of a condition to a particular sex, for example colour blindness and haemophilia in humans.

If two dihybrid heterozygous parents are crossed, and the genes are independently inherited (i.e. they are on separate chromosomes), then a 9 : 3 : 3 :1 ratio would be expected. However, if the two genes are linked (by being on the same chromosome) then the expected ratio would be 3 : 1.

The Chi-squared test – testing for goodness of fit

There are times when it is not clear if the ratio of offspring produced in a genetic cross actually fits the ratio you expect. The **chi-squared (X^2) test** is an appropriate test to confirm if the results of a cross actually fit the ratio predicted.

You will be familiar with the common genetic ratios (for example 9 : 3 : 3 : 1 or 3 : 1) but actual offspring ratios are seldom exact. The chi-square test provides information as to whether any deviation from the expected ratio is significant.

The term '**significance**' is a statistical term – a significant difference is where the difference between data sets (in genetics, usually the difference between the observed and expected results) is due to more than random variation alone. When comparing observed and expected ratios in genetics, if the differences between the two sets of results are **significant**, then you **cannot** assume that any differences are due to chance (i.e. the variation produced by the random mixing of gametes). We will revisit significance later.

In the chi-squared test it is important to work out the expected frequencies, based on the data presented and then carry out a series of calculations based on the expected and observed data.

In the chi-square table below, the first column is

the **category**, for example the different genetic traits – in a 9 : 3 : 3 : 1 ratio there would be 4 traits (so 5 rows including the title row), then there are columns for the **observed** and **expected** results (**O** and **E** respectively) – then a row for the number of observed **minus** the number of expected results **(O – E)** then the **square** of this value $\mathbf{(O - E)^2}$ and finally the square of the difference divided by the expected results for that trait $\mathbf{(O - E)^2 \div E}$. To get the X^2 value you add the values in this final column $\mathbf{((O - E)^2 \div E)}$ together.

The table below shows a typical table used in a chi-square test. In our worked example near the start of the dihybrid section we got a 1 : 1 : 1 : 1 ratio. Supposing in that cross we had 100 offspring plants in the numbers shown in the observed (O) column, then assuming the 1 : 1 : 1 : 1 ratio the expected (E) results would be as shown. The rest of the table can be worked out as shown.

Category	Observed (O)	Expected (E)	(O – E)	$(O - E)^2$	$\frac{(O - E)^2}{E}$
Tall plants that produce round seeds	23	25	–2	4	0.16
Tall plants that produce wrinkled seeds	28	25	3	9	0.36
Short plants that produce round seeds	27	25	2	4	0.16
Short plants that produce wrinkled seeds	22	25	–3	9	0.36
					X^2 = **1.04**

Tip: You will almost always be given the actual (the observed) results from a cross (O). From this you can work out (or you will be given) the total number of offspring. Again, from this you can work out the expected numbers for each category. For example, if there are 60 offspring and the predicted genetic ratio is 1 : 1 (i.e. the offspring from a monohybrid cross between a heterozygous parent and a parent with two recessive alleles), then the expected values would be 30 and 30 (were the ratio of offspring to work out exactly).

Tip: Although there can be negative values in the (O – E) column, when squared in $(O - E^2)$, these will become positive.

What do we then do with the X^2 value (for example the 1.04 calculated in the table above)?

In terms of the chi-squared test, **probability** is a measure of how likely a deviation between the expected and the observed results are due to chance (i.e. random variation). For example, a probability value of 0.10 means there is 10% chance that the difference between the expected and the observed results are due to chance – another way of looking at this is saying that there is a 90% chance that the differences are significant, i.e. there is a 90% chance the difference is significant, i.e. the results do not agree with the predicted ratio.

Critically, the 0.05 probability level is the cut off in statistics – if the p value is greater than 0.05 (5%) (written as $p > 0.05$) this means that statistically the possibility of the difference between the observed and expected being due to chance is high enough to accept the predicted ratio – if the p value is lower ($p < 0.05$) than this then the possibility that the difference between the observed and the expected results being due to chance is so low that the predicted ratio cannot be accepted.

The following table shows some probability (p) values and whether the predicted genetic ratio fits the results.

p value	*p* = 0.10	0.05	0.01	0.001
Probability that difference between the observed and expected results is due to chance (can be explained by random variation)	10%	5%	1%	0.1%
Probability that the difference between the observed and expected results is significant (cannot be explained by random variation)	90%	95%	99%	99.9%

Probability values in the blue part of the table mean that there is not a significant difference between the observed and expected results (i.e. the observed results are a good fit to the expected results or any difference between the observed and expected results is not significant) – probability values in the green part of the table show that the difference is significant, i.e. the actual (observed) results do not fit the predicted (expected) results.

How do we find the probability levels? Consider the chi-square table earlier and note that the X^2 value is 1.04. To make sense of this value you need a table of X^2 values – you will be provided with this in an exam. There is a table of chi-square values and associated probability values on page 176. The left (first) column of this table is the degrees of freedom (d.f.) column and this helps you decide which row of the table you should use. The d.f. value is the number of categories/traits minus one – for example, if there are three categories, such as you get with a 1 : 2 : 1 phenotypic ratio then there are 2 d.f. and you use this row.

However, in our chi-square table, we have 4 categories, so we have 3 degrees of freedom. Using this row our value of 1.04 lies between the 0.9 and the 0.5 probability values. This can be written as $0.9 > p > 0.5$ which is well to the left of the critical 0.05 level (i.e. the possibility of the differences being due to chance are between 90% – 50%) therefore our conclusion is that the **observed results are a good fit to the expected ratio or the differences between the observed and expected results are not significant** (so you can accept the predicted ratio).

Tip: In this example, if the X^2 value had been the value at a 0.05 level of probability, i.e. 7.81 (or higher, i.e. further to the right in the table) our conclusion would have been that the observed results were not a good fit to the expected ratio or the differences between the observed and expected results were significant (i.e. the predicted ratio does not hold true based on the observed results).

Tip: In an exam question, you may be asked to state which two probability levels your calculated X^2 value falls between, rather than asked to express your answer in terms of > *p* >. In this case, you just read off the two probability values at the top of the table.

Questions

1. (a) Define the term haploid cell. [1]

   (b) Name the stages of meiosis where:
   - crossing over occurs
   - independent assortment occurs [2]

   (c) The diagram below represents a stage of meiosis. (For simplicity, not all the chromosomes are shown).

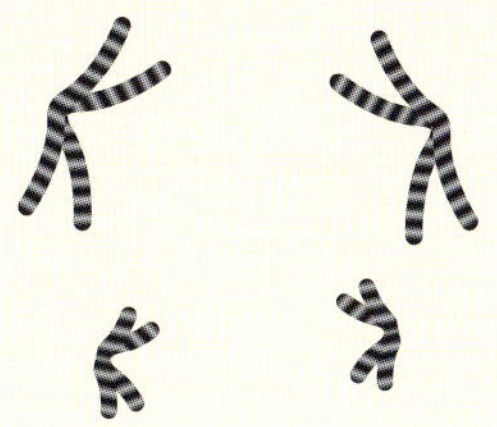

   Identify the division and stage of meiosis shown. Explain your answer. [3]

2. An individual can be blood group **A**, **B**, **AB** or **O**. **A** and **B** are codominant and each are dominant to **O**.

   (a) (i) Using the information provided, state the genotype(s) for blood group **O**. [1]

   (ii) State all the possible genotypes for blood group **B**. [1]

   (b) Using a Punnett square show the possible blood groups that there can be in the children of a parent who has blood group **AB** and a parent who is blood group **O**. [3]

3. (a) Haemophilia is a sex-linked condition in which affected individuals are missing components necessary for effective blood clotting. The haemophilia allele is recessive to the allele for normal blood clotting. The genotype for a normal female is $\mathbf{X^HX^H}$.

   (i) Explain what is meant by the term sex-linked. [1]

   (ii) Using the format above, state the genotype for a male who does not have haemophilia. [1]

   (iii) Using the information provided, use a Punnett square to show how it is possible for two parents neither of whom have haemophilia to have a child who has the condition. [3]

(b) Huntington's disease is a neurological degenerative condition caused by a single defective allele. The defective disease-causing allele is dominant to the normal allele. (Let N = Huntington allele and n = normal allele).
The gene for Huntington's disease is on an autosome (non-sex chromosome).
Use a Punnett square to show the genotypes and phenotypes of the offspring produced by a female parent who does not carry the haemophilia allele nor the Huntington allele (genotype X^HX^H nn) and a male parent who has haemophilia and is heterozygous for the Huntington's gene. [5]

4. (a) (i) Describe what is meant by the term independent assortment. [1]
(ii) State the division and stage of meiosis during which independent assortment occurs. [1]

(b) In the fruit fly *Drosophila*, the genes for body colour and wing type are located on separate chromosomes. Normal body colour is dominant to ebony body colour and normal wing is dominant to vestigial (reduced) wing.
(Let **C** = normal body colour and **W** = normal wing).
(i) State the genotype(s) that will give flies with normal body colour and vestigial wing. [1]
(ii) In terms of alleles present, state the gametes produced by flies with ebony body colour and vestigial wings. [1]
(iii) Using a Punnett square, work out the offspring genotypes and phenotypes of a cross between a fly heterozygous for each gene and a fly heterozygous for the body colour gene but homozygous recessive for the wing gene. [4]

(c) In a separate cross, flies that were heterozygous for each of the wing and body colour genes were interbred (i.e. crossed with flies of the same genotype).
(i) Using your understanding of typical genetic ratios, predict the offspring phenotype ratio produced by this cross. [1]
The table below shows the phenotypes of offspring produced from the cross described above. A total of 1600 offspring flies were produced.

Category	Observed (O)	Expected (E)	(O – E)	$(O – E)^2$	$\frac{(O – E)^2}{E}$
Normal body, normal wing	917				
Normal body, vestigial wing	288				
Ebony body, normal wing	305				
Ebony body, vestigial wing	90				

(ii) Using your answer to part (i), copy the table and complete the (numbers for the) expected column. [1]
(iii) Complete the rest of the table and calculate the X^2 value. [2]

The table below gives the probability values for use with the Chi-squared test. The degrees of freedom (d.f.) is calculated as $n - 1$ where n is the number of categories.

d.f.	probability = 0.900	0.500	0.100	0.050	0.010	0.001
1	0.016	0.455	2.71	3.84	6.63	10.83
2	0.211	1.39	4.61	5.99	9.21	13.82
3	0.584	2.37	6.25	7.81	11.34	16.27
4	1.06	3.36	7.78	9.49	13.28	18.47

(iv) On the basis of your calculated X^2 value, and using the table above, state the following:
- the degrees of freedom for the test;
- the probability value [2]

(v) Explain the outcome of your Chi-squared test. [1]

17: THE APPLICATION OF GENETIC ENGINEERING AND GENE THERAPY

Students should be able to:

11.4.1 demonstrate an understanding of the fact that human insulin is a protein made in the pancreas;

11.4.2 demonstrate an understanding of how insulin is involved in the regulation of blood sugar levels but in diabetes mellitus there is a deficiency;

11.4.3 recall that insulin is extracted from natural sources such as cattle and pigs but that this insulin is not identical to human insulin and extraction of the hormone is very difficult;

11.4.4 describe how insulin can be obtained from bacteria and recall that Humulin is a licensed drug made from genetically modified *E. coli* bacteria;

11.4.5 discuss the advantages of using insulin from genetically modified organisms, including:
- fewer adverse reactions;
- larger quantities being made;
- low production costs; and
- fewer ethical or religious issues, such as objections to using animals;

11.4.6 discuss how haemophiliacs suffer from a defective gene that fails to produce factor VIII or IX, which is an important agent in blood clotting; and

11.4.7 recall that factor VIII was obtained from natural sources such as blood serum but this posed other major risks such as viruses, which previously resulted in many haemophiliacs contracting HIV/AIDS.

11.5.1 evaluate and compare genetic engineering and traditional breeding in animals;

11.5.2 explain the impact of genetic engineering, with reference to:
- exponential world population growth;
- the amount of available land;
- its potential to increase yields; and
- its potential to make therapeutic chemicals in other animals, for example human serum albumin to treat burns;

11.5.3 discuss ethical issues relating to genetically modified or transgenic organisms;

11.6.1 explain what gene therapy is;

11.6.2 discuss initial attempts at gene therapy, including attempts to treat cystic fibrosis in humans; and

11.6.3 explain the cause and symptoms of cystic fibrosis and the associated gene therapy treatment;

11.7.1 discuss treating a genetic disease by altering an individual's natural genotype by:
- germ cell therapy of sperm, egg or early embryo; and
- somatic cell therapy;

11.7.2 recall that gene therapy can work in three ways:
- by repairing the defective gene;
- by replacing the faulty gene with a normal one; and
- by adding a normal gene, leaving the defective one in position;

11.7.3 explain the use of gene therapy to supplement defective genes;

11.7.4 demonstrate knowledge and understanding of the polymerase chain reaction (PCR);

11.7.5 recall that DNA sequencing and the polymerase chain reaction (PCR) are used to produce DNA probes that can screen patients for clinically important genes; and

11.7.6 recall that this information is used in genetic counselling, for example:
- in family planning for parents who are both carriers of defective genes; and
- in the case of oncogenes, in deciding the best course of treatment for cancers.

11.1.19 demonstrate an understanding that many human diseases result from mutated genes or from genes that are useful in one context but not in another, for example sickle cell anaemia and aneuploidy;

Insulin

Insulin as a hormone

Insulin is a **protein** made in the **pancreas** – specifically the **β-cells** in the **Islets of Langerhans** – and plays an important part in the regulation of blood sugar levels. You will remember that you covered insulin in the section on homeostasis (2.4) at AS level.

Tip: You should remember that insulin is a **hormone** and that hormones are chemical messengers that travel in the blood to bring about a response in one or more target organs.

Insulin serves to stop blood glucose (sugar) levels getting too high – this is most likely to occur after taking food rich in carbohydrate. Therefore, it is not surprising that blood insulin levels rise and peak as glucose (from carbohydrate in the diet) is absorbed from food and enters the blood, as shown in the following graph.

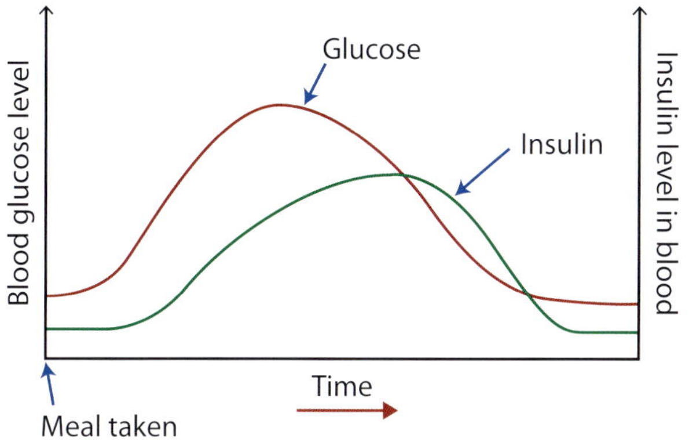

Insulin works by **lowering** blood glucose levels – the responses insulin brings about all act to reduce blood glucose – through the following processes.

- increasing the uptake of glucose into body cells;
- increasing the rate at which glucose is used in respiration in cells;
- increasing the rate at which glucose is converted to glycogen for storage in the liver and in the muscles; and
- (when glycogen stores are full) increasing the rate at which glucose is converted to fat.

Diabetes

Diabetes mellitus is a condition in which the regulation of blood glucose fails to work properly. This can be caused by the pancreas failing to produce any (or enough) insulin, as occurs with **type 1 diabetes**, or by the body cells becoming resistant to the effects of insulin as happens with **type 2 diabetes**. Patients with type 1 diabetes need to take injections of insulin to stop their blood glucose levels rising too high.

Worked example

(a) Diabetes is usually diagnosed by the blood glucose (sugar) level being higher than it should be. Explain why a high blood sugar level can be used in the diagnosis of diabetes.

(b) Type 1 diabetes is often diagnosed in children. In the period up to diagnosis, these children often lose weight rapidly. Explain why.

Answer

(a) Too little or no insulin is being produced/or it fails to work effectively. Therefore, the body is not able to reduce blood sugar levels by increasing uptake into body cells/ increasing respiration/converting to glycogen or fat (resulting in the high blood glucose level).

(b) The blood glucose cannot be taken up into cells. The body uses (stored) fat for respiration, therefore causing the weight loss.

For many years the injected insulin came from the pancreases of animals such as cattle and pigs when the animals were in abattoirs for slaughter. Over the last few decades, the insulin used in treating type 1 diabetes has been produced by genetically engineered bacteria.

Genetically engineered organisms

Genetically engineered insulin

Genetically engineered microorganisms are microbes which have had their DNA altered, usually by the addition of DNA from another 'foreign' organism (i.e. from a different species). In the case of insulin production, the human gene for insulin is inserted into recipient microorganisms and then the microorganisms (bacteria) start producing the insulin.

Tip: Organisms which have DNA added to their genome from another species are referred to as **transgenic**.

Humulin is an example of a genetically engineered insulin and it is typically made by the genetic manipulation of *E. coli* bacteria. There are two key stages in manipulating these microorganisms:

- extracting the (insulin) gene from humans; and
- inserting the human DNA into the DNA of the microbe in such a way that it will continue to code for (and produce) protein (in this case insulin).

Extracting the desired (insulin) gene from human cells and inserting it in bacterial DNA

Once the position of the desired gene has been identified in human cells, special enzymes called **restriction endonucleases** are used to cut out this gene. Restriction enzymes work in such a way that they cut out the genes but leave what are called '**sticky ends**' at either end.

Restriction endonucleases cut DNA at specific sequences of bases called recognition sequences. The restriction endonuclease enzyme **EcoR1** has a recognition sequence of GAATTC and the enzyme cuts between the G and A bases at the ends of this sequence as shown in the following diagram. The result is that on either side of the cut the two DNA ends have 'sticky ends' that consist of a single extending DNA strand containing exposed bases.

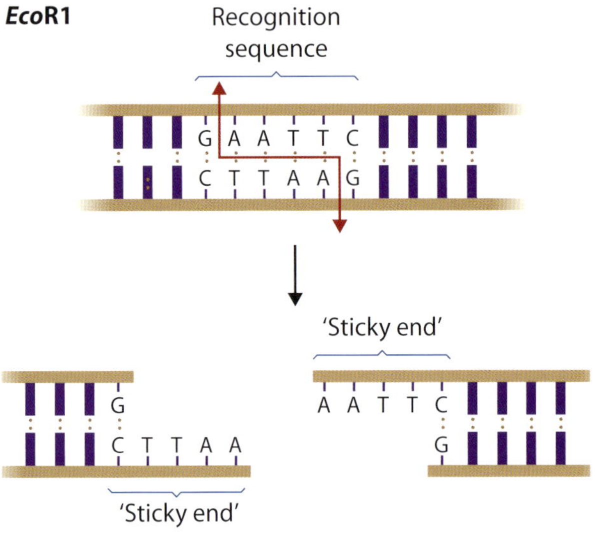

Restriction enzymes and sticky ends'

> **Tip:** Other restriction enzymes have different recognition sequences and therefore cut the DNA at different places and so produce sticky ends with different sequences of exposed bases.

Bacteria have their DNA in a single large continuous loop rather than in a series of chromosomes as in mammals. Additionally, they have a number of very small loops of DNA called **plasmids**. Plasmids are easily extracted from bacteria and are relatively easy to incorporate back in. Taking account of this, genetic engineers use the plasmids as **vectors** – a method of getting the insulin into the host bacteria.

As the plasmids are closed loops, they must be cut open before inserting the insulin gene. This is done using the same restriction endonuclease enzyme that is used to cut out the insulin gene from human DNA. The advantage of using the same enzyme is that the bases of the sticky ends produced on the plasmid will be complementary to the bases on the insulin sticky ends.

Therefore, the insulin gene, including its sticky ends, will make a perfect join and hydrogen bonds form between the matching base pairs on each end of the cut plasmid. Once the bases have paired up, the enzyme **DNA ligase** is used to join the DNA backbones together – the joining of the complementary sticky ends is a process referred to as **annealing**. The removal of a human gene and its insertion into a plasmid is summarised in the following diagram.

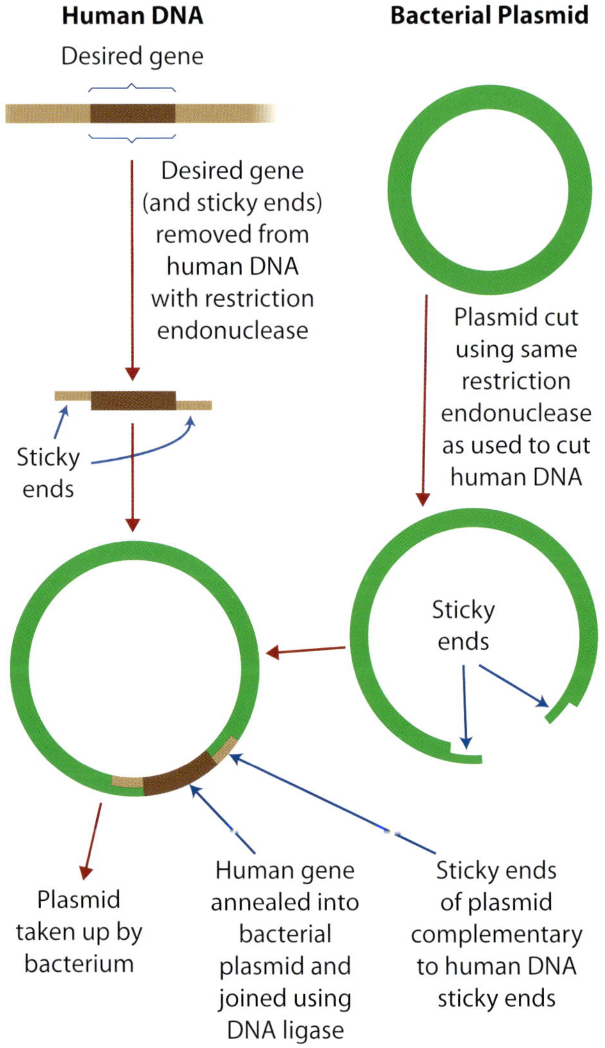

Extracting a human gene and inserting it into a bacterial plasmid

Once the plasmid vector has had the foreign (human) gene inserted, the bacterium is encouraged to take up the vector. There are several ways this is done, including heat treatment. Once this is done, the bacteria **replicate (multiply)** and the large number produced are cultured in fermenters to produce large quantities of the desired product (for example Humulin) which is then **purified and packaged**.

Advantages of genetically engineered insulin

The advantages of using genetically engineered insulin rather than extraction from dead animals include:

- **non-human insulin** is slightly **different** to human insulin and therefore has the potential to cause allergic reactions or not work as efficiently – cow insulin differs from human insulin by three amino acids and pig insulin differs by one amino acid – therefore, there are **fewer adverse reactions** with genetically engineered insulin such as Humulin;
- genetically engineered insulin can be produced in **high quantities** to meet the growing demand created by the rapidly increasing number of people with diabetes;
- the **extraction of insulin** from the pancreases of dead animals **is difficult** (and not cost effective);
- the **production cost** of producing insulin by genetic engineering is **low** (once the technique has been refined) – making genetically engineered insulin less expensive;
- there are **fewer ethical or religious issues**; and
- **Humulin** is absorbed more rapidly into the bloodstream and can reduce blood glucose levels in a **shorter time**.

> **Tip:** It is important to understand that many different types of bacteria could be used to make insulin – the process is basically the same.

Other examples of genetic engineering

Making Factor VIII

As discussed in the previous chapter, haemophilia is a sex-linked genetic condition which mainly affects males. People with haemophilia have a defective allele (gene) which fails to produce **factor VIII** or **IX**, important components in the process of blood clotting. Individuals (men) who have haemophilia are referred to as haemophiliacs and they are at risk of major blood loss should they have a cut. For many years they were given blood transfusions (serum) which contained the missing factors so that their blood would clot normally as necessary.

However, these transfusions posed other problems such as the **transfer of viruses** from donors to the haemophiliac recipients. An example is the transfer of **HIV** from donors who were HIV positive. The consequence of this was that many haemophiliacs who had been given contaminated blood developed **AIDS** and many died as a result. Today, this problem is largely avoided by the screening of blood products. However, a difficulty is that even after screening blood for harmful microbes and viruses, some viruses are so small that they can still get through and infect the donor.

> **Tip:** Treatment aimed at producing the missing blood factors in individuals with haemophilia now focuses on gene therapy (by replacing the missing gene; see later in this chapter) rather than giving patients infusions of genetically engineered products.

Making other drugs or substances useful to humans

Microorganisms and other larger organisms have been genetically modified to produce large quantities of medical, pharmaceutical and industrial substances by genetic engineering such as **factor VIII**, **enzymes**, **hormones** and **anti-cancer drugs**. In the case of genetically modified (GM) plants, the plants themselves are often the desired outcome (see below). Additionally, it is now possible to replace or repair damaged genes.

Transgenic animals, for example, **chickens** have been used to produce **antibodies** for medical use, **sheep** for **Factor VIII** as described above, and **cows** that produce milk with **reduced lactose content**. As well as the production of specific chemicals, a key focus of genetic engineering is to produce animals that grow faster and larger to meet the demands of a growing population.

GM (transgenic) plants

To genetically modify a plant, 'gene guns' can be used to shoot the desired genes into the cells of young plants. Alternatively, the DNA can be added to isolated plant cells and the plants grown from tissue culture. GM crops such as maize (corn) have been grown in many parts of the world, although Europe has largely opposed their use, particularly if it is likely to be involved in the human food chain. Some of the advantages of GM crops are summarised in the table below.

Tip: As with transgenic animals, it is important to understand that a general goal with GM plants is to **increase productivity (yield)**.

Tip: Although some forms of genetic engineering can increase the ecological range of crop and domestic animals, this is offset by the increased urbanisation that results from a rapidly growing human population and the desertification of vast quantities of land (previously used for agriculture) as a result of global warming.

The social, ethical and economic implications of genetic engineering

Before the use of genetic engineering to improve yield, **traditional breeding** was used to improve the quality of crops and domestic animals. The principle underpinning traditional breeding is that the 'best' individuals are interbred, with 'poorer quality' individuals not used for breeding. This '**selective breeding**' takes place over many generations to produce the highest quality stock and produce. Virtually all our common crops and farm animals have been selectively bred over many years to produce the stock we have today. For most domestic stock and crops, current species are very different to their ancestors. To give one example, modern wheat produces more grain and has shorter stems of more even height. The advantage of the extra grain is obvious, but shorter stems reduce the likelihood of wind damage and the more even height facilitates harvesting using modern machinery.

There are two obvious **advantages with genetic engineering** of crops and animals compared with traditional breeding:

- the desired changes will be achieved in a **shorter time** – using traditional breeding it takes many years and many breeding cycles for the desired changes to take place, particularly so in animals, which have longer life cycles than most crops;
- genetic engineering can produce changes or products which would **not occur by traditional breeding alone**, for example sheep producing Factor VIII and the production of 'golden' rice.

When looking at the overall benefits of genetic engineering it is important to include the direct manipulation and **replacement of faulty disease-causing genes** whether by adding the normal gene (see the next section) or by actually amending the genes in-situ.

Genetic engineering and genetic manipulation have their opponents and **arguments against** include

Feature	Benefit
Nutritional enhancement	This involves modifying the plants so that they are very rich in certain vitamins, minerals or other food type. 'Golden rice' is a form of GM rice with enhanced levels of vitamin A and iron.
Greater ecological range	Many plant species have been developed that can grow in a greater ecological range than normal – for example, ryegrass species have been developed which have had a drought tolerance gene added from another species meaning that it can now grow in places which were previously too dry (but see the second tip below).
Greater productivity (yield)	Genetically engineered crops could help produce the extra food required to feed a growing world population through the greater yields produced through faster and greater growth and the greater ecological range as described above.
Herbicide and pesticide resistance	This allows herbicides (weed killer) and pesticides to be used with the result that weeds and harmful pests can be destroyed without harming the GM crop itself.

the following:

- some people are worried that it is 'playing God' and is unnatural, and they have **ethical and/or religious** issues with it;
- the potential of producing '**designer babies**' which have DNA manipulated by man to produce individuals with a range of 'desirable' properties;
- a worry that manipulating DNA may have **consequences, that as yet, are unknown**;
- a worry that GM crops or other GM products could cause **allergies**;
- the creation of '**superweeds**' as a consequence of developing GM crops.

However, most scientists accept that **genetic engineering can bring huge medical and other benefits, as long as it is careful regulated**. Another clear benefit arising from genetic engineering is gene therapy, which is the topic of the next section.

Gene Therapy

It is now known that many human diseases are a result of a mutated (defective) gene, for example Huntington's disease, cystic fibrosis, Tay Sachs and many others where one or more mutated genes cause a particular disease or give individuals a predisposition for a disease such as with some forms of cancer.

Gene therapy is the process by which functional genes are added to body cells to replace or compensate for defective genes or the defective genes are repaired. The type of gene therapy used in medicine is **somatic gene (cell) therapy** where the functional genes are added to affected tissues only.

Before gene therapy is used it is important to identify which genes are defective. For some relatively common diseases, such as cystic fibrosis, the faulty gene was identified many years ago and its position in the genome known.

A mutated or defective gene can remain at a relatively high level in the human population in environmental settings where it can be beneficial, whereas in other environmental settings it has no benefit and therefore tends to be in very low frequency as a result of selection. One example is **sickle cell anaemia**. Sickle cell anaemia is a blood disorder which is particularly common in some parts of Africa and some Mediterranean countries.

The condition causes the haemoglobin to be a 'sickle' shape that flows through small blood vessels less well leading to affected individuals suffering from anaemia. Individuals who are homozygous for this gene (i.e. two defective alleles) often die at a young age. However, those who are heterozygous have sickle cell 'trait' where the haemoglobin is less efficient in transporting oxygen, but the benefit is that these individuals are protected against malaria to some extent. Not surprisingly, the incidence of sickle cell anaemia is highest in those regions where the disease malaria is common.

Tip: The distribution of sickle cell trait across the globe is an example of natural selection. The heterozygous genotype is only advantageous in regions where malaria is common, so it is only common in these regions – there are very few sickle cell alleles in the population in areas where there is no malaria.

Worked Example

The table below shows the proportions of people in a number of countries who do not have the sickle cell allele (normal phenotype), have sickle cell trait (heterozygotes), and have sickle cell disease. In these countries, malaria (often a fatal disease) is a common illness.

Phenotype	Genotype	Percentage
normal	HbAHbA	28
sickle cell trait	HbAHbS	64
sickle cell anaemia	HbSHbS	8

(a) What percentage of individuals in the table have homozygous phenotypes?

(b) Using the information provided and your knowledge, explain the results for individuals with sickle cell anaemia.

(c) Using the information provided and your knowledge, describe and explain the results for normal and sickle cell trait phenotypes.

Answer

(a) 36

(b) Individuals with sickle cell anaemia (often) die young (therefore there will be relatively few in the population).

(c) There are more individuals with sickle cell trait than normal phenotypes. Sickle cell trait helps protect against malaria (whereas normal trait does not) (or converse).

Sometimes mutations involve having one (or more) fewer or extra (entire) chromosomes rather than just a single gene being affected. The addition or loss of one or more chromosomes is referred to as aneuploidy.

Tip: As with gene mutations, aneuploidy often has harmful consequences but can, occasionally, bring advantages – aneuploidy has been an important aid to horticulturists in plant breeding.

Gene therapy as a medical procedure has had a difficult beginning. Around the year 2000, when gene therapy was being developed as an experimental treatment, a number of patients died in early trials. It is thought that the process involving the addition of 'foreign' genes disrupted the normal working of the DNA to such an extent that this triggered leukaemia in some patients, and in others it put their immune systems into 'overdrive' causing very severe reactions within the body. However, the process has been refined and gene therapy is now a successful treatment for a growing number of medical conditions.

Gene therapy works in three main ways:

- by **repairing** the defective gene;
- by **replacing** the faulty gene with a normal one;
- by **adding** a normal gene, leaving the defective one in position.

Cystic fibrosis

Many human medical conditions are caused by the presence of a single defective gene (allele). **Cystic fibrosis** is an example of a genetically inherited condition where, if an individual possesses two defective alleles, he or she will have the condition (i.e. the cystic fibrosis allele is recessive to the 'normal' allele). In Europe, approximately 1 in 2500 people are affected. The condition is due to the malfunctioning of the protein produced by the faulty gene which is responsible for keeping cell membranes lining the digestive and respiratory systems in good condition. This protein is the **trans-membrane-conductance regulator (CFTR)** protein and is involved in secreting chloride ions out of cells.

In an individual with cystic fibrosis, the protein will not function as normal and the membranes become covered with **thick sticky mucus**. This is a consequence of water not moving out of cells by osmosis (in these cells in individuals who do not have cystic fibrosis the water dilutes the mucus surrounding the membranes). This affects several parts of the body including:

- **the lungs** – the build-up of mucus in the lungs affects **gas exchange** (leading to shortness of breath) and leads to a much higher risk of **lung infection** (as a result of microbes becoming trapped in the mucus and the body being unable to expel them); and
- **the digestive system** – the build-up of mucus in the **pancreatic duct** prevents the pancreatic enzymes reaching the gut, leading to problems with **food digestion**.

Gene therapy and cystic fibrosis

Gene therapy has been used to **improve lung function** in cystic fibrosis patients. Two types of vectors have been used to deliver the functional genes into the cells lining the lung air passages. These two vectors are as follows:

- **Adenoviruses** – these are viruses which cause respiratory infections so are adapted in being able to penetrate the cells lining the lung air passages. However, before they can carry out their role as vectors in gene therapy, they need to have their 'harmful' disease-causing genes removed as well as having the functional CFTR gene spliced in.
- **Liposomes** – these are small vesicles ('packages') formed of fat (lipid) which contain the donor DNA. The lipid coating helps the DNA gain entry to the affected cells more easily.

However, irrespective of the method used to insert genes into cells, there are difficulties in getting the DNA into the cell nucleus (where the host DNA is) and getting the DNA to function as normal without causing disruption to the host genome.

Tip: Liposomes are less effective at getting the donor DNA into the host cell nucleus compared to viruses but they are often safer in that they do not have some of the problems associated with deliberately inserting viruses into human cells (for example, infection, allergies and other immune responses).

While there have been great strides made in treating cystic fibrosis with gene therapy there have also been some significant problems. These include the following:

- while it is relatively easy to use aerosols to get functional genes into the airways of the lungs, it is much more difficult to access the pancreatic duct;
- new cells produced by the body will still contain the defective gene;
- the aerosol may not reach all parts of the lung;
- the use of viruses may cause infections, immune responses or allergies;
- immune reactions may destroy the virus vectors before they can deliver their DNA;
- the added gene may not become incorporated into the host DNA therefore repeat treatments are necessary and the defective gene will still pass on to offspring.

As stated previously, the gene therapy used to treat genetic disease described in the sections above is referred to as **somatic** gene therapy. **Germ cell therapy** (also known as germline gene therapy) involves **manipulating the genome in the male sperm, female egg or early embryo**. With this type of gene therapy all the cells of the developing (new) individual are normal for the gene(s) under consideration, and there is no issue with having to get replacement genes into cells in inaccessible parts of the body. Additionally, with germ cell therapy the defective gene will not pass on to any offspring as any gametes subsequently produced in the new individual will not contain the defective gene. Germ cell therapy presents many moral and ethical issues and is currently illegal in humans.

Gene therapy – the current position

Where it is possible, gene therapy now involves replacing or fixing the defective gene. For example, sickle cell anaemia can be treated by removing bone marrow from affected individuals and then 'editing' the relevant gene in the bone marrow stem cells. When the bone marrow is returned to the patient it will contain the edited gene, meaning that all new haemoglobin produced will be normal rather than sickle. Treating some forms of leukaemia by this method has had up to a 90% success rate.

Tip: Gene therapy is particularly effective in treating blood diseases such as sickle cell anaemia and leukaemia as the bone marrow (containing the cells producing blood) can be removed from the body and edited – it is much more difficult to treat cells that are more widely dispersed within the body.

New technologies such as **CRISPR/cas9** allow scientists to remove and replace defective genes, or even small sections of DNA, with the normal functional form. These new techniques can accurately pinpoint small sections of DNA and then cut out and replace the targeted section with the normal DNA sequence.

Tip: CRISPR/cas9 is particularly effective in that it is able to target and replace defective genes or sections of DNA with accuracy.

Gene therapy is now being used to treat some forms of disease that affect the retina in the eye. The eye is relatively accessible, making it easier to replace damaged genes.

Genetic Screening, PCR, DNA Probes and Genetic Counselling

Genetic screening

Scientists have now mapped the human genome, so they know where particular genes are located. Research has also enabled scientists to distinguish between normal and defective genes. This is the basis of **genetic screening**. It is now possible to analyse DNA to screen individuals for many genetic conditions, often well before the symptoms of the condition become apparent. While the extent of genetic testing has increased dramatically in recent years, the principle has been around for a long time. An obvious example is screening mothers at risk of having a child with Down's Syndrome. Individuals with Down's Syndrome have 47 chromosomes in each cell rather than the standard 46. For many years screening has involved removing foetal cells from the mother's amniotic fluid during pregnancy and counting the number of chromosomes in these cells.

Tip: Down's Syndrome is an example of aneuploidy, i.e. the presence or absence of one or more entire chromosomes in each cell.

A lot of research has gone into genes linked to cancer. **Oncogenes** are genes which stimulate cell growth and division and, if defective, can cause cells to grow out of control, causing cancer. Other genes can lead to cancer if defective, including those important in DNA repair. Two highly researched genes are the **BRCA1** and **BRCA2** genes which have been clearly linked to breast and ovarian cancer in women and prostate cancer in men. A female with the BRCA1 allele has a very high probability of having breast cancer in her lifetime – the harmful allele is dominant to the non-harmful recessive allele. As a consequence, some women who have tested positive for this gene allele have their breasts removed as a pre-emptive measure.

Tip: It is not that the BRCA genes actually cause cancer – they are tumour-suppressor genes that can repair damage to DNA (damage which could lead to cancer). The problem is that if this repair system isn't working, then cancer is much more likely to develop.

Tip: Research has shown that 400 or more genes are associated with cancer in some way.

Investigation into these genes has involved the **polymerase chain reaction (PCR)**.

The polymerase chain reaction (PCR)

The polymerase chain reaction (PCR) is a mechanism which massively increases the number of copies of a (targeted) sequence of DNA (or RNA). The PCR technique is a modified version of the process of DNA replication which takes place in cells naturally and has several distinct stages as follows:

1. The DNA section to be amplified is **heated to around 95°C**. This breaks the hydrogen bonds holding the two strands together, causing them to separate.
2. The DNA is **cooled to 40–60°C**. This cooling allows the **primers** to bind (anneal) to each strand at specific points (this would not happen if the temperature had remained at 95°C). The primers are short chains, approximately 20 nucleotides long, which are complementary to the bases in the part of the DNA selected. The primers have a number of functions:
   - they stop the two DNA strands rejoining;
   - they bracket the section of DNA to be copied;
   - DNA replication can only start within a double stranded region.

   In addition to primers being added, free nucleotides and the enzyme DNA polymerase are added to complete the copying process.
3. The mixture is **heated again, this time to around 70°C. DNA polymerase** copies each strand, starting with the primers. Special thermostable (heat stable) DNA polymerase is used which can work at temperatures of around 70°C.
4. The two DNA molecules formed following the PCR process are used as templates and the process is repeated. Millions of copies of DNA can be produced in a very short time.

The diagram opposite summarises the PCR process. As described above, PCR is a process that amplifies (makes many copies of) a section of DNA. The DNA produced can then be used to make DNA probes for a particular gene or section of DNA or used in a range of ways to investigate gene mutations.

Tip: In addition to helping with the study of mutations, PCR is used in many other ways. These include forensic science, paternity disputes, pedigree animal analysis and the identification of human remains following an air crash or other disaster. PCR has also been used in the identification of individuals infected with Covid-19 and, also, identifying which strains (variants) are causing the infection.

Tip: PCR is usually a very important precursor to the use of genetic fingerprinting. It is the production of enough of a particular section (or sections) of DNA that enables genetic fingerprinting to take place – genetic fingerprinting is discussed in more detail in the next chapter.

Tip: The key feature of PCR is that it accurately copies sections of DNA and can produce a sufficient quantity for analysis.

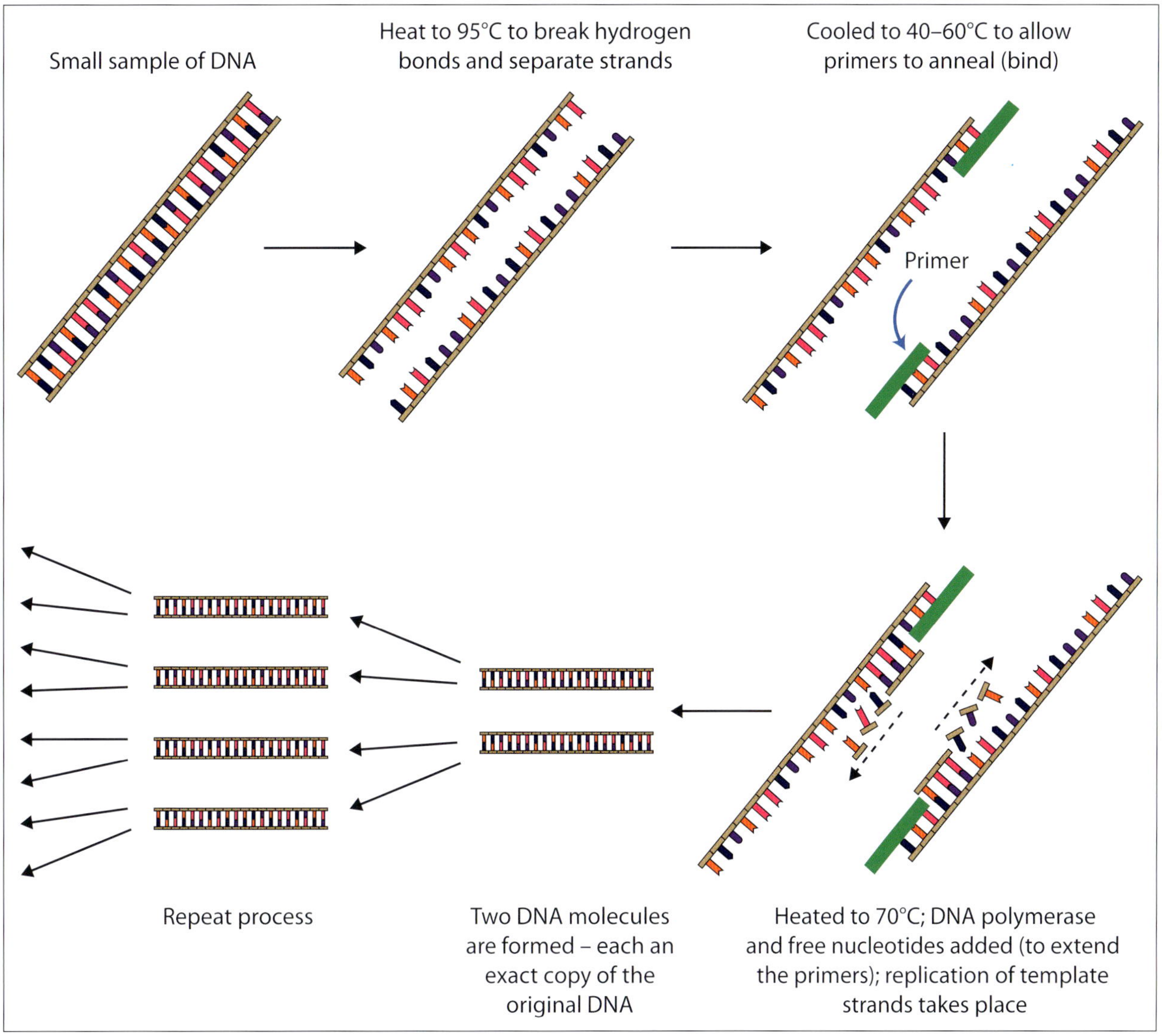
Small sample of DNA
Heat to 95°C to break hydrogen bonds and separate strands
Cooled to 40–60°C to allow primers to anneal (bind)
Primer
Repeat process
Two DNA molecules are formed – each an exact copy of the original DNA
Heated to 70°C; DNA polymerase and free nucleotides added (to extend the primers); replication of template strands takes place

DNA probes

A **DNA probe** is a single strand of DNA which has complementary bases to the disease-causing gene. In genetic screening using probes, if the probe is complementary to the 'normal' unaffected gene then it will bind to normal genes, but not the defective disease-causing genes.

The following diagram shows the key features of a DNA probe.

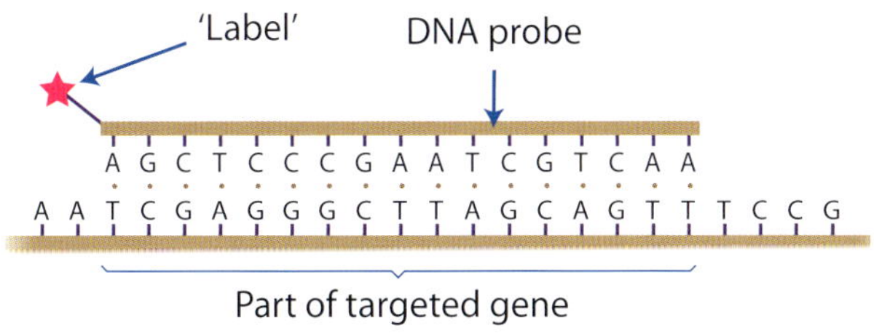
'Label'
DNA probe
A G C T C C C G A A T C G T C A A
A A T C G A G G G C T T A G C A G T T T C C G
Part of targeted gene

A DNA probe

The probe is 'labelled' chemically or in a way that will fluoresce under UV light so that it can be identified as having combined (or not) with the gene.

Tip: Obviously probes can be made to be complementary to either a normal or a defective gene, depending on the type of screening involved.

Tip: It was only when the human genome was sequenced (i.e. the order of bases in DNA was established) that DNA probes could be produced. This is because it is only possible to work out the sequence of bases in a DNA probe if the sequence of bases that it is complementary to is known.

Some genes, such as the BRCA or the CFTR genes, are clearly associated with cancers or other medical conditions. For other genes, the link is much less clear and with many medical conditions, such as Type 2 diabetes, many genes are involved and often the genes only give a predisposition for getting the disease rather than directly causing it.

Genetic counsellors can help people understand the **risk** (probability) of them developing a disease due to defective genes and even the possibility of parents having a child affected by a disease based on the genomes of the parents. By understanding the risk of having a genetic disease (or a condition with even a small genetic component), individuals can make suitable choices in advance – these can include an understanding of what treatment options are available, the possibility of starting treatment earlier or having further tests, or in the case of prospective parents, the very difficult decision of whether or not to have children.

Questions

1. (a) Name the medical condition caused by the failure of the pancreas to produce insulin. [1]
   (b) The following diagram summarises the process of genetically engineering bacteria to produce insulin.

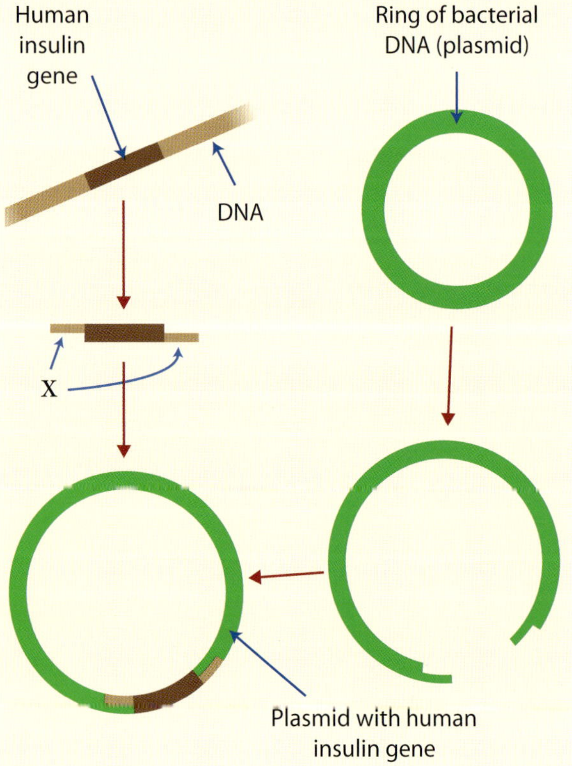

   (i) Name the extensions of the DNA labelled **X**. [1]
   (ii) Name the type of enzyme that produces these extensions. [1]
   (iii) Explain fully the advantage of cutting the DNA in such a way as to leave these parts. [3]
   (iv) Describe what occurs after the final stage shown in the diagram. [2]
   (d) Give **two** advantages of using human insulin to treat patients rather than insulin extracted from animals such as pigs or cows. [2]

2. (a) Describe what causes haemophilia. [2]
   (b) (i) Describe how individuals with haemophilia were treated before the introduction of genetic engineering. [1]
   (ii) Give one disadvantage with this early form of treatment. [1]

3. (a) Outline the main differences between the techniques involved in traditional breeding of animals and the development of transgenic animals. [4]
   (b) In terms of world population growth and the amount of available land for food production, explain the benefits of genetic engineering. [3]

4. Cystic fibrosis is caused by the presence of a mutation in a gene. In recent years, gene therapy has been used as one line of treatment for the condition.
   (a) Describe what is meant by the term 'somatic cell (gene) therapy'. [1]
   (b) Give **two** reasons why the treatment of cystic fibrosis by gene therapy has not been as successful as initially hoped. [2]

5. The following diagram summarises the polymerase chain reaction (PCR).

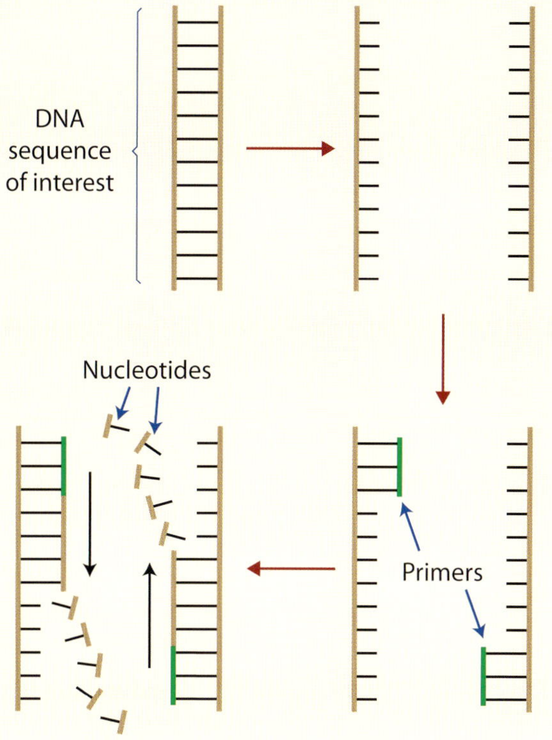

(a) At the start of the process, what causes the double stranded DNA to split into two single strands? [1]
(b) Using the diagram and your knowledge, give **two** functions of the primers. [2]
(c) Name the enzyme involved in bonding nucleotides to each other at the final stage. [1]
(d) A sample contains one DNA molecule. Calculate the number of DNA molecules that will be present after 4 cycles of PCR. [1]

18: GENE CLONING, GENETIC FINGERPRINTING AND STEM CELL TECHNOLOGY

Students should be able to:

11.8.1 discuss gene cloning technologies that allow for the study and alteration of gene function in order to:
- understand organism function better; and
- design new industrial and medical processes;

11.8.2 evaluate the ethical, moral and social issues associated with the use of recombinant technology in agriculture, in industry and in medicine;

11.8.3 discuss the humanitarian aspects of recombinant DNA technology and the opposition from environmentalists and anti-globalisation activists;

11.9.1 demonstrate an understanding that an organism's genome contains many repetitive, non-coding base sequences and that the probability of two individuals having the same repetitive sequences is very low;

11.9.2 evaluate the technique of genetic fingerprinting (using bars on DNA fingerprints) in analysing DNA fragments that have been cloned by PCR;

11.9.3 evaluate the use of genetic fingerprinting in determining genetic relationships and the genetic variability within a population;

11.9.4 explain the biological principles that underpin genetic fingerprinting techniques;

11.9.5 interpret data showing the results of gel electrophoresis to separate DNA fragments; and

11.9.6 explain why scientists might use genetic fingerprints in the fields of forensic science, medical diagnosis, and animal and plant breeding.

11.10.1 discuss what stem cells are and why they are important;

11.10.2 describe and explain the unique properties of stem cells;

11.10.3 explain how stem cells differ from all other cells;

11.10.4 describe what embryonic stem cells are and explain how embryonic stem cells are stimulated to differentiate by differential gene expression;

11.10.5 describe what adult stem cells are, where they are found and what they normally do;

11.10.6 describe and explain the similarities and differences between embryonic and adult stem cells; and

11.10.7 evaluate and discuss the ethical issues raised through the use of stem cell technology.

Stem cells

What are stem cells?

Stem cells are cells that can give rise to **other types** of cells. The zygote is the first cell formed at fertilisation by the fusion of a sperm and an egg. Clearly, this cell and the cells this cell produces following cell division then go on to produce the full range of cells found in humans. The diagram below shows how stem cells can give rise to:

- **more stem cells;**
- **differentiated (specific types of) cells.**

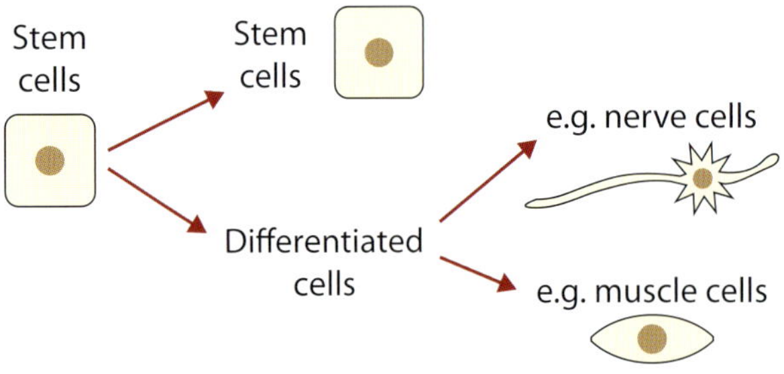

A very young embryo contains **embryonic stem cells** and these cells (and the cells they produce) are responsible for producing virtually all the cell types in the human body. Most cell types in the body, for example skin or nerve cells, can produce other cells of the same type. For example, skin cells can give rise to other similar skin cells but not to other types of cells, such as nerve cells.

The early embryo cells which can give rise to all the cell types in the body are described as being **pluripotent**.

Tip: Stem cells are **not differentiated**. Other cells in the body, such as nerve cells or muscle cells, are described as **differentiated** as they have already formed into particular types of cell with particular functions.

Tip: Stem cells give rise to other stem cells **and** cells which become differentiated.

Embryonic stem cells are most versatile very early in embryonic development (3 to 5 days). While all embryonic stem cells are undifferentiated, with the ability to form a wide range of cell types, it is obvious that some stem cells give rise to different cell types compared to others. How do they do this?

The phenomenon can be explained by **differential gene expression** – in effect, some genes are more switched on (or are more active) in some of the stem cells than in others. For example, in those stem cells which produce skin cells, the genes which produce the proteins important in skin cells are active (or expressed) whereas others that might be more important in other cell types are not expressed.

In addition to embryonic stem cells, there are also **adult stem cells**. As their name suggests, these cells are also present in adults. Where they differ from embryonic stem cells is that they only can produce **a limited range of cell types**, described as being **multipotent**. For example, adult stem cells in the bone marrow can produce the different types of blood cell, but they cannot produce the wide range of non-blood cells required by the body. Other examples of adult stem cells include those which produce new nerve cells in the brain and those in the testes which produce sperm.

Stem cells and medicine

An understanding of the function of stem cells has led scientists to harness their potential in medicine. For example, transfusions of stem cells (from another individual with a close tissue match) into a patient's bone marrow have been used to treat leukaemia and other blood disorders.

Tip: In treating some blood cancers, the process involves killing or removing the patient's own (cancerous) stem cells in the bone marrow and replacing them with donor stem cells.

As scientists now have the gene editing skills to edit mutated genes in the bone marrow cells of affected people (see previous chapter), this can help cure or alleviate many other medical conditions.

There are many other examples of stem cells being used in medical treatment. For example, stem cells are used to replace and repair sections of the eye cornea and they are used to replace damaged skin tissue (for example, skin grafts following severe burns, where sheets of skin can be grown in laboratories).

It is hoped that, in future, stem cell cloning will be used to grow replacement organs or, at the very least, replacement **parts** of organs, including replacement pancreases for diabetes patients.

Stem cells also have a role in drug development as stem cells can be used to produce large quantities of the cell type being investigated.

A major drawback has been that the most potent stem cells (embryonic stem cells) are only obtained by being removed from a young embryo (leading to the destruction of the embryo). Aborted embryos or embryos that are no longer needed in IVF clinics can be used but this, of course, creates ethical issues for many people.

Stem cells and ethics

Research and development involving stem cells has been slower than in many other areas of biology, largely due to the ethical issues that it raises. The use of embryos as the (only) source of pluripotent stem cells has been hotly contested. Arguments along the lines of life starting at conception are central to those who argue that embryos should not be used.

The counterargument is that aborted or 'extra' and unused embryos from fertility clinics would never lead to the development of a human anyway. Furthermore, stem cell research has led to successful treatments for many medical conditions including some forms of cancer (e.g. leukaemia). In summary, the potential of stem cell research in future medical advances is huge.

The development of a new type of stem cell has been very important in progress in this area. Scientists are now able to 'reprogram' differentiated cells, such as skin cells, to give them the properties of embryonic stem cells. These reprogrammed cells have the expression level of a number of genes altered with some having higher expression levels and others lower levels – the actual genetic engineering will depend on the type of differentiated cell involved. Genes with an increased expression level are more active and produce more protein; the opposite if the expression level is reduced. These cells are referred to as **induced pluripotent stem (iPS) cells**. The process is summarised in the following diagram.

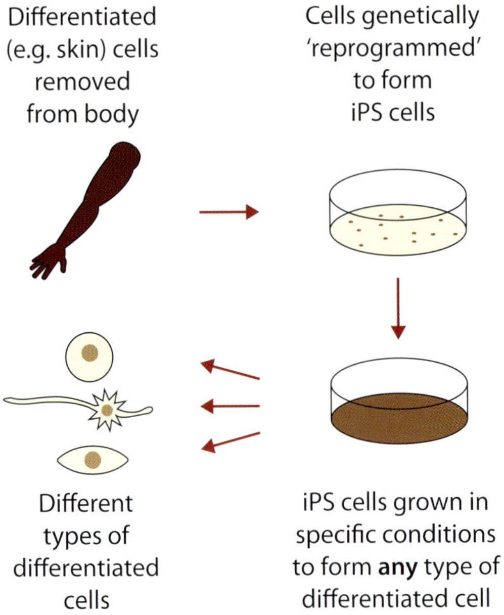

The iPS stem cells have two obvious advantages:

- by using skin (or other) cells the ethical issues associated with using embryos are avoided; and
- if the (skin) cells to be reprogrammed as iPS are removed from the patient into which the differentiated cells will be used, there are no issues with tissue rejection.

Worked Example

(a) Name the two types of stem cells in the body.

(b) Stem cells can be used to produce skin cells for the treatment of burns. However, progress in using stem cells to produce replacement organs such as pancreases for diabetes patients has been much slower. Suggest a reason for this.

(c) The diagram in the section on induced pluripotent cells (immediately before this worked example), refers to differentiated cells being 'genetically reprogrammed'. Outline what 'genetic reprogramming' involves.

Answer

(a) Embryonic and adult stem cells.

(b) Skin involves a smaller range of cells types/ an organ has many different types of cell/ skin cells are less complex/other appropriate response.

(c) The expression level of some genes is changed.

Genetic (DNA) fingerprinting

Around 2% of the genome codes for protein, and while some of the rest involves gene regulation – i.e. switching genes on and off and controlling their level of expression (activity) – much of the genome has no obvious function (or at least some functions are not fully worked out yet). Nonetheless, around 98% of DNA in the genome does not directly code for protein.

In places, this non-coding DNA contains many repetitive sequences of bases (e.g. the bases AGATA), where these base sequences are repeated over and over again many times. The number of repeat sequences can vary from a small number to several hundred (i.e. the sequence AGATA is repeated one after another for up to several hundred times).

Each of these repetitive sequences is referred to as a **microsatellite repeat sequence** (MRS) or **short tandem repeat (STR)**.

An important point is that the number of repeats varies between individuals – this is the basis of genetic fingerprinting.

Tip: It is important to remember that it is the number of repeats that differ between individuals, it is not that the sequences of bases being repeated change.

Process of genetic fingerprinting

Genetic fingerprinting involves the following steps:

1. As often only a small amount of DNA is available, e.g. at a crime scene, the **polymerase chain reaction** (PCR) is used to provide an increased quantity for analysis.
2. **Restriction endonuclease** enzymes are used to cut out the repetitive sequences at each end.
3. The (MRS) fragments of DNA (repetitive sequences) are then placed in a 'well' in a **gel**

electrophoresis tank. In gel electrophoresis, an electrical current flows in a buffer solution, through agarose gel, between the cathode and the anode electrodes. The current carries the DNA fragments towards the anode with the smaller fragments (i.e. fewer bases in length) travelling faster and further in the gel than the longer fragments. The DNA is stained to make it visible in order that the final position of the fragments can be seen. The process of gel electrophoresis (genetic fingerprinting) is summarised in the following diagram.

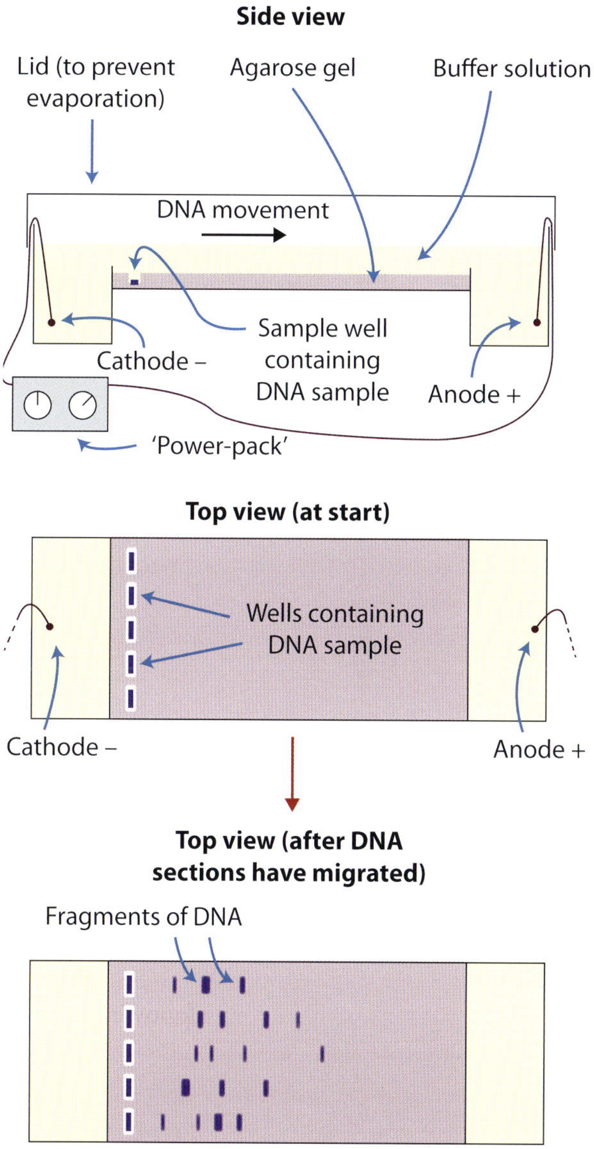

Gel electrophoresis and the separation of DNA fragments

4. The process described above is carried out on ten to fifteen different MRSs which differ significantly between individuals. Using ten or more MRSs decreases the possibility of any two individuals having the same fingerprint, ensuring than any one individual's genetic fingerprint is unique.

Tip: It is important to remember that it is only by using a number of repetitive sequences in genetic fingerprinting that each individual's genetic fingerprint is unique.

Applications of genetic fingerprinting

Genetic fingerprinting has many uses. These include:

- medicine and medical research – by identifying different species/strains of bacteria and viruses causing disease and in identifying the link between genome and disease susceptibility;
- crime scene investigation;
- paternity disputes;
- checking pedigree status in plants, racehorses and pets;
- identifying human remains (for example, in air crash disasters); and
- identifying relationships between groups of organisms – DNA fingerprinting has even been used on fossil humans to identify how closely related they are to each other, and also to check if they are possible ancestors to modern humans.

Tip: Issues that have arisen over the use of genetic fingerprinting usually involve the possibility of contamination with other DNA – not its concept.

Worked Example

The diagram below represents part of the genetic fingerprint of an individual.

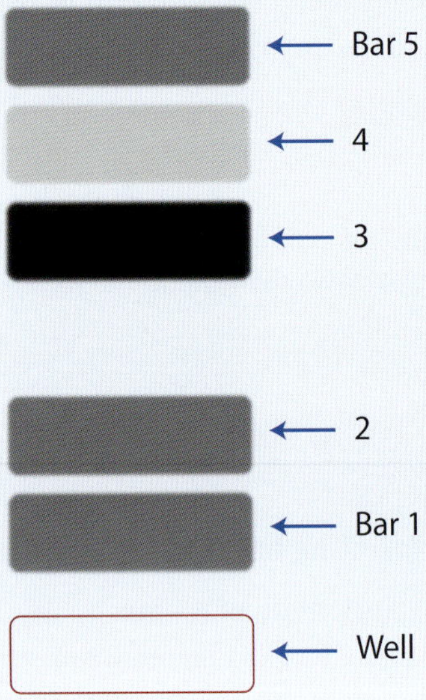

(a) In terms of the DNA present within each of the bars, describe and explain the difference between bars 1 and 5.

(b) Bar 3 is much darker than bar 4. State the reason for this.

(c) Explain how the genetic fingerprints of a brother of the individual tested and an individual of no relation would be expected to compare with the individual tested.

Answers

(a) The DNA (fragments) in bar 5 are smaller than in 1 and so they have been able to travel faster and further in the gel.

(b) There are more DNA fragments in bar 3 than in bar 4.

(c) The banding for the brother would be very similar, but not exactly the same (in terms of position and/or number and/or density of bars). There would be many more differences in the fingerprint of the individual who is no relation.

The ethics of gene technology in general

As we have seen, stem cells have always been a hot ethical area, but what about gene technology in general?

The first commercial product produced by a transgenic organism was insulin, which was produced by genetically modified bacteria which had the human insulin gene inserted into their genomes. This has had major medical benefits to millions of diabetes patients.

Tip: The advantages of using GM bacteria to produce human insulin is discussed in more detail in the previous chapter.

Genetically engineered microbes (bacteria and yeast) have been producing products useful in medicine and industry for years and these have met with relatively little opposition from the general public, and there is no doubt this type of progress has brought massive benefits to the human population.

However, transgenic domestic animals and GM plants have met with much more opposition, perhaps because the general public has a greater awareness of these species. Nonetheless, transgenic plants – including tomatoes with a longer shelf life, vitamin A enhanced rice (miracle rice), drought-resistant maize and wheat plants with a higher yield – all have massive advantages, particularly with the rapidly growing world population and the issues associated with climate change.

While many countries in the world such as the USA and Argentina have embraced the use of GM crops, there is still considerable opposition in Europe, although this opposition is likely to soften over time as wider science understanding replaces myth and lack of understanding. Nonetheless, in Europe, GM crops are more widely used for animal feed than in human food products, as this is considered more acceptable to public opinion. Many members of the public still have concerns about 'superweeds', allergies being caused by transgenic organisms and native crops being outcompeted, but, in reality, the safeguards in place make these claims largely unfounded.

Genetic fingerprinting has also met with considerable opposition, again partially due to a lack of understanding but also because of fears concerning data protection and the use of extensive data banks storing personal information.

As the development of GM crops is expensive and they are developed over long time scales, large multinational companies, such as Monsanto, are involved and this has led to considerable opposition from anti-globalisation activists. Monsanto and other companies have been accused of putting 'profit before people', creating 'frankenfoods' and harming the environment.

Although there may be PR battles still to be fought and won, a majority of scientists fully support the increasing role that genetic engineering has in medicine, industry and agriculture.

It is in medicine where genetic engineering is likely to impact most on people in the British Isles. The production of GM insulin, an essential medicine for millions of people with diabetes, has already been covered, and many other essential medical products are being produced by genetic engineering.

Gene therapy, after an indifferent period at the start of the twenty first century, is proving very successful in treating a range of medical conditions and the range of diseases being treated (or cured) is increasing all the time.

The working out of the human genome (by gene sequencing) has increased our understanding of the link between genes and disease – a much more common link than originally anticipated. This has led to an increase in genetic screening for disease and the development of cures in some cases and better treatment in others with the introduction of 'personalised' medicine. PCR and genetic fingerprinting play a large part in this field. Nonetheless, there are also issues in this area with many concerned that screening and genetic 'enhancement' could lead to 'designer babies', where even features such as hair colour could be manipulated in advance.

Tip: Many of the issues surrounding genetic engineering are also covered in the previous chapter.

Questions

1. (a) Give one difference between embryonic and adult stem cells. [1]

   (b) iPS are a particular type of stem cell. The diagram below summarises how they are produced from differentiated cells.

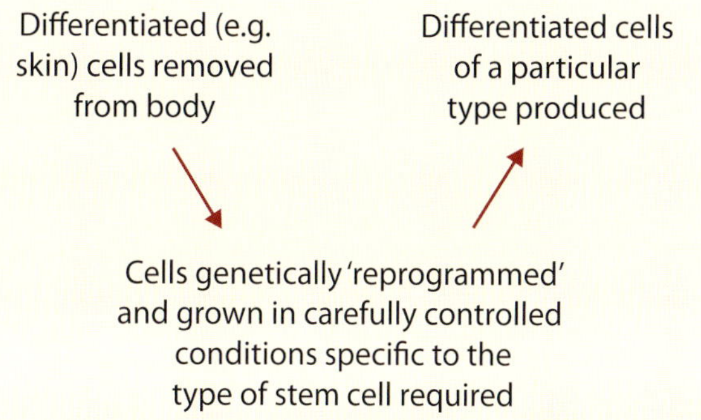

   (i) Suggest what is meant by 'genetically reprogramming' the skin cells. [1]

   (ii) Give **one** advantage of using these cells rather than embryonic stem cells. [1]

   (iii) Give **one** example of the use of stem cells in medicine. [1]

2. (a) DNA evidence is often left in very small (trace) amounts at a crime scene.

   (i) Name the technique that is used to amplify the DNA to produce sufficient quantities for genetic fingerprinting. [1]

   (ii) In genetic fingerprinting, state the function of restriction enzymes. [1]

   (b) The diagram below represents part of a DNA fingerprint from an individual who has a genetic disease (Lane **2**) and a fingerprint from two individuals who do not have that condition (Lanes 1 and 3).

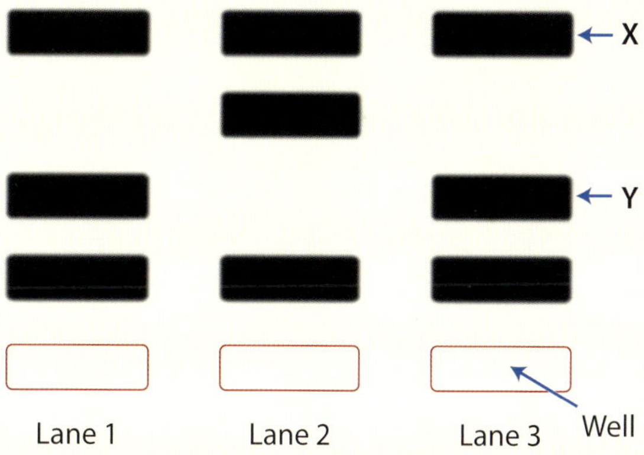

   (i) State why the DNA fragments in band **X** have travelled further than the fragments in **Y**. Explain your answer. [2]

   (ii) Summarise the results shown. [2]

   (iii) Suggest a possible reason for the differences between the affected individual and the two individuals without the condition. Explain your answer. [2]

Answers

Note: The marks for each answer are for guidance only. Mark allocation may vary depending on the questions in the exam.

Unit A2 2: Organic Chemistry

1: NOMENCLATURE, STRUCTURE AND ISOMERISM IN ORGANIC COMPOUNDS

1.

n	Name of alkane	Molecular formula	Name of alkene	Molecular formula
2	ethane	C_2H_6	ethene	C_2H_4
3	propane	C_3H_8	propene	C_3H_6
6	hexane	C_6H_{14}	hexene	C_6H_{12}

[1] per row **[3]**

2.

Homologous series	General formula	Name of functional group	Hydrocarbons?
alkanes	C_nH_{2n+2}	------	yes
alkenes	C_nH_{2n}	carbon carbon double bond	yes
alcohols	$C_nH_{2n+1}OH$	hydroxyl	no

[1] per row **[3]**

3.

	Name	Molecular formula	Name of functional group
Alkane with 1 carbon	methane	CH_4	none
Alkene with 3 carbons	propene	C_3H_6	carbon carbon double bond
Alcohol with 3 carbons	propanol	C_3H_7OH	hydroxyl
Alkene with 2 carbons	ethene	C_2H_4	carbon carbon double bond
Alkane with 5 carbons	pentane	C_5H_{12}	none
Alcohol with 1 carbon	methanol	CH_3OH	hydroxyl
Alkane with 6 carbon atoms	hexane	C_6H_{14}	none

[1] per row **[6]**

4. **(a)** C_nH_{2n+2} [1]
(b) Successive members differ by CH_2 [1]
(c) Gradation in physical properties [1] Mpt increases down group/ bpt increases down group [1]
(d) C_7H_{16} [1] Higher boiling point [1] **[6 marks]**

5. **(a)** CH_2 [1] **(b)** CH_3CH_2OH/C_2H_6O [1]
(c) C_3H_8 [1] **(d)** CH_4 [1]
(e) CH [1] **(f)** CH_2O [1] **[6 marks]**

6. **(a)** $CH_2O = 30$
$(CH_2O)n = 120$; $30n = 120$; $n = 4$. So: $C_4H_8O_4$ [1]

(b) $(C_2H_6O)n = 46$; $(24 + 6 + 16)n = 46$; $n = 1$.
So: C_2H_6O [1]

(c) a formula which shows the actual number of atoms of each element in a molecule [1]
a formula which shows the simplest whole number ratio of atoms of each element in a compound [1] **[4 marks]**

7. Moles C = $\frac{2.88}{12} = 0.24$ [1] moles H = 0.36 [1]

Ratio 1 : 1.5
2 : 3

C_2H_3 [1] **[3 marks]**

8.

Element	C	H
Mass (g)	81.8	18.2
Moles	81.8 ÷ 12 = 6.82 [1]	18.2 ÷ 1 = 18.2 [1]
Divide by smallest	1	2.67
Multiply till whole	3	8

C_3H_8 [1]
Note: 2.67 = 2⅔, so multiply by 3 to get a whole number. **[3 marks]**

9. Moles C = $\frac{70.6}{12} = 5.86$ [1]

Moles H = $\frac{13.7}{1} = 13.7$ [1]

Moles O = $\frac{15.7}{16} = 0.98$ [1]

Ratio 6 : 14 : 1
$C_6H_{14}O$ [1] $C_{12}H_{28}O_2$ [1] **[5 marks]**

10. (a) Moles of carbon = $\frac{1.08}{12} = 0.09$ [1]

Moles of hydrogen = $\frac{0.21}{1} = 0.21$ [1]

Ratio C : H is 0.09 : 0.21; 1 : 2.33; 3 : 7
C_3H_7 [1]

(b) $(C_3H_7)n = 86$
$(12 \times 3 + 7)n = 86$
$43n = 86$; $n = 2$; C_6H_{14} [1] **[4 marks]**

11.

	C	F	H	O
Moles	$\frac{24}{12} = 2$	$\frac{66.5}{19} = 3.5$	$\frac{1.5}{1} = 1.5$	$\frac{8}{16} = 0.5$
Divide by	$\frac{2}{0.5}$	$\frac{3.5}{0.5}$	$\frac{1.5}{0.5}$	$\frac{0.5}{0.5}$
Smallest ratio	4	7	3	1

[2] for Moles row.
$C_4F_7H_3O$ [1] **[3 marks]**

12. (a)

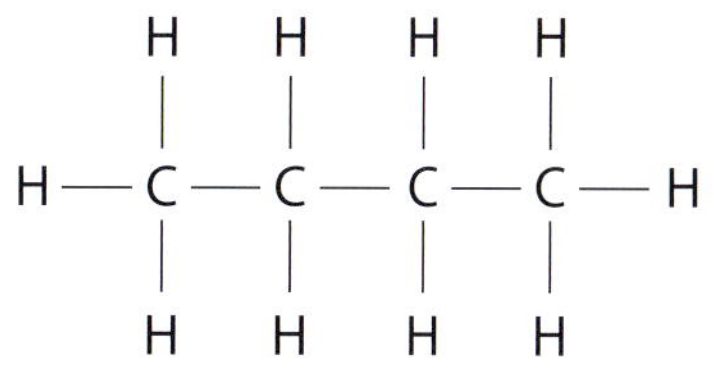

$CH_3CH_2CH_2CH_3$

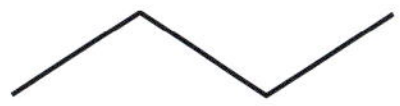

(b)

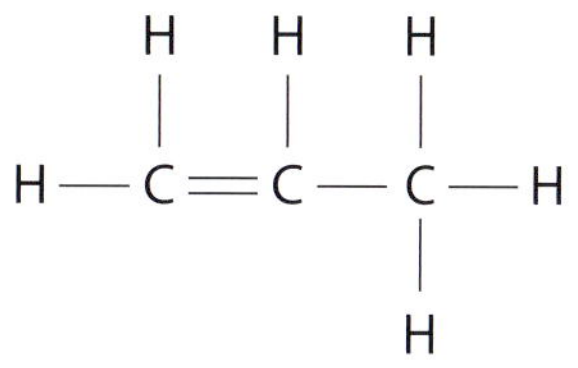

CH_2CHCH_3

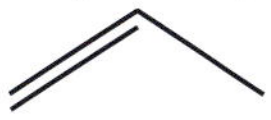

(c)

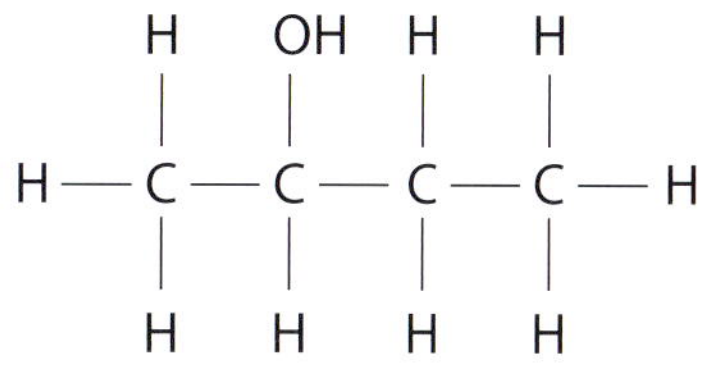

$CH_3CH(OH)CH_2CH_3$

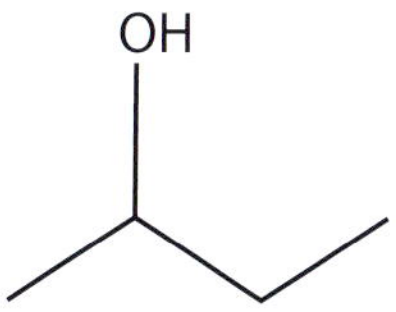

(d)

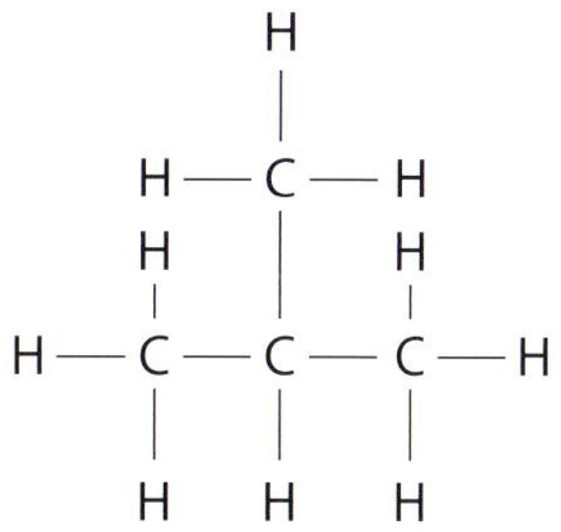

$CH_3CH(CH_3)CH_3$

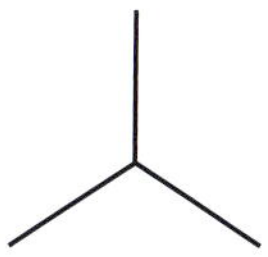

(e)

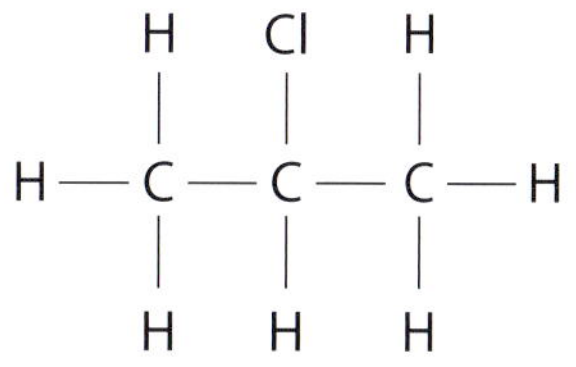

$CH_3CHClCH_3$

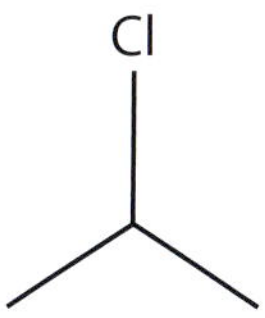

12. (f)

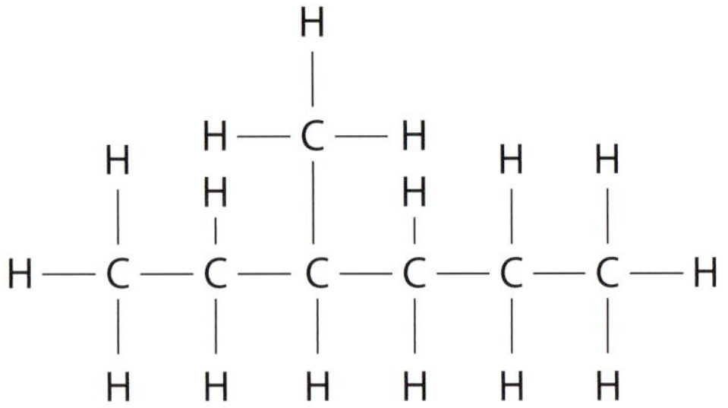

$CH_3CH_2CH(CH_3)CH_2CH_2CH_3$

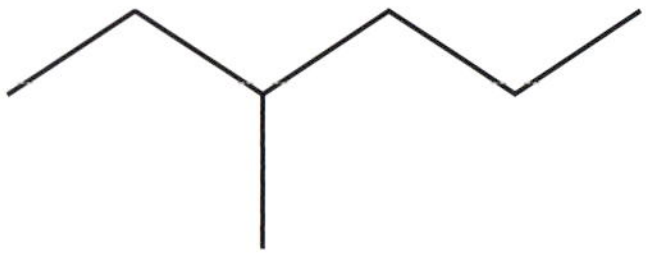

(g)

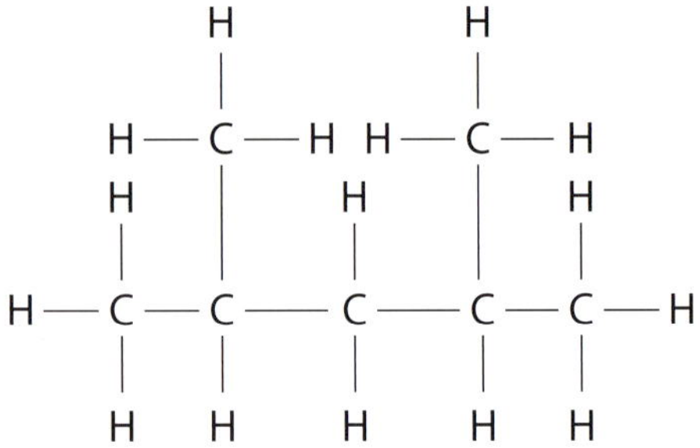

$CH_3CH(CH_3)CH_2CH(CH_3)CH_3$

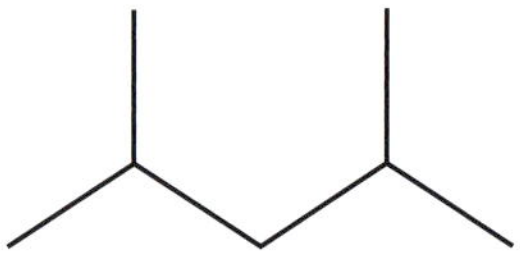

(h)

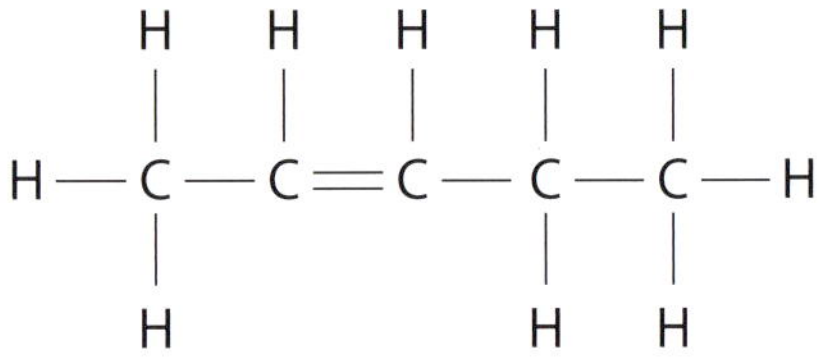

$CH_3CHCHCH_2CH_3$

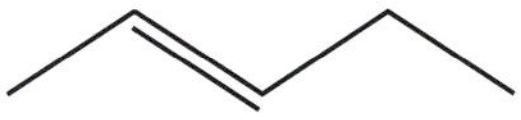

(i)

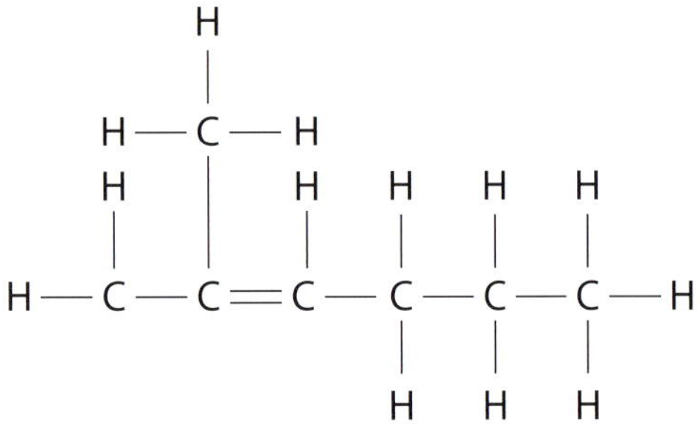

$CH_3C(CH_3)CHCH_2CH_2CH_3$

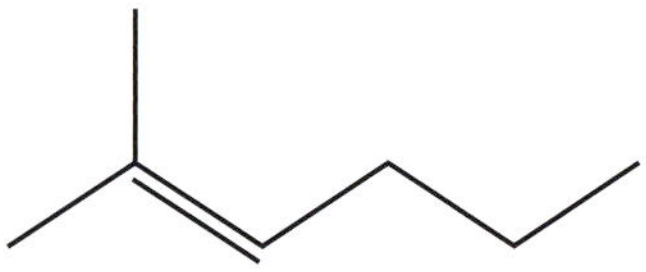

[3] each **[27 marks]**

13. (a) propane **(b)** 1,3-dibromopropane.
(c) 1-bromobutane **(d)** (2-)methylpropane
(e) 2-chloro-2,3,3-trimethylpentane
(f) 3-bromo-2-methylpentane
(g) 1,2-dichloropropane
(h) propan-2-ol **(i)** (2,2-)dimethylpropane
(j) 2-methylpentane **(k)** butan-1-ol
(l) 3-chloro-2,2,4-trimethylhexane
(m) but-2-ene **(n)** 2-methylpent-1-ene
(o) pent-2-ene **(p)** (2-)methylpropene
(q) 3,3-dimethylpent-1-ene
(r) butanoic acid **(s)** 2-bromobut-1-ene
(t) propan-2-ol

[1] each **[20 marks]**

2: ALKANES

1. (a) Saturated means that a molecule contains only single C–C bonds and no C=C or C≡C bonds. [1] Hydrocarbon means that the molecule contains carbon and hydrogen only. [1]

(b)  [1]

(c) Structural isomers – Molecules which have the same molecular formula but a different structural formula. [2]

(d)

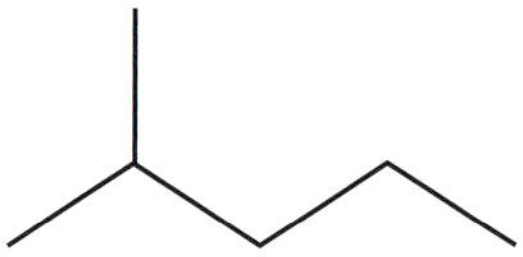

2-methylpentane

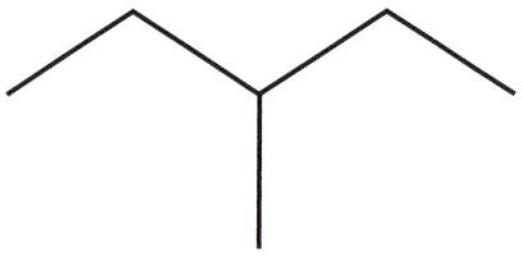

3-methylpentane

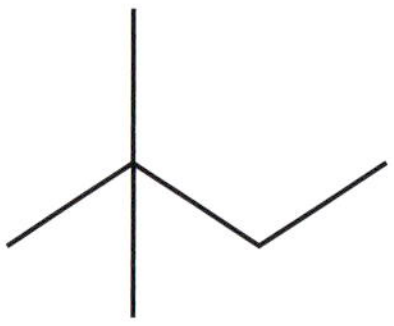

2,2-dimethylbutane

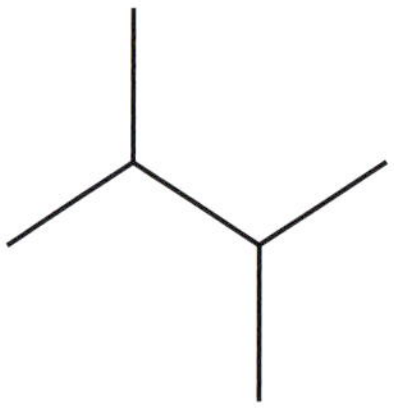

2,3-dimethylbutane

[1] mark for name [1] for structure
Any 2 of the above.

(e) $C_6H_{14} + 9½O_2 \rightarrow 6CO_2 + 7H_2O$ [2]

(f) carbon monoxide [1] carbon [1]

(g) C_6H_{12} [1]

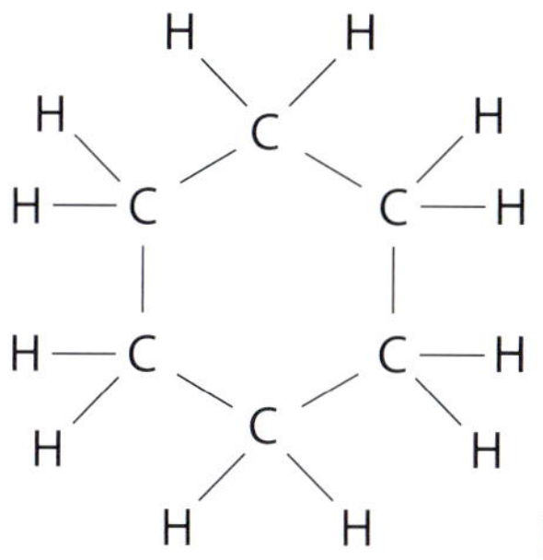
[1]
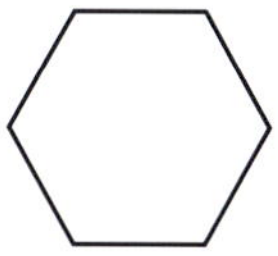
[1]

[16 marks]

2. (a) 1-chlorobutane / 2-chlorobutane / 1-chloro-2-methylpropane / 2-chloro-2-methylpropane Any [2]
   (b) pentane / (2-)methylbutane / (2,2-)dimethylpropane Any [2]
   (c) propan-1-ol [1] propan-2-ol [1] **[6 marks]**

3. (a) Crude oil is heated and the vapour is passed into a fractionating column. [1] As the vapour moves up the column it gets cooler. [1] Different chain lengths condense at different boiling points. [1]
   (b) Don't burn well / less flammable [1]
   (c) To provide shorter more useful hydrocarbons. [1]
   (d) Reforming is a process in which the hydrocarbon molecules of petroleum are rearranged to improve their properties, usually with the loss of a small molecule such as hydrogen. [2]
   (e) $C_6H_{14} \rightarrow C_6H_6 + 4H_2$ [1]
   (f) (i) $C_7H_{16} \rightarrow C_2H_4 + C_5H_{12}$ [1]
   (ii) $C_{10}H_{22} \rightarrow C_3H_6 + C_7H_{16}$ [1]
   (iii) $C_{16}H_{34} \rightarrow 2C_2H_4 + C_4H_8 + C_8H_{18}$ [1]
   [10 marks]

4. (a) Combustion is the reaction of fuels with oxygen, forming oxides and releasing heat energy. [2]
   (b) carbon dioxide [1] water [1]
   (c) carbon monoxide water carbon. [2] One wrong. [1]
   (d) $C_3H_8 + 3½O_2 \rightarrow 3CO + 4H_2O$ [2] **[8 marks]**

5. (a) Nitrogen from the air reacts with oxygen / $N_2 + O_2 \rightarrow 2NO$ [1] at high temperature and pressure in the engine. [1] Carbon monoxide is formed when the fuel burns incompletely. [1]
   (b) Nitrogen oxides react with unburned hydrocarbons to produce photochemical smog. [1] Carbon monoxide prevents the blood from carrying oxygen. [1]
   (c) $2NO \rightarrow N_2 + O_2$ [1]
   $2CO + O_2 \rightarrow 2CO_2$ [1]
   (d) beaches destroyed / wildlife killed / feathers coated in oil and birds cannot fly. Any [2]
   [7 marks]

6. (a) (i) $N_2 + O_2 \rightarrow 2NO$ [1]
   (ii) $N_2 + 2O_2 \rightarrow 2NO_2$ [1]
   (iii) $N_2 + 2O_2 \rightarrow 2NO_2$ [1]
   (b) platinum/rhodium [1] Pt/Rh [1]
   (c) (i) Carbon dioxide and water [1]
   (ii) Carbon dioxide [1]
   (iii) Nitrogen and oxygen [1]
   (iv) Nitrogen and oxygen [1]
   (d) (i) Reduction is a reaction in which hydrogen is gained or oxygen is lost. [1]
   (ii) $2NO \rightarrow N_2 + O_2$ [1]
   (e) Once used it cannot be replaced in a human lifetime [1]
   (f) ethanol [1] biodiesel [1]
   (g) They are renewable and can be replaced [1] they are carbon neutral [1] **[16 marks]**

7. (a) Breaks the bond in chlorine and starts the reaction [1]
   (b) methane + chlorine → chloromethane + hydrogen chloride [1]
   (c) $CH_4 + Cl_2 \rightarrow CH_3Cl + HCl$ [1]
   (d) A hydrogen in methane is replaced by a chlorine [1] **[4 marks]**

8. (a) $CH_4 + 2Cl_2 \rightarrow CH_2Cl_2 + 2HCl$ [1]
   (b) $CH_4 + 4Cl_2 \rightarrow CCl_4 + 4HCl$ [1]
   (c) $CH_4 + Br_2 \rightarrow CH_3Br + HBr$ [1]
   (d) $CH_4 + 4F_2 \rightarrow CF_4 + 4HF$ [1] **[4 marks]**

9. (a) UV light [1]
   (b) $CH_4 + 4Cl_2 \rightarrow CCl_4 + 4HCl$ [1]
   (c) Hydrogen chloride tetrachloromethane [1]
   [3 marks]

3: ALKENES

1. (a) hex-2-ene [1]
   (b) 2-methylhex-2-ene [1]
   (c) 2-chloropent-2-ene [1]
   (d) 3-methylbut-1-ene [1]
   (e) 2-chloropent-1-ene [1]
   (f) buta-1,2-diene [1] **[6 marks]**

2. (a) A covalent bond formed by the linear overlap of atomic orbitals [1]
   (b) A covalent bond formed by the sideways overlap of p orbitals [1]
   (c) carbon carbon double bond [1]
   (d) 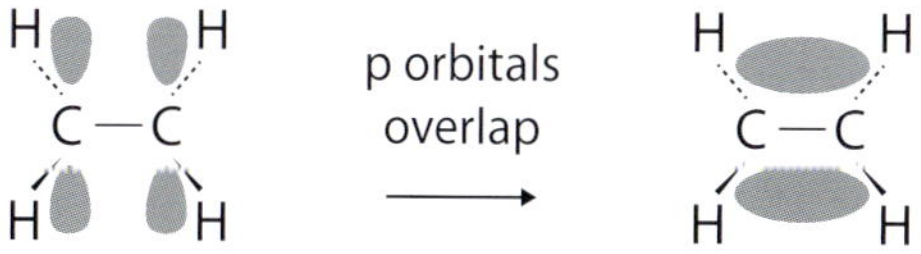

   [2]
   (e) Contains carbon and hydrogen only [1] Contains a carbon carbon double or carbon carbon triple bond [1]

(f) C=C in ethene composed of sigma and pi [1]
C–C in ethane composed of sigma [1]

(g) [1] per row [2]

Compound	Structural formula	Number of pi bonds present in compound	Number of sigma bonds present in compound
ethene	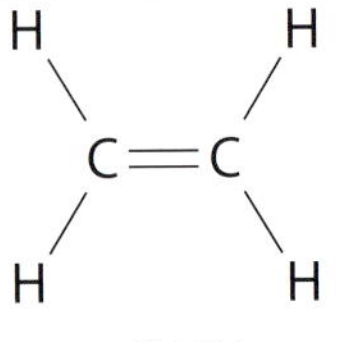 or CH_2CH_2	1	5
ethane	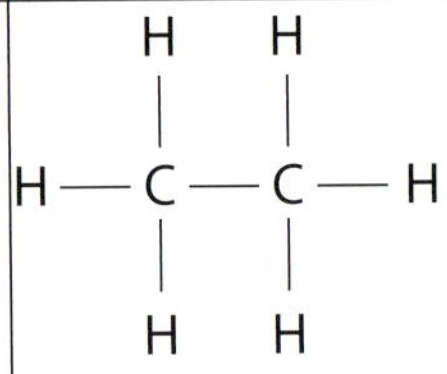 or CH_3CH_3	0	7

(h) pi bond has high electron density /project out of plane of molecule [1] prone to attack by electrophiles [1] **[13 marks]**

3. B [1] **[1 mark]**

4. **(a)**

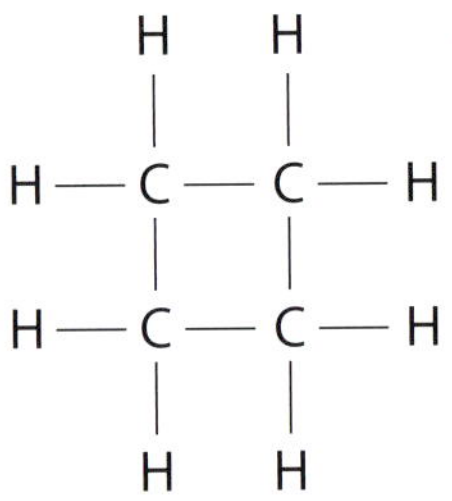

cyclobutane [1]

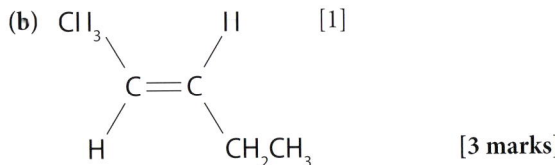

(b)

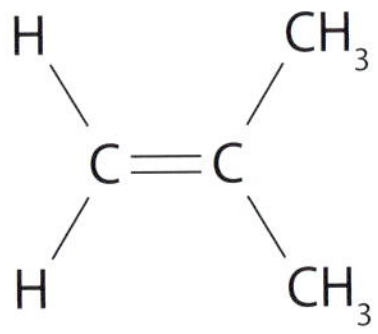

2-methylpropene [1] **[2 marks]**

5. **(a)** It has an energy barrier to rotation about a double bond [1] it has two different groups/atoms on the carbons of the double bond [1]

(b)

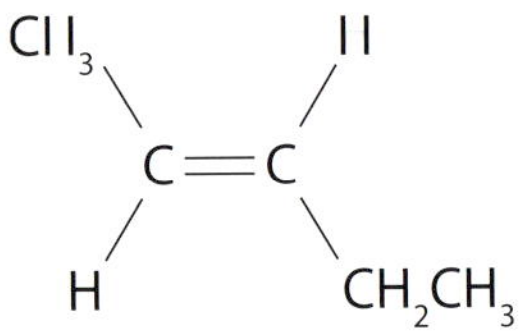

[1] **[3 marks]**

6. **(a)** hydroxyl OH [1]
Carbon carbon double bond / C=C [1]

(b)

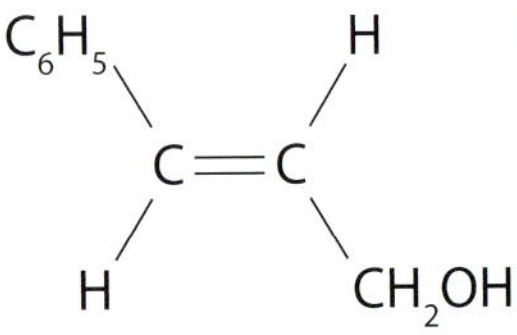

[1] **[3 marks]**

7. **(a)** $CH_3C(CH_3)CHCH_3 + H_2 \rightarrow CH_3C(CH_3)HCH_2CH_3$ [1] 2-methylbutane[1]

(b) $C_2H_4 + HBr \rightarrow C_2H_5Br$ [1] bromoethane [1]

(c) $C_2H_4 + Cl_2 \rightarrow C_2H_4Cl_2$[1] 1,2-dichloroethane[1]

(d) $C_2H_4 + H_2O \rightarrow C_2H_5OH$ [1] ethanol [1]

(e) $C_3H_6 + Cl_2 \rightarrow C_3H_6Cl_2$ [1] 1,2-dichloropropane [1] **[10 marks]**

8. **(a)** $C_2H_4 + 3O_2 \rightarrow 2CO_2 + 2H_2O$ [2]

(b) $C_4H_8 + 6O_2 \rightarrow 4CO_2 + 4H_2O$ [2] **[4 marks]**

9. **(a)** 1,2-dichlorobutane [1]

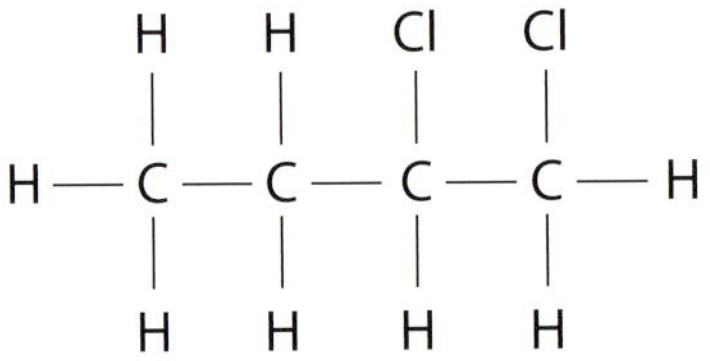

[1]

(b) 2,3-dichloropentane [1]

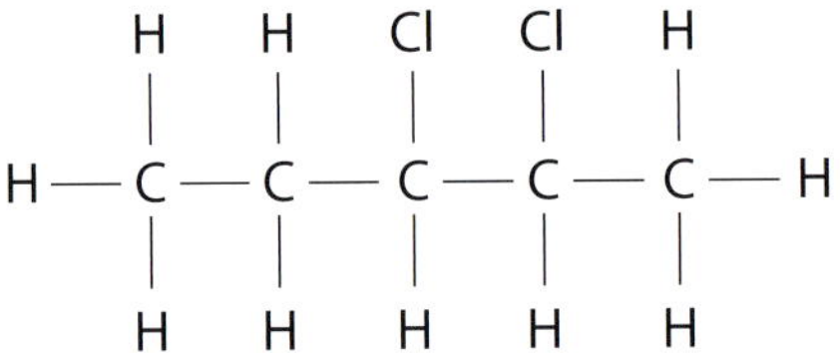

[1]

(c) 2-chloropentane [1]

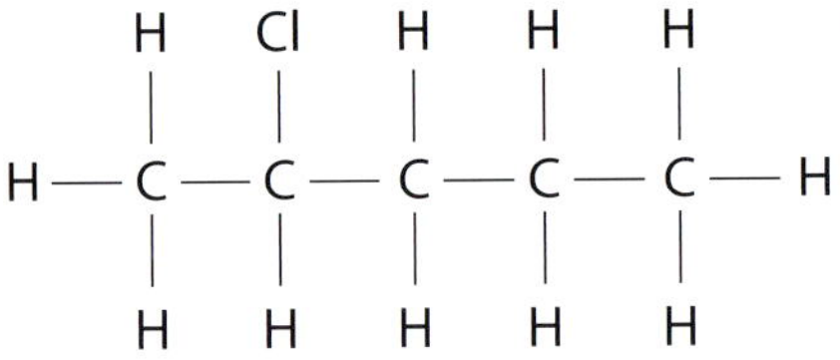

[1] **[6 marks]**

10. **(a)** Addition of a hydrogen molecule across a double bond [1]

(b) finely divided nickel [1] 140–160°C [1]

(c) $C_5H_{10} + H_2 \rightarrow C_5H_{12}$ [1] pentane [1]

(d) $CH_3(CH_2)_7CH{=}CH(CH_2)_7COOH + H_2 \rightarrow CH_3(CH_2)_7CH_2CH_2(CH_2)_7COOH$ / $CH_3(CH_2)_{16}COOH$ [1] **[6 marks]**

11. Indicative content:

Ethane:
- Bromoethane;
- hydrogen bromide;
- mixture of brominated alkanes may form due to chain reaction
- UV light
- substitution

Ethene:
- addition;
- 1,2-dibromoethane;
- room temperature / bromine water

Marks awarded as follows:

Candidates provide an excellent comparison with at least 5 indicative content points. They use excellent spelling, punctuation and grammar and the form and style are of an excellent standard. [5] – [6]

Candidates provide a good comparison with at least 3 indicative content points. They use good spelling, punctuation and grammar and the form and style are of a good standard. [3] – [4]

Candidates provide a limited comparison with at least 2 indicative content points. They use satisfactory spelling, punctuation and grammar and the form and style are of a basic standard. [1] – [2] **[6 marks]**

12. **(a)** A 2-methylpropene [1]
B 1,2-dibromo-2-methylpropane [1]

(b) No, as the same atom (H) on one carbon of double bond / or same group (CH_3) on one carbon of double bond [1]

(c) orange/yellow/brown to colourless [1]

(d) electrophilic addition [1]

(e)

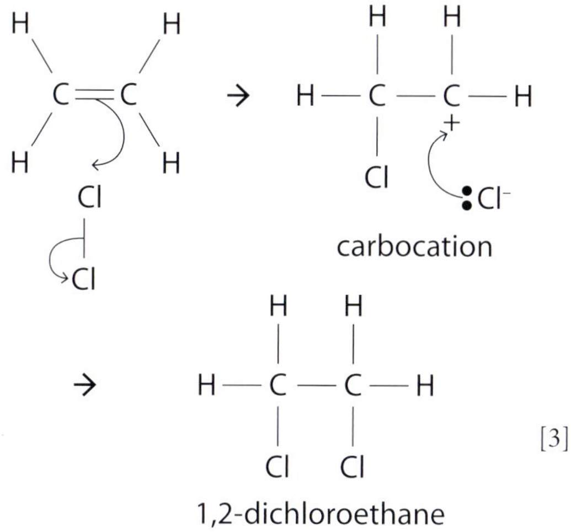

[3]

(f) $CH_3CH_2CH_2CH_2CH_2Cl$ [1] 1-chloropentane [1] **[9 marks]**

13. **(a)** An ion or molecule that attacks a region of high electron density. [1]

(b) Carbon carbon double bond. [1]

(c) 3-methylpentane [1]

(d) $CH_3CHClCHClCHClCHCl_2$ [1]

(e) Higher priority group on LHS is $CH_3CH_2CH_2$ [1]
Higher priority group on RHS is CH_2Br [1]
Both are on same side so Z isomer. [1] **[7 marks]**

4: POLYMERS

1. **(a)** A polymer is a large molecule formed when monomers join together. [1]

(b) A monomer is a small molecule that joins with other monomers to make a polymer. [1]

(c) C=C / carbon carbon double bond [1]

(d)

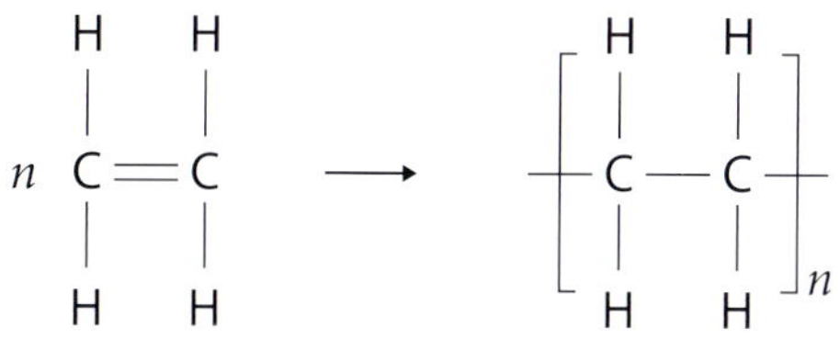

[3]

(e) poly(styrene) [1]

(f) bromoethene [1]

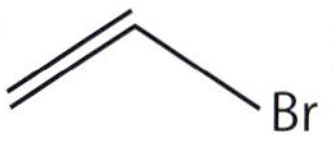

[1] **[9 marks]**

2. **(a)**

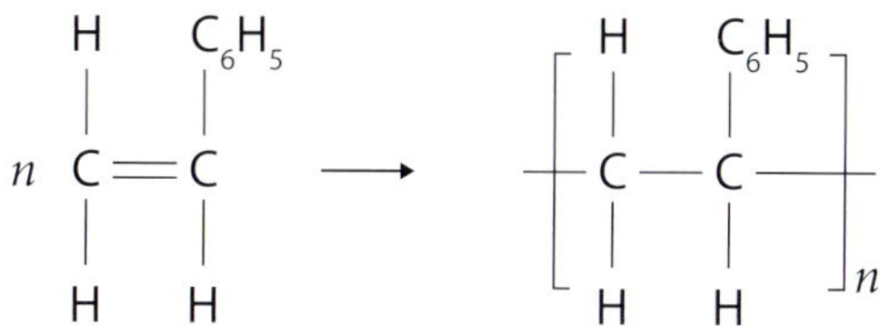

[3]

(b)

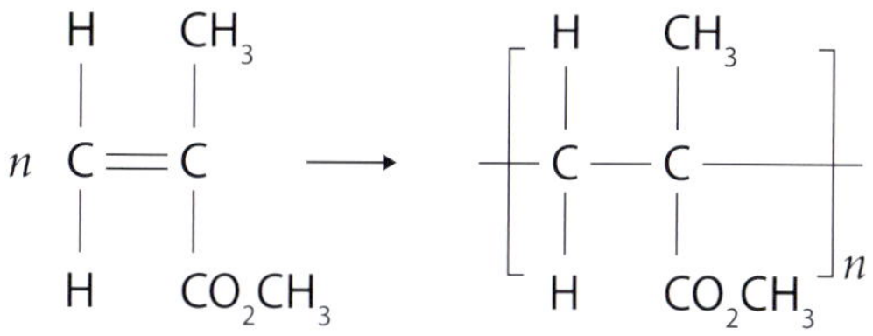

[3]

[6 marks]

3.

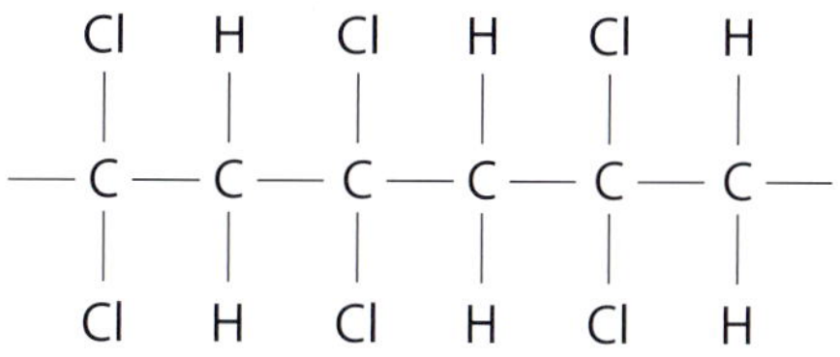

[2]

[2 marks]

4. (a)

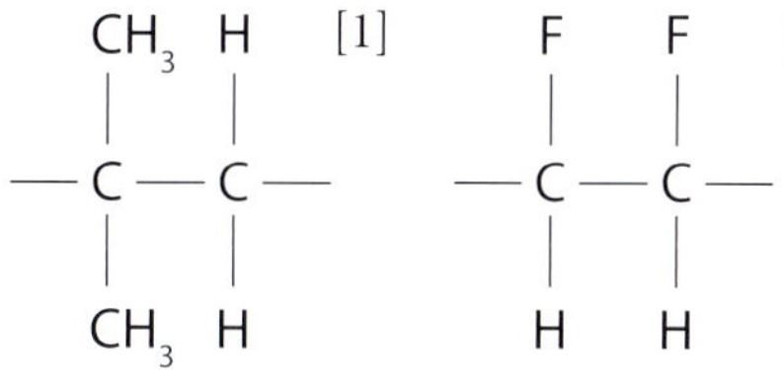

[1] [1]

(b)

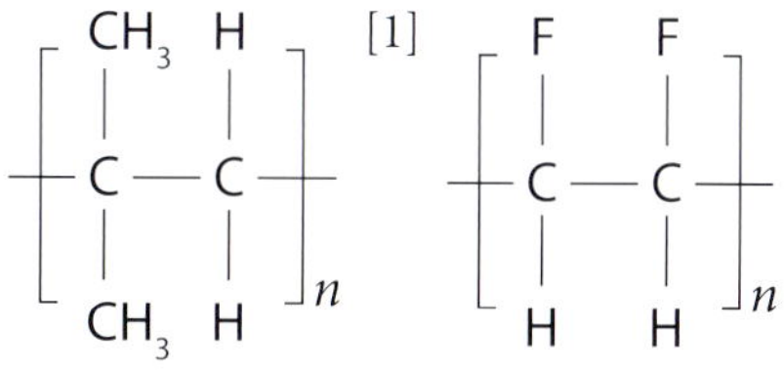

[1] [1]

[4 marks]

5. **(a)**

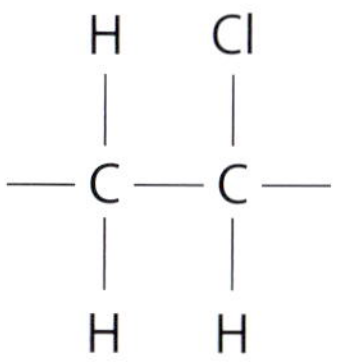

[1]

(b)

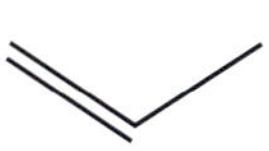

[1]

(c) No as it contains chlorine and not just carbon and hydrogen. [1]

(d) acidic hydrogen chloride gas released / carbon dioxide contributes to global warming [1]

(e) removing toxic waste gases caused by the incineration of plastics; [1] developing biodegradable polymers [1] **[6 marks]**

6. (a) addition [1] polymerisation [1]
(b) polythene/poly(ethene) [1]
(c) the number of monomers [1]
(d) Incineration in a power station [1] using the energy released to generate electricity/heat homes [1] **OR** Recycling [1] conserves crude oil resources [1] **OR** Using it as a feedstock (raw material) for cracking [1] conserves crude oil resources. [Any 2 strategies] **[8 marks]**

7. Indicative content:

- polythene is made by addition polymerisation;
- nylon is made by condensation polymerisation;
- polythene is made from one monomer;
- polythene is made from ethene monomer;
- nylon is made from two monomers;
- nylon is made from an acid/acyl chloride and 1,6-diaminohexane;
- in the polymerisation to make polythene there is one product, the polymer;
- in the polymerisation to make nylon there are two products, the polymer and water/hydrogen chloride;
- in condensation polymersation a small molecule is removed eg water/ hydrogen chloride;
- in addition polymerisation the double bond breaks and molecules add together.

Marks awarded as follows:

Candidates provide an excellent comparison with at least 7 indicative content points. They use excellent spelling, punctuation and grammar and the form and style are of an excellent standard. [5] – [6]

Candidates provide a good comparison with at least 4 indicative content points. They use good spelling, punctuation and grammar and the form and style are of a good standard. [3] – [4]

Candidates provide a limited comparison with at least 2 indicative content points. They use satisfactory spelling, punctuation and grammar and the form and style are of a basic standard. [1] – [2] **[6 marks]**

8. (a) It can be hydrolysed [1]
(b)

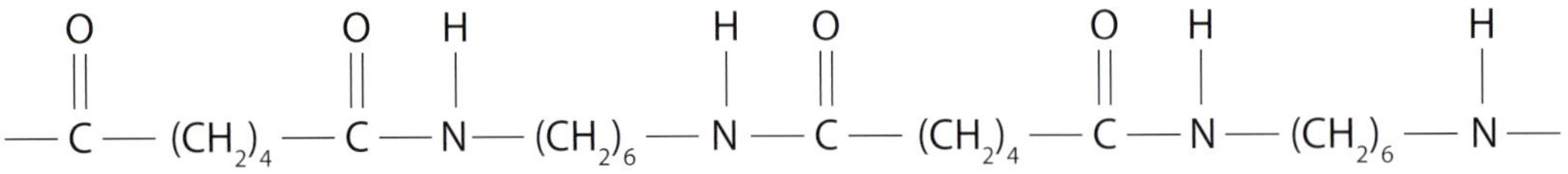

[2]

(c) Condensation polymers are polymers formed by the elimination of small molecules such as hydrogen chloride or water when monomers bond together. [2] **[5 marks]**

9. (a)

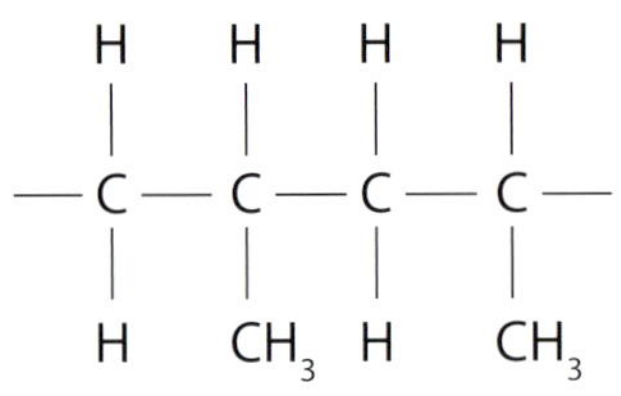

[1]

(b) condensation [1]
(c) Dissolve 1,6-diaminohexane in deionised water in a beaker. [1] Dissolve decanedioyl dichloride in cyclohexane in another beaker. [1] Pour the decanedioyl dichloride solution onto the solution of 1,6–diaminohexane [1] ensuring that mixing of solutions is minimised by pouring down the wall of the beaker/glass rod. [1] Use tweezers to pull out the nylon formed and wind around a glass rod. [1]
(d) One monomer has 6 carbons the other has 10. [1] **[8 marks]**

5: ALCOHOLS

1. (a) propan-1-ol (b) (2-)methylpropan-1-ol
(c) butan-2-ol
(d) 1-chloro- 4-methylpentan-2-ol
(e) methanol (f) propan-2-ol
(g) (2-)methylpropan-2-ol
(h) hexan-2-ol (i) (2-)methylpropan-1-ol.
[1] mark each **[9 marks]**

2. (a) primary (b) primary
(c) secondary (d) secondary
(e) primary (f) secondary
(g) tertiary (h) secondary
(i) primary [1] mark each **[9 marks]**

3. (a) P (b) P (c) T (d) T (e) T (f) P (g) P (h) S **[8 marks]**

4. (a) Reactive group within a compound [1]
(b) hydroxyl [1]
(c) No as it contains oxygen and not just carbon and hydrogen [1]
(d) $C_nH_{2n+1}OH$ [1]
(e) similar chemical reactions [1] successive members differ by CH_2 [1] physical properties show a gradation down the group [1]
(f) $C_2H_5OH + 3O_2 \rightarrow 2CO_2 + 3H_2O$ [2]
(g) carbon monoxide, carbon/soot, water. [2] One wrong = [1]
(h) An alcohol which has three carbons atoms directly bonded to the carbon atom that is bonded to the –OH group. [1] **[12 marks]**

5. (a) Molecules which have the same molecular formula but a different structural formula. [2]

(b) 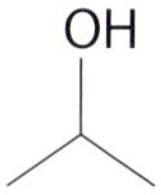

propan-2-ol [1]

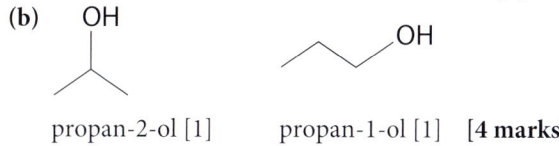

propan-1-ol [1] **[4 marks]**

6. A pentan-3-one $CH_3CH_2COCH_2CH_3$ [1]
B butanal $CH_3CH_2CH_2CHO$ [1]
C hexanoic acid $CH_3CH_2CH_2CH_2CH_2COOH$ [1]
[3 marks]

7.

Name	Structure	Classification – primary, secondary or tertiary
butan-1-ol	**$CH_3CH_2CH_2CH_2OH$**	**primary**
butan-2-ol	**$CH_3CH_2CH(OH)CH_3$**	**secondary**
2-methylpropan-2-ol	$CH_3C(OH)(CH_3)CH_3$	**tertiary**
2-methylpropan-1-ol	**$CH_3CH(CH_3)CH_2OH$**	primary

[6]

(b) 2-methylpropan-2-ol [1]
(c) orange to green [1]
(d) $CH_3CH_2CH_2CH_2OH + 2[O] \rightarrow CH_3CH_2CH_2COOH + H_2O$ [2]
butanoic acid [1] **[11 marks]**

8. C **[1 mark]**

9. (a) Repeated boiling and condensing of a (reaction) mixture [1] to ensure the alcohol is fully oxidised [1]
(b) $CH_3CH_2CH_2OH + 2[O] \rightarrow CH_3CH_2COOH + H_2O$ [2]
(c) acidified potassium dichromate (VI) [1]
Orange to green [1]
(d) change apparatus for distillation / condenser sidewards / add a stillhead / add a thermometer / add a collection flask. Any [3]
(e) propan-2-ol [1]
(f) (i) stays blue [1]
(ii) red ppt [1] **[12 marks]**

10. Indicative content:

- Take separate test tubes of butan-2-ol and 2-methyl propan-2-ol;
- add a few drops of acidified potassium dichromate(VI);
- Warm in a hot water bath;
- There is a colour change from orange to green with the butan-2-ol;
- This is because it is a secondary alcohol and can be oxidised;
- The acidified potassium dichromate (VI) stays orange in the 2-methylbutan-2-ol;
- This is because it is a tertiary alcohol and cannot be oxidised.

Marks awarded as follows:

Candidates provide an excellent comparison with at least 5 indicative content points. They use excellent spelling, punctuation and grammar and the form and style are of an excellent standard. [5] – [6]

Candidates provide a good comparison with at least 3 indicative content points. They use good spelling, punctuation and grammar and the form and style are of a good standard. [3] – [4]

Candidates provide a limited comparison with at least 2 indicative content points. They use satisfactory spelling, punctuation and grammar and the form and style are of a basic standard. [1] – [2] **[6 marks]**

11. (a) An elimination reaction is one where a small molecule is removed from a larger molecule. [1]
(b) $C_3H_7OH \rightarrow C_3H_6 + H_2O$ [1]
Conc sulfuric/phosphoric acid catalyst [1]
170 °C [1]
(c) orange to colourless [1] **[5 marks]**

12. (a) $C_2H_5Br + NaOH \rightarrow C_2H_5OH + NaBr$ [1]
(b) substitution [1]
(c) promotes smooth boiling [1]
(d) upright [1]
(e) alcohol is flammable [1]
(f) Add anhydrous calcium chloride / sodium sulfate [1] until changes from cloudy to clear. [1] Filter off the drying agent. [1]
(g) Some product is lost in distillation. [1] Reaction is not complete / some side reactions occur. [1]
(h) $CH_2{=}CH_2$ / $C_2H_4 + H_2O \rightleftharpoons C_2H_5OH$ [1]
conc phosphoric acid [1] **[12 marks]**

6: SPECTROSCOPIC TECHNIQUES

1. (a) No strong absorption between 3200–3500 cm^{-1} for OH of alcohol. [1] No absorption between 1650 and 1800 for C=O of aldehyde or ketone. [1]
(b) Absorption at 2850 to 3000 cm^{-1} due to C–H bond of hydrocarbons. [1] **[3 marks]**

2. (a) 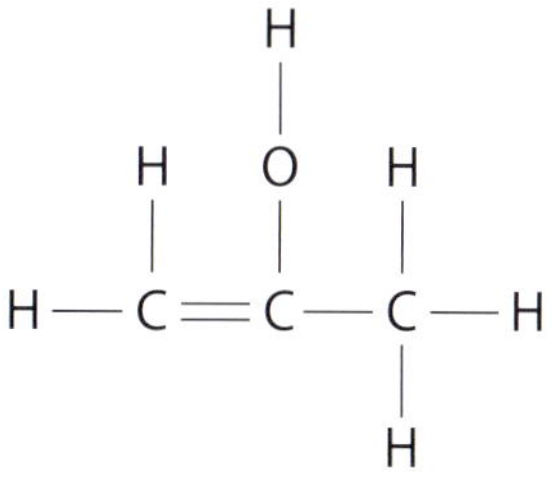

[1]

(b) C=C 1600–1700 cm^{-1} [1]
O–H 3200–3500 cm^{-1} [1] **[3 marks]**

3. (a) O–H [1]

(b) A = butan–1–ol [1] B = butan–2–ol [1]
(c) 2–methylpropan–2–ol [1]
$CH_3C(OH)(CH_3)CH_3$ [1]
(d) **(i)** 2–methylpropan–1–ol [1]
$CH_3CH(CH_3)CH_2OH$ [1]
(ii) E has CHO [1] F has COOH [1]
(iii) Still contains peak at 3200–3500 cm^{-1} due to O–H/alcohol. [1] Does not contain peak at 2500–3200 cm^{-1} due to O–H/carboxylic acid. [1] Does not contain peak at 1650–1800 cm^{-1} due to C=O. [1] Any [2] **[11 marks]**

4. **(a)** Absorption at 3200–3500 cm^{-1} [1] due to O–H [1]
(b) Match with a database spectra [1]
(c) The peak with the highest m/z ratio gives the relative formula mass [1]
(d) Run a spectrum on the reaction mixture at different times. It is complete when there is an absence of OH absorption [1] at 3200–3500 cm^{-1} [1]
(e) Acidified potassium dichromate(VI) [1] Warm [1]
(f) Same bonds present/C–C, C–H, C–O and O–H so same absorptions [1] **[9 marks]**

5. **(a)** abundance [1]
(b) mass/charge ratio [1]
(c) It is given by the value of the major peak with highest m/z value (46) [1]
(d) $C_2H_5^+$ or CHO^+ [1] CH_2OH^+ [1] $C_2H_5O^+$ [1]
(e) 31 [1] **[5 marks]**

6. D **[1 mark]**

7: MAKING AND PURIFYING ORGANIC COMPOUNDS – THE PREPARATION OF ASPIRIN

1. **(a)** $C_6H_4(OH)COOH$ or 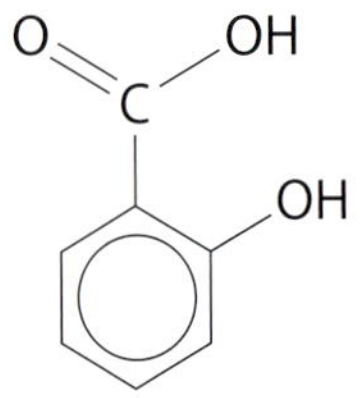 [1]

(b) Indicative content:

- Place salicylic acid in a flask;
- Add ethanoic anhydride;
- Slowly;
- Add some drops of conc phosphoric(V) acid;
- Heat/reflux;
- Add water;
- Pour the mixture unto crushed ice in a beaker cool;
- The solid product is removed by suction filtration.

Marks awarded as follows:
Candidates provide an excellent description with at least 6 indicative content points. They use excellent spelling, punctuation and grammar and the form and style are of an excellent standard. [5] – [6]

Candidates provide a good description with at least 4 indicative content points. They use good spelling, punctuation and grammar and the form and style are of a good standard. [3] – [4]

Candidates provide a limited comparison with at least 2 indicative content points. They use satisfactory spelling, punctuation and grammar and the form and style are of a basic standard. [1] – [2]

(c) Dissolve the aspirin in the minimum volume [1] of hot ethanol/water. [1] Filter when hot by gravity filtration, using a hot funnel, [1] allow filtrate to cool and crystallise [1] and filter off the crystals using suction filtration.
(d) Place some solid in a capillary tube/melting point tube sealed at one end. [1] Heat slowly (using melting point apparatus). [1] Record the temperature at which the solid starts and finishes melting. [1] Compare the temperature(s) with known values in a data book / if there is a small range or sharp melting point it is pure. [1]
(e) Add a few drops of ferric chloride / iron(III) chloride. [1] It remains yellow if there are no impurities. [1] It changes to a purple colour if impurities are present. [1]
(f) Moles of salicylic acid = 10.0 ÷ 138 = 0.07246
Moles of aspirin formed = 0.07246
Theoretical yield = 0.07246 × 180 = 13.0 g
Percentage yield = 9.1 ÷ 13.0 × 100 = 70% [3]
[21 marks]

2. **(a)** catalyst [1]
(b) slowly [1] wear gloves and goggles [1]
(c) repeated boiling a liquid and condensing the vapour [1]
(d) ethanoic anhydride [1] ethanoic acid [1]
(d) to form crystals [1]
(e) faster / gives a drier product [1]
(f) breaking up molecules by reaction with water [1]
[9 marks]

3. Moles of butanol = 5 ÷ 74 = 0.06757
Moles of bromobutane = 0.06757
Mass = 0.06757 × 137 = 9.3 g
$\% = \frac{6.4}{9.3} \times 100 = 69\%$ **[3 marks]**

4. Moles ethanol = mass ÷ M_r = 23 ÷ 46 = 0.5
Moles ethyl ethanoate = 0.5
Mass = moles × M_r = 0.5 × 88 = 44 g
$\% = \frac{33}{44} \times 100 = 75\%$ **[5 marks]**

5. Moles phenol = 50.0 ÷ 94 = 0.532
Moles TCP = 0.532
Mass TCP = 0.532 × 197.5 = 105.1 g theoretical yield
$\% = \frac{97.6}{105.1} \times 100 = 93\%$ **[5 marks]**

6. $d = \frac{m}{v}$, $m = d \times v = 0.8 \times 8.0 = 6.4$ g
Moles of butanol = 6.4 ÷ 74 = 0.08649
Moles of bromobutane = 0.08649
Mass = 0.08649 × 137 = 11.8 g
$d = \frac{m}{v}$, $v = \frac{m}{d} = \frac{11.8}{1.3} = 9.1\ cm^3$
$\% = \frac{3.7}{9.1} \times 100 = 41\%$ **[4 marks]**

Unit A2 3: Medical Physics

8: PHYSIOLOGICAL MEASUREMENTS TO MONITOR HEALTH

1. (a) (i) Hypothermia occurs when the body cannot produce enough heat and the core temperature falls to dangerous levels. [1]
(ii) Hyperthermia occurs when the body cannot dissipate enough heat through the normal biological processes causing the core temperature to rise to dangerous levels. [1]
(iii) Above 44°C, below 26°C. [2]
(b) There is a danger of breaking the glass stem and mercury is very poisonous. Better alternative thermometers are always available in the UK. [2]
(c) Child is admitted to hospital after a road accident with serious facial and arm injuries / other appropriate answer. [1] **[7 marks]**

2. (a) (i) Sphygmomanometer – to measure blood pressure [2]
(ii) Stethoscope [1]
(b) (i) Unit is mm of mercury (mm Hg). [1]
(ii) Hypotension is low blood pressure – considered to be 90/60 mm Hg or lower. [1]
(iii) Patient B appears to be suffering from hypotension at the time of measurement. [1]
(iv) Patient D appears to have hypertension. [1]
(c) See text on page 76. {QWC Question} [6] **[13 marks]**

3. (a) fMRI is functional magnetic resonance imaging. [1]
(b) (i) Unsuitable patients include those with metal implants in their bones, those with a heart pacemaker and those unable to remain totally still for considerable time (comprehensive list given on page 78). [3]
(ii) radio waves [1]
(iii) brain tumours / cancer, strokes, brain haemorrhages [3]
(c) MRI is very expensive to purchase, maintain and operate. [1] **[9 marks]**

4. (a) EEG is electroencephalograph(y) or electroencephalogram. [1] MEG is magnetoencephalograph(y) or magnetoencephalogram. [1]
(b) (i) brain [1]
(ii) MEG measures changes in the magnetic activity in the brain. EEG measures changes in the electrical activity in the brain. [2]
(c) (i) Time interval AB is approx. 0.1 s [1]
Frequency is approx. $\frac{1}{\text{period}}$ [1]
$= \frac{1}{0.1} = 10$ Hz [1]
(ii) Alpha wave and patient is relaxed [2] **[10 marks]**

9: DIAGNOSTIC IMAGING TECHNIQUES

1. (a) (i) Electrons [1]
(ii) There is a high voltage between B and C, with B positive with respect to C. [1]
(iii) Most of the kinetic energy (>99%) is converted into heat, the rest (<1%) is converted into X-rays. [1]
(iv) The target becomes very hot. [1] Copper is a very good conductor of heat – it conducts heat away from the tungsten target. [1]
(v) The oil is used as a coolant – to remove heat from the copper. [1]
(vi) Any gas present would slow down the accelerated electrons by collisions between the electrons and gas molecules. [1]
(vii) A: (Glass) X-ray tube lined with lead on the inside [1] B: Anode [1] C: Cathode [1]
(viii) Lead lining on the inside of the glass tube absorbs the X-rays. [1]
(ix) The aluminium absorbs the "soft", low energy X-rays which are not required. [1]
(b) (i) X-rays are electromagnetic waves of high energy / frequency. [1]
(ii) Since bones are better absorbers of X-rays than flesh, [1] fewer X-rays reach the detector, (so that region is white). [1] Most X-rays hitting the flesh pass straight through without absorption (so that region appears black). [1]
(iii) Ionising radiation causes some of the atoms / molecules through which they pass to become ions by collision processes. [1] This is

done by causing them to lose one or more electrons. [1]

(iv) Ionisation in cells disrupts DNA and can cause cancer. [1] **[19 marks]**

2. (a) Computed Tomography [1]

(b) In a conventional X-ray: both the patient and the source are stationary [1] and the dose is relatively small. [1] In a CT scan: the X-ray emitter and/or the detector rotate around the patient [1] and the dose is large. [1]

(c) Similarity: Both form a shadow image. [1] Difference: Conventional X-ray is a still 2D image. CT scan is a dynamic [2] image OR it is in 3D OR it gives more detail than a conventional X-ray image.

(d) Possible reason: Woman may be pregnant. [1] Alternative: MRI scan. [1] [10 marks]

3. (a) (i) Ultrasound is sound with a frequency greater than 20 kHz. [1]

(ii) Medical ultrasound uses frequencies between 1 MHz and 18 MHz (approx). (Some texts quote a range from 1 MHz to 15 MHz.) [1]

(iii) An A-scan (or amplitude scan) is one used to find the depth of a structure, rather than to produce an image. A B-scan (or brightness scan) produces a static, visual image of internal body structures, such as the image of a kidney OR a dynamic image such as the opening of valves in the heart. [2]

(b) (i) Ultrasound relies on the detection of an echo from a structure. The pulse must, therefore, be short enough to ensure the leading edge of the pulse returns well after the trailing edge departs. [2]

(ii) Not all of the sound energy is reflected from a structure – some of it is absorbed. As the reflected pulse passes through tissue it is attenuated – that is, some of its energy is absorbed. [2]

(c) (i) Pulse A represents the echo received from the inner abdominal wall. Pulse B is the echo received from the left boundary of the organ. Pulse C is the echo received from the right boundary of the organ. Pulse D is the echo received from the vertebra. [4]

(ii) The bony vertebra reflects a much greater proportion of the incident sound than the softer tissue on the right side of the organ. [1]

(iii) Width of organ = ½ × (speed in organ × time from left to right to left)

= ½ × (1200 × (0.27 ms – 0.12 ms))

= ½ × 1200 × 0.15×10^{-3}

= 0.09 m (or 9 cm) [4] **[17 marks]**

4. (a) (i) A radioisotope is an isotope that changes to a more stable state by emitting radiation. OR It consists of unstable nuclei that undergo radioactive decay emitting alpha, beta or gamma radiation. [1]

(ii) Positron Emission Therapy [1]

(b) Time difference is at a maximum when emission comes from edge of head. One detector triggers almost instantly, the delay to the other triggering is T = distance ÷ speed = 0.18 m ÷ 3×10^{8} m s^{-1} = 0.6 ns [4] **[6 marks]**

5. Intensity reflected = 0.0625%, so reflection coefficient = 6.25×10^{-4}

If Z = acoustic impedance of tissue, then:

$$\left(\frac{1.64\times10^{6} - Z}{1.64\times10^{6} + Z}\right)^{2} = 6.25\times10^{-4}\ [1]$$

Taking the square root of both sides gives:

$$\frac{1.64\times10^{6} - Z}{1.64\times10^{6} + Z} = 2.5\times10^{-2}\ [1]$$

$2.5\times10^{-2} \times (1.64\times10^{6} + Z) = 1.64\times10^{6} - Z$

$41\,000 + 2.5\times10^{-2}Z = 1.64\times10^{6} - Z$

$Z = (1.64\times10^{6} - 41\,000) \div (1 + 2.5\times10^{-2})$ [1]

$Z = 1.56\times10^{6}$ kg m^{-2} s^{-1} [1] **[4 marks]**

10: MEDICAL USES OF RADIATION

1. (a)

	alpha (α)	beta (β)	gamma (γ)
Nature	helium nucleus (particle)	fast electron β^{+} (or positron β^{+}) (particle)	high frequency electromagnetic wave / photon
Relative charge*	+2	–1 (or +1)	none
Relative mass*	4	$\frac{1}{2000}$	none
Radiation range	0.1 mm aluminium, or thin paper, or a few cm of air	a few mm of aluminium	a few cm of lead

*relative to the proton [12]

(b) Alpha is the most ionising of the nuclear radiations, but its range is very small. Inside the body its effects are catastrophic because its ionising ability makes it a powerful carcinogenic agent. Outside the body it causes ionisation in air, but it is easily stopped by clothing or the skin. [2]

(c) (i) The physical half-life of a radioactive substance is the time taken for its activity to decrease to half of its original value. [1]

(ii) The biological half-life of a radioactive substance is defined as the time taken for half of that radioactive substance to be removed from the body by natural metabolic processes. [1]

(d) (i) Half-life of ^{32}P is 0693 ÷ λ = 0.693 ÷ 0.0475 = 14.589 days or approximately 14.6 days [1]

(ii) Urination (OR respiration OR defecation) [1]

(iii) $(T_{effective})^{-1} = (14.6)^{-1} + (1455)^{-1} = 0.06918$

$T_{effective} = 0.06918^{-1} = 14.5$ days [1]

(e) $\lambda = 0.693 \div T_{½} = 0.693 \div 2.5 = 0.2772\ h^{-1}$ [1]

$\ln A = \ln A_0 - \lambda t$ [1]

$t = (\ln A_0 - \ln A) \div \lambda$

= (ln 1000 – ln 100) ÷ 0.2772 = 8.307 hours = 8 h 18 min [1] So earliest departure time = 4:18 pm on the same day [1] **[23 marks]**

2. (a) See text on page 98. {QWC Question} [6]

(b) (i) At $t = 0$, $\ln A = 7.30$, so $A = e^{7.30} = 1480$ Bq [1]

At $t = 720$, $\ln A = 0$, so $A = e^0 = 1$ Bq [1]

(ii) λ = – gradient = 7.30 ÷ 720 = 0.0101 s^{-1} [1]

$T_{½} = 0.693 \div \lambda = 0.693 \div 0.010168.4$

= 68.4 seconds [1]

(iii) $t = (\ln A_0 - \ln A) \div \lambda$

= (ln 1480 – ln 500) ÷ 0.0101

= 107.4 seconds [2]

(c) Corrected activity is the measured activity minus the background radiation activity. [1] **[13 marks]**

3. (a) Comparison: electron and positron have the same mass. Contrast: electron is a particle, positron is an anti-particle (antimatter); electron has a relative charge of –1, positron +1 [2]

(b) On collision, a positron and an electron annihilate each other and produce two γ-ray photons of the same energy which separate in opposite directions. [2]

(c) Cardiac perfusion imaging is the testing of blood flow to the muscles of the heart as part of an ischemic study, usually involving the positron emitter, rubidium-82, and a γ-ray camera to obtain moving images. [1]

(d) **Collimator**: a lead block with holes in it through which gamma rays pass. Its purpose is to obtain spatial information about the gamma-ray emissions from the imaging subject, by tracing the gamma rays back to their source.

Scintillant: a material, such as sodium iodide, which gives out a flash of visible light when struck by high energy radiation, such as a gamma ray. Its purpose is to detect the γ-rays.

Photomultiplier tubes: these amplify the signal produced when the visible light from the scintillant produces a single electron on collision with a photocathode by photoelectric emission.

Computer: in the context of a PET scan, the computer analyses the signals from the photomultiplier array to produce an image. [8] **[13 marks]**

4. (a) See text on page 102. {QWC Question} [6]

(b) (i) Radiopharmaceuticals are radioactive substances which are administered to patients in the course of their diagnosis or treatment. [1]

(ii) Iodine-131 is a radioactive isotope of iodine with a half-life of 8 days. It decays by β^- (and gamma) emissions and is taken by mouth. Iodine accumulates in the thyroid gland and the radioactive emissions from the drug kill cancerous cells there. [2] **[9 marks]**

5. (a) Medical = 100% – (10% + 11.5% + 50% + 14% + 0.5%) = 14% [1]

(b) CT scans and γ-ray scans [2]

(c) See text on page 96. {QWC Question} [6] **[9 marks]**

6. (a) Thallium is used to obtain a detailed image of an organ. [1]

(b)
- Thallium emits gamma radiation which can readily pass through the body – this makes it suitable for use with a gamma-ray camera for imaging purposes.
- The gamma rays emitted by thallium are weakly ionising, so that the least amount of radiological damage is done to the tissues.
- It is generally given as an intravenous injection, so there is minimal discomfort to the patient and its use is less invasive than other techniques.
- Its short biological half-life means that it is rapidly excreted from the body (in urine) and the patient does not remain radioactive for long – the patient can usually be treated as a day-patient.
- It may not be suitable for pregnant women (because of the danger to the foetus) or for young children (because of their small body mass).
- There is always risk of cell damage or cancer to any patient having this therapy – this risk is minimised by using as small a dose as possible and carrying out the procedure as quickly as it can be done.

{QWC Question} [6] **[7 marks]**

11: WAVES

1. (a) (i) Electromagnetic: gamma rays, x-rays, visible light, infrared, microwaves [5]
   Longitudinal: ultrasound [1]

   (b) (i) Amplitude: 1.5 nm [1]

   (ii) Wavelength: 4 cm [1]

   (iii) P leads Q by 270° [2]

   (iv) Period $T = \frac{1}{f} = \frac{1}{7.5\times10^{9}} = 1.33\times10^{-10}$ s
   Speed $= f\lambda = 7.5\times10^{9} \times 4\times10^{-2}$
   $= 3\times10^{8}$ m s^{-1} [2]

   (v) Microwaves [1] **[13 marks]**

2. Speed of first wave in bone $= f\lambda$
   $= 1.5\times10^{6} \times 1000\times10^{-6} = 1500$ m s^{-1}
   Wavelength = speed ÷ frequency = 1500 ÷ 2×10^{6}
   $= 7.5\times10^{-4}$ m = 750 µm [4] **[4 marks]**

3. Peaks all occur at 0.6 cm and troughs all at –0.6 cm {6 small squares above (and below) horizontal axis}. [1]
   Graph passes through (–0.04, 0), (0.02, 0.6), (0.08, 0), (0.14, –0.6), (0.20, 0), (0.26, 0.6), (0.32, 0) [3]
   [4 marks]

4. (a)

C	X-rays	B	Visible light	A	Microwaves	D

   [4]

   (b) A: infrared, B: ultraviolet, C: γ-waves, D: radio waves [4] **[8 marks]**

5. (a) Standing waves are formed when two waves of the same frequency and speed (and amplitude) travelling in opposite directions superpose in time and space. [2]

   (b) [2]

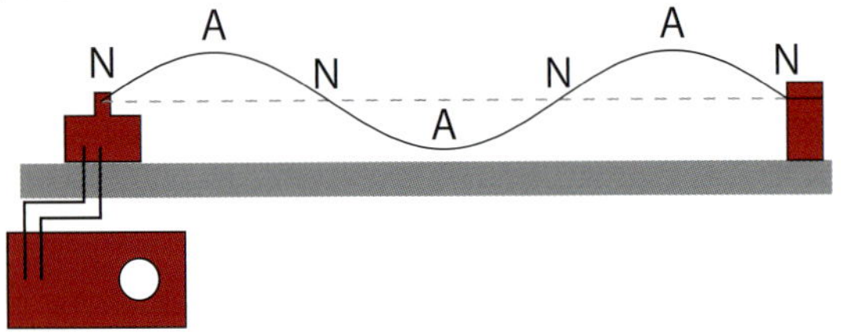

   (c) Third harmonic [1]

   (d) Length of wire = 1.5 wavelengths = 90 cm [1]
   Wavelength = 60 cm [1]

   (e) $v = f\lambda = 250$ Hz × 0.6 m = 150 m s^{-1} [2]

   (f) If the same pattern is obtained the wavelength is the same. [1] If the speed has increased, then the frequency must also do so. [1] The operator should slowly increase the frequency of the oscillator. [1] **[12 marks]**

6. (a) Sound is at its loudest. [1]

   (b) [1] and (c) [2]:

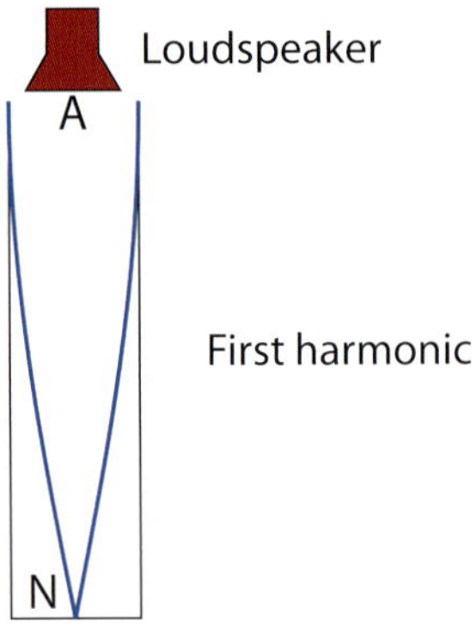

   (d) Slowly increase the length of the air column while maintaining the same note from the loudspeaker, until, once again, the sound is at its loudest. [3]

   (e) A second harmonic would have a node at the speaker. But the speaker is in the air where there will be an antinode, not a node. [1]

   (f) At the first harmonic:
   $\lambda = 4L = 4 \times 0.42 = 1.68$ m [1]
   $f = 336 \div 1.68 = 200$ Hz [1]
   At third harmonic:
   $f = 3 \times$ frequency at first harmonic
   $= 3 \times 200 = 600$ Hz [1] **[11 marks]**

7. At fundamental, $\lambda = 4L = 4 \times 0.026$ m = 0.104 m [1]
   $f = v \div \lambda = 338 \div 0.104$ [1] = 3250 Hz = 3.25 kHz
   [2 marks]

8. • Select the tuning fork with the lowest frequency marked on it.
   • Sound the fork on a rubber bung and hold it over the open end of the resonance tube.
   • Starting with the air column as small as possible, slowly raise the inner tube and the fork together, maintaining a distance of about 1 cm between the end of the tube and the fork.
   • Continue raising them both until the sound heard from the tube is at its loudest.
   • Clamp the inner tube and measure the distance, L, from the surface of the water to the end of the inner tube using a metre stick.
   • Repeat all of the above steps for all forks whose frequencies are known, in order of increasing frequency.
   • Plot a graph of L against $\frac{1}{f}$ and draw the straight line of best fit through the data points.
   • Now find the distance, L, for the fork whose frequency is to be found.
   • Using the graph, read and record the frequency, f, for this value of L.
   • This value of f is the frequency of the unknown fork.
   {QWC Question} [6] **[6 marks]**

12: THE EAR AND HEARING

1. A: Auditory canal – funnels sound toward the ear drum – protects the ear drum from injury.
B: Tympanic membrane – sound causes the membrane to vibrate – vibrations pass from the membrane to the ossicles.
C: Eustachian tube – keeps the air pressure equal on either side of the ear drum – keeps the middle ear free of mucus and less susceptible to infection.
D: Cochlea – in the cochlea vibrations move the cilia of the organ of Corti, which then sends electrical impulses via the auditory nerve to the brain.
E: Stapes – the third of three bones in the middle ear which amplifies vibrations and passes them via the oval window to the cochlea. [10] **[10 marks]**

2. **(a)** The semi-circular canals are three tiny, fluid-filled tubes in the inner ear which control a person's sense of balance. When a person moves, the liquid inside the semi-circular canals also moves, like water in a bottle. Tiny hairs that line each canal translate the movement of the liquid into electrical impulses that are sent to the brain via the auditory nerve. The brain then interprets these signals and can tell the rest of the body how to stay balanced. [4]
(b) Each canal is responsible for monitoring movement in one of the three dimensions in space. [1] **[5 marks]**

3.

Outer ear	pinna	auditory canal	tympanic membrane	
Middle ear	malleus	incus	stapes	eustachian tube
Inner ear	oval window	cochlea	auditory nerve	semi-circular canals

[½] per correct answer; round up **[6 marks]**

4. The pinna funnels sound through the auditory canal. The sound causes the tympanic membrane (ear drum) to vibrate. The vibrations pass through the ear drum to the malleus bone in the middle ear. The malleus is one of three ossicles (the others are the incus and the stapes) which amplify the vibrations. The vibrations pass through the oval window to the cochlea. The oval window separates the liquid-filled inner ear from the air-filled middle ear. Different parts of the cochlea respond to different frequencies. The cochlea changes mechanical vibrations into electrical signals. The electrical signals pass along the auditory nerve (to the brain). {QWC Question} [6] **[6 marks]**

5. **(a)** **(i)** A sound intensity of 2.4×10^{-4} W m^{-2} means that 2.4×10^{-4} J of sound energy is incident (at right angles) on a surface of 1 m^2 every second. [1]
(ii) The non-logarithmic form of the decibel equation is: $I = I_o \times 10^{\frac{\text{dB level}}{10}}$
An intensity level of 88.8 dB corresponds to an intensity of $I = I_o \times 10^{8.88}$, where I_o represents the threshold intensity of human hearing, 1×10^{-12} W m^{-2} [1]
(b) Intensity of chimes
$= I = I_o \times 10^{8.88} = 7.586\times10^{-4}$ W m^{-2}
Intensity level (dB level) of clock alone
$= 10 \log_{10} \frac{I}{I_o} = 10 \log_{10} \frac{2.4\times10^{-4}}{1\times10^{-12}}$
$= 10 \log_{10} 2.4\times10^{8} = 83.8$ dB [2]
(c) Intensities (but not intensity levels) simply add:
Total intensity $= 2.4\times10^{-4}$ W m^{-2} $+ 7.586\times10^{-4}$
$= 9.986\times10^{-4}$ W m^{-2} [1]
(d) Combined intensity level
$= 10 \log_{10} \frac{9.986\times10^{-4}}{1\times10^{-12}} = 90$ dB
When the clock chimes, the total intensity increases by more than a factor of 4, but the decibel level rises by a little over 6 dB. [1]
[6 marks]

6. **(a)** **(i)** 1×10^{-12} W m^{-2}
(ii) 0 dB [2]
(b) The threshold intensity is less than 1×10^{-12} W m^{-2} [1]
(c) $I = I_o \times 10^{\frac{\text{dB level}}{10}} = 1\times10^{-12} \times 10^{\frac{-25}{10}}$
$= 1\times10^{-12} \times 10^{-2.5} = 3.16\times10^{-15}$ W m^{-2} [3]
(d) Human upper frequency limit = 20 kHz
Upper frequency limit of dog
$= 3 \times 20$ kHz $= 60$ kHz [1] **[7 marks]**

7. • Connect an oscillator to a loudspeaker and adjust the oscillator frequency to 1000 Hz.
• With the alarm sounding adjust the amplitude of the oscillator until the user indicates that the sound from its speaker and that from the alarm are equally loud.
• Switch off the alarm and, using a decibel meter, measure the sound intensity level (dB level) from the speaker attached to the oscillator.
• The numerical value of the dB level on the decibel meter is the loudness of the alarm (in phons). [4]
[4 marks]

8. **(a)** 1000 Hz [1]
(b) None – they are all equally loud as they are all on the 100 phon equal loudness curve. [1]
(c) D would be perceived as being louder. [1] C has a loudness of 100 phon and a sound intensity level around 90 dB. [1] D is at the same frequency as C, but has a higher dB level (100 dB), [1] so it will appear louder than the 90 phon sound of C.
[5 marks]

13: LIGHT IN COMMUNICATION AND RADIO WAVES

1. (a) (i) refraction
   (ii) air
   (iii) No refraction when the angle of incidence is 0° [3]
   (b) The critical angle is the angle of incidence in the glass for which the angle of refraction in the air is 90°. [1]
   (c) The light must be travelling from a material of high refractive index towards a material of lower refractive index. The angle of incidence in the material of higher refractive index is greater than the critical angle. [2] **[6 marks]**

2. See the method described on page 128. {QWC Question} [6] **[6 marks]**

3. (a) [3]

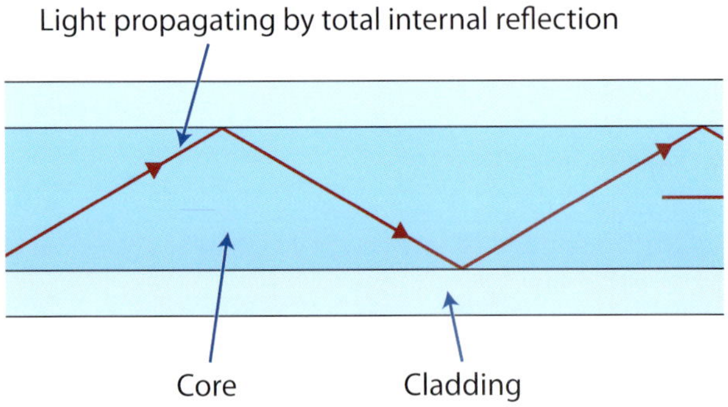

Speed of light is greatest in the cladding.

   (b) The core of a single mode fibre has a smaller diameter than a multi-mode fibre. [1]
   (c) A step-index fibre is one in which the core is of a uniform refractive index and there is a sharp decrease in the refractive index at the cladding. [2]
   (d) Advantage: A single mode fibre-optic cable can be used for long range communication (> 2 km), for example a WAN (wide area network), whereas a multi-mode fibre is restricted for use over much shorter distances. Disadvantage: Single mode fibres are more expensive than multi-mode fibres. [2] **[8 marks]**

4. (a) The signal passing along the axial path takes a shorter time to pass through the fibre than that by repeated total internal reflection. When these signals come together there is dispersion and the image obtained will be blurred or distorted. [2]
   (b) To reduce dispersion a systems designer might reduce the data transmission rate or reduce the distance over which the signal has to travel. [2] **[4 marks]**

5. (a) Microwaves [1]
   (b) The Doppler effect is the changing in frequency of a signal reflected from a moving object. [1]
   (c) Radar waves are transmitted by (radar) dish / antenna. [1] Radar waves are reflected off aircraft. [1]Reflected radar waves return to dish / antenna. [1]
   (d) The frequency (of the returning wave) is compared to the original frequency. [1] If higher, then the aircraft is moving towards the airport. [1] If lower, then the aircraft is moving away from the airport. [1] The larger the change in frequency, the faster the aircraft is moving. [1]
   (e) Ultrasound is too slow. [1] Ultrasound would not have the range required in air. [1] **[11 marks]**

6. (a) Oscillator; microphone; modulator; aerial [4]
   (b) (i) Wavelength $\lambda = v \div f = 3\times10^8 \div 3\times10^8 = 1$ m [1] Each rod is a quarter of a wavelength. [1] Each rod is 25 cm long. [1]
   (ii) 300 MHz [1]
   (c) Associated with all electromagnetic waves are oscillating electric and magnetic fields, which are at right angles to each other and to the direction of propagation of the wave. [2] **[10 marks]**

7. (a) Wireless headphones; wireless mouse; wireless keyboard [3]
   (b) There needs to be wireless communications between the two devices. [1]
   (c) Range (or power). [1] **[5 marks]**

8. The sound wave emitted by the whistle has a wavelength of 0.5 m. [1] While the train approaches the observer:
   - the sound detected has a wavelength less than 0.5 m [1]
   - its intensity increases [1]

   When the train is beside the observer, the intensity is a maximum. [1]
   While the train is moving away from the observer:
   - the sound detected has a wavelength less than 0.5 m [1]
   - its intensity decreases [1] **[6 marks]**

14: THE EYE

1. (a) [12]

Part	Name	Function
A	cornea	to refract light entering the eye
B	pupil	the "hole" through which light enters the eye
C	iris	controls the amount of light entering the eye
D	lens	brings light to a sharp focus on the retina
E	retina	an area rich in photo-receptive nerve cells which respond to light
F	optic nerve	nerve which transmits image information to the brain

(b) [7]

Statement	Rods	Cones
There are more than 120 million of these cells in the retina.	√	
They are used for our peripheral vision and are concentrated in the outer edges of the retina.	√	
They are responsible for straight-ahead vision.		√
They allow us to see colour.		√
They are only found in the fovea.		√
They cannot discern sharp images or perceive fine detail.	√	
They are responsible for sensing motion.	√	
They cells are needed for the perception of light and darkness and adapting to night-time vision.	√	

[19 marks]

2. (a) (i) When viewing a distant object, the eye lens is relaxed, thin and at its weakest. As the object moves closer the ciliary muscles cause the lens to become thicker and stronger in order to maintain a sharp image on the retina. There comes a point, known as the near point, beyond which this cannot occur without eye strain. [3]
(ii) Accommodation [1]
(b) (i) Stereoscopic vision is the ability of our eyes to see the same object as one image and to create a perception of depth. [1]
(ii) Stereoscopic vision is only possible because we have two eyes. [1] **[6 marks]**

3. (a) (i) A person is said to have long sight (hypermetropia) if their near point is further away than 25 cm. A long-sighted eye has no difficulty focusing on far away objects but cannot produce enough converging power to create a focused image of nearby objects. [1]
(ii) [3]

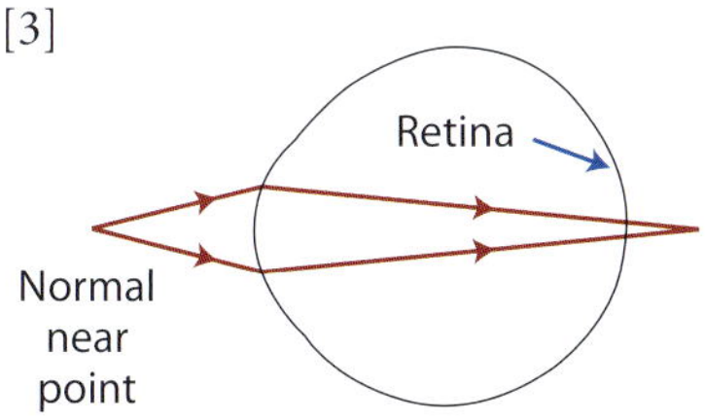

(b) (i) Long sight (hypermetropia) [1]
(ii) A lens of power +2.5 D is converging with a focal length 40 cm. [1]
With an object 25 cm from the lens, a virtual image is formed at the old near point.

$\frac{1}{u} + \frac{1}{v} = \frac{1}{f}$ [1]

$\frac{1}{25} + \frac{1}{v} = \frac{1}{40}$ [1]

$\frac{1}{v} = \frac{5}{200} - \frac{8}{200} = -\frac{3}{200} = -66.7$

v is negative because the image is virtual.
So near point without glasses = 66.7 cm. [1]
[9 marks]

4. (a) The lens is thinner when viewing distant objects. [1]
(b) (i) $P = \frac{1}{u} + \frac{1}{v}$ [1] $= \frac{1}{0.25} + \frac{1}{0.02} = +54$ D [1]
(ii) Unaided $P = \frac{1}{2} + \frac{1}{0.02}$ [1] = +50.5 D
(iii) Power of lens required = 54 – 50.5 = +3.5 D [1] **[5 marks]**

15: DNA AND THE GENETIC CODE

1. (a) Adenine; [1]
(b) 4; [1]
(c) Hydrogen; [1] **[3 marks]**

2.

Researchers(s)	Methodology
	X-ray crystallography; [1]
Watson and Crick; [1]	
Chargaff; [1]	

[3 marks]

3. (a) (i) mRNA is single stranded; [1] therefore the bases are not paired; [1] [2]
(ii) Adenine, cytosine, guanine and uracil; [1]
(iii) (Each strand of) mRNA represents a gene and there are many genes in a chromosome; [1] DNA extends along the full length of a chromosome/a strand of DNA includes many genes; [1] [2]
(b) Combines with a specific amino acid; [1] to bring it to the correct codon/position on the mRNA; [1] [2] **[7 marks]**

4. (a) Watson and Crick; [1]
(b) (i) The two DNA strands separate and each acts as a template; [1]
for bases to attach using base pairing rules to form two double strands (identical to each other and to the parent DNA); [1] [2]
(ii) DNA helicase breaks the hydrogen bonds between base pairs; [1]
thus enabling the two DNA strands to separate; [1]
DNA polymerase joins adjacent nucleotides (on the same strand)/joins deoxyribose (sugar) and phosphate together; [1]
by phosphodiester bonds; [1] [4]
(c) There would be two bands of DNA; [1]
one in same position as in tube 1 and one in same position as in tube 3; [1]
tube 3 DNA (containing template strands for DNA in tube 4) has half the strands ^{14}N and half ^{15}N; [1]

therefore 50% of tube 4 DNA strands will contain only ^{14}N and half will contain a mixture of ^{14}N and ^{15}N; [1] [4] **[11 marks]**

16: MEIOSIS AND GENETICS

1. (a) A cell which has only one chromosome from each homologous pair; [1]
   (b) Crossing over – prophase I; [1]
   Independent assortment – metaphase I; [1] [2]
   (c) Anaphase I; [1]
   anaphase as chromosomes are being pulled to opposite poles (sides) of the cell; [1]
   division I as the two chromatids of each chromosome are still attached; [1] [3] **[6 marks]**

2. (a) (i) OO; [1]
   (ii) BB and BO; [1]
   (b)

	A	B
O	AO	BO
O	AO	BO

Possible blood groups: A and B
([1] for gametes; [1] for cross and [1] for identifying the possible blood groups as A and B) [3] **[5 marks]**

3. (a) (i) A sex-linked condition is more likely to occur in a particular sex/a condition determined by a gene on the X chromosome; [1]
   (ii) X^HY; [1]
   (iii) Parents: X^HX^h **x** X^HY

	X^H	X^h
X^H	X^HX^H	X^HX^h
Y	X^HY	X^hY

X^hY is the genotype for haemophilia in this cross. ([1] for correct gametes; [1] for correct cross and [1] for identifying the individual with haemophilia.) [3]

(b) X^hY Nn (male parent) **x** X^HX^H nn (female parent)

	X^h N	X^h n	YN	Yn
X^Hn	X^HX^h Nn	X^HX^h nn	X^HY Nn	X^HY nn

Genotypes	Phenotypes
X^HX^h Nn	No haemophilia (carrier) and will develop Huntington's disease
X^HX^h nn	No haemophilia (carrier) and will **not** develop Huntington's disease
X^HY Nn	No haemophilia and will develop Huntington's disease
X^HY nn	No haemophilia and will **not** develop Huntington's disease

([1] for correct parent genotypes; [1] for correct gametes; [1] for correct cross and [2] for matching correct phenotypes to genotypes (delete [1] for each mistake) [5]

[10 marks]

4. (a) (i) During the formation of gametes/meiosis the segregation (separation) of the alleles of one gene is independent to the segregation (separation) of the alleles of any other gene/ the separation of the chromosomes from one homologous pair into gametes is independent to the separation of the chromosomes in any other homologous pair; [1]
   (ii) Metaphase I; [1]
   (b) (i) CC ww and Cc ww; [1]
   (ii) cw; [1]
   (iii) Parents: Cc Ww × Cc ww

	CW	Cw	cW	cw
Cw	CC Ww	CC ww	Cc Ww	Cc ww
cw	Cc Ww	Cc ww	cc Ww	cc ww

Genotype(s)	Phenotypes
CC Ww and Cc Ww	Normal body colour and normal wing (3/8)
CC ww and Cc ww	Normal body colour and vestigial wing (3/8)
cc Ww	Ebony body and normal wing (1/8)
cc ww	Ebony body colour and vestigial wing (1/8)

([1] for correct gametes; [1] for correct cross and [2] for matching correct phenotypes to genotypes (delete [1] for each mistake) [4]

(c) (i) 9 : 3 : 3 : 1; [1]
   (ii)

Category	Observed (O)	Expected (E)	(O–E)	(O–E^2)	$\frac{(O-E)^2}{E}$
Normal body normal wing	917	900			
Normal body vestigial wing	288	300			
Ebony body normal wing	305	300			
Ebony body vestigial wing	90	100			

[1]

(iii)

Category	Observed (O)	Expected (E)	(O–E)	(O–E²)	$\frac{(O-E)^2}{E}$
Normal body normal wing	917	900	17	289	0.32
Normal body vestigial wing	288	300	–12	144	0.48
Ebony body normal wing	305	300	5	25	0.08
Ebony body vestigial wing	90	100	–10	100	1.0

$X^2 = 1.88$

([1] for table completed correctly and [1] for calculation of X^2) [2]

(iv) degrees of freedom 3 (4 – 1); [1]
probability value 0.900 to 0.500; [1] [2]

(v) There is no significant difference between the observed and expected values/the results are a good fit to the ratio of 9 : 3 : 3 :1; [1]

[15 marks]

17: THE APPLICATION OF GENETIC ENGINEERING AND GENE THERAPY

1. **(a)** Diabetes mellitus; [1]
   (b) **(i)** Sticky ends; [1]
   (ii) Restriction endonucleases; [1]
   (iii) DNA bases are exposed (in the sticky ends); [1]
   if the same restriction endonuclease/enzyme is used in cutting out the human gene and the plasmid/bacterial DNA then complementary bases will be present in the two structures; [1]
   allowing the human gene to anneal/bond with the plasmid/bacterial DNA; [1] [3]
   (iv) The plasmid is placed back into the bacterium; [1]
   which then multiply to produce many bacteria carrying the human insulin gene; [1] [2]
   (c) Any **two** from:
   fewer adverse reactions/more effective [1]
   larger quantities being made [1]
   lower production costs [1]
   fewer ethical or religious issues [1]
   extraction from animals is difficult (and very time consuming) [1] [2] **[10 marks]**

2. **(a)** Presence of a defective allele/gene; [1]
   leading to the failure to produce factor VIII or IX (which are important agents in blood clotting); [1] [2]
   (b) **(i)** Blood/serum transfusion containing the missing clotting factors; [1]
   (ii) The serum/blood transferred was often contaminated with viruses/HIV; [1]
   [4 marks]

3. **(a)** In traditional breeding only the animals with the best characteristics are selected for breeding (or converse); [1]
   this process of selective breeding is repeated over many generations/breeding cycles; [1]
   in transgenic animals a beneficial gene is added to the animals' genome (usually at a very early stage of development); [1]
   enabling the animals to produce substances it otherwise would not or possess features it otherwise would not; [1] [4]
   (b) The world population is increasing rapidly at the same time as the area of available land for food production is decreasing; [1]
   genetic engineering can increase yields/nutrient status/allow crops to grow in areas previously unusable/can increase the ecological range of crops; [1]
   to compensate for the reduced available land; [1] [3] **[7 marks]**

4. **(a)** Somatic cell (gene) therapy is the process whereby functional genes are added to cells in the body to replace or compensate for defective genes; [1]
   (b) Any **two** from:
   not all parts of the body are equally accessible [1]
   the aerosol may not reach all parts of the lung [1]
   new cells produced in the body will still contain the defective gene [1]
   the use of viruses (as vectors) may cause infections, immune responses or allergies [1]
   immune reactions may destroy virus vectors (before the DNA is delivered in the affected cells) [1]
   the added gene may not become incorporated into the host DNA/it may be damaged during the process of delivery [1] [2]
   [3 marks]

5. (a) Heating the double stranded DNA to (approximately) 95°C; [1]
   (b) Any **two** from:
   stops the DNA strands from re-joining [1]
   brackets the section to be copied [1]
   DNA replication only starts with double stranded section [1] [2]
   (c) DNA polymerase; [1]
   (d) 16; [1] **[5 marks]**

18: GENE CLONING, GENETIC FINGERPRINTING AND STEM CELL TECHNOLOGY

1. (a) Embryonic stem cells can give rise to a very wide range of cell types (virtually all the cells in the body)/are pluripotent/adult stem cells can give rise to a limited range of cell types/are multipotent; [1]
   (b) (i) Altering the expression level of particular genes/increasing and/or decreasing the expression levels of other genes; [1]
   (ii) More easily available/fewer ethical issues/can reduce issues with tissue rejection (if the reprogrammed cells are obtained from the same individual into which the cells will be added); [1]
   (iii) Treatment of leukaemia/cancer/other appropriate response; [1] **[4 marks]**

2. (a) (i) Polymerase chain reaction (PCR); [1]
   (ii) Cutting out targeted (repetitive sequences of) DNA; [1]
   (b) (i) The DNA fragments in X move faster/more easily through the gel; [1]
   as they are shorter in length; [1] [2]
   (ii) The individual with the genetic disease has a (targeted) section of DNA different to that in healthy individuals; [1]
   and does not have a (targeted) section of DNA present in the genetic fingerprint of healthy individuals [1] [2]
   (iii) One of the sequences targeted by the restriction enzyme(s) used has a different number of bases than the sequence in healthy individuals; [1]
   as the sequence has travelled further through the gel (due to it being shorter), this suggests that a number of bases are missing in the affected individual/bases deleted; [1][2]
   [8 marks]